Treating the Trauma of Rape:
Cognitive-Behavioral Therapy for PTSD

TREATMENT MANUALS FOR PRACTITIONERS
David Barlow, *Editor*

Recent Volumes

Treating the Trauma of Rape
Cognitive-Behavioral Therapy for PTSD

EDNA B. FOA, PhD
BARBARA OLASOV ROTHBAUM, PhD

Series Editor's Note by David H. Barlow

THE GUILFORD PRESS
New York   London

© 1998 The Guilford Press
A Division of Guilford Publications, Inc.
72 Spring Street, New York, NY 10012
www.guilford.com

Printed in the United States of America

This book is printed on acid-free paper.

Last digit is print number: 9 8 7 6 5 4 3 2 1

Library of Congress Cataloging-in-Publication Data

Foa, Edna B.
    Treating the trauma of rape : cognitive-behavioral therapy
for PTSD / Edna B. Foa and Barbara Olasov Rothbaum.
        p.   cm.—(Treatment manuals for practitioners)
    Includes bibliographical references and index.
    ISBN 1-57230-178-3 (hard)
    1. Rape trauma syndrome—Treatment.   2. Cognitive therapy.
I. Rothbaum, Barbara Olasov.   II. Title.   III. Series
    [DNLM: 1. Rape—rehabilitation.   2. Rape—psychology.
3. Stress Disorders, Post-Traumatic—therapy.   4. Cognitive
Therapy—methods. WM 401 F649t 1998]
RC560.R36F6   1998
616.85'21—dc21
DNLM/DLC
for Library of Congress   97-30807
                                                                CIP

Permission to reprint the following material is gratefully acknowledged: Chapter 4 is
adapted from Foa and Meadows (1997). *Annual Review of Psychology* (Vol. 48, pp. 449-
480). © 1997 by Annual Reviews. Chapter 5 is adapted from Foa and Jaycox (in press).
Psychotherapeutic Frontiers: New Principles and Practices. © by the American Psychiatric
Association. The case of Susan in Chapter 10 (pp. 168-172) is adapted from Rothbaum
and Foa (1992b). © 1992 by the Association for Advancement of Behavior Therapy.

To Charles, Yael, and Michelle, with love.

—E. B. F.

To John, Alex, and Jake, the loves of my life.

—B. O. R.

To all the brave women who have taught us about helping them.

—E. B. F. and B. O. R.

Acknowledgments

Many people helped to bring this book about, and we would like to acknowledge their contribution. First, we would like to thank the staff of the Violence and Traumatic Stress Program at the National Institute of Mental Health (NIMH). Since 1986, when we received the first grant to study treatments for rape victims with posttraumatic stress disorder (PTSD), they have all been extremely supportive. It was then, in 1986, that we went to the Medical University of South Carolina in Charleston to learn how to treat rape victims with Stress Inoculation Training (SIT). Dean Kilpatrick, PhD, Connie Best, PhD, and their colleagues were exceedingly hospitable and helpful during this training period.

This book is the outcome of collaborative work shared by many colleagues, research assistants, and trainees from the PTSD project in the Center for the Treatment and Study of Anxiety at Allegheny University of the Health Sciences. In particular, we would like to thank Blanche Freund, Constance Dancu, Elizabeth Hembree, Diana Hearst-Ikeda, Lisa Jaycox, and Elizabeth Meadows, who helped develop our treatments and write the treatment manuals. We also want to thank David Clark for teaching us how to conduct cognitive therapy and for his help in writing cognitive components of the manuals. The book is largely based on these manuals. David Riggs, Michael Kozak, and Lisa Jaycox have contributed to the conceptualization of PTSD that we offer here, and we thank them for their input. Our special gratitude is extended to Dottie Marano for her patience in typing and retyping the manuscripts and in compiling the references.

At Emory University School of Medicine, we would like to thank Barbara's colleagues for supporting her work there, including this book. They include Charles B. Nemeroff, MD, PhD, Philip T. Ninan, MD, and Bettina Knight, RN.

We also want to acknowledge Barbara Watkins, our editor at The Guilford Press, who has worked with us closely throughout the laborious process of completing this manuscript. Her penetrating criticism and constructive suggestions greatly enhanced the book.

Most of all, we would like to thank the survivors we have worked with over the years, who have allowed us to glimpse their personal nightmares of PTSD. Through them, we learned, we gathered data, we tested techniques, and we grew as therapists, scientists, and people. We appreciate their courage and their willingness to share.

Series Editor's Note

Few problems confronted by mental health professionals present with the anguish and tragedy inherent in rape. Its shockingly high prevalence and the resulting all too frequent development of chronic posttraumatic stress disorder make this problem one of the most acute and wrenching disorders with which mental health clinicians must deal. For too long, society's reaction to this event was to ignore it and to instruct the victim to do likewise. Revelation of the rape often did as much harm as the event itself. As a result, we are still discovering and uncovering the tragic consequences of this trauma. For example, despite the fact that rape-induced traumas have occurred for millennia, we have only recently discovered the phenomenon of rape-induced paralysis, which seems to be a manifestation of an ancient defensive reaction in most mammals referred to as tonic immobility (Suarez & Gallup, 1979; Barlow, 1988). In many cases, this serotonergically mediated defensive reaction was misinterpreted by some as acquiescence to the rape, which, of course, only compounded the trauma.

It is now becoming more acceptable to not only report the assault but also to seek professional help for the aftermath of the rape. With this societal sea change has come the demand for treatments that are truly effective in alleviating the enormous emotional suffering connected with this trauma. Fortunately, several programs now exist that have met the test of efficacy, and perhaps none has received more attention than the superb program presented in this book, originated by Drs. Foa and Rothbaum, two of the leading clinicians and clinical scientists working in this area. As the authors point out, lack of knowledge of these effective treatments on the part of mental health practitioners only compounds the tragedy of rape. The purpose of this book is to facilitate dissemination of this valuable and important treatment program so that practitioners can more effectively and more quickly relieve the enormous suffering connected with this trauma.

DAVID H. BARLOW
Boston University

References

Barlow, D. H. (1988). *Anxiety and its disorders: The nature and treatment of anxiety and panic*. New York: Guilford Press.
Suarez, S. D., & Gallup, G. G., Jr. (1979). Tonic immobility as a response to rape in humans: A theoretical note. *Psychological Record, 29,* 315–320.

Preface

Epidemiological studies underscore the grave effects of experiencing trauma. According to the *Diagnostic and Statistical Manual of Mental Disorders*, fourth edition (DSM-IV; American Psychiatric Association [APA], 1994), a "trauma" is defined as an event that involves perceived or actual threat and elicits an extreme emotional response. Thus, a trauma victim has experienced or witnessed a situation involving actual or threatened death or bodily injury (a threat to the physical integrity of self and other). The person's response to the trauma involves helplessness, horror, or intense fear. The psychological syndrome most often observed following such an experience is called Posttraumatic Stress Disorder (PTSD).

Research clearly demonstrates that traumatic life events, especially sexual and other criminal assault, occur in significant numbers. The psychological sequelae of these traumas (and especially of rape) are vast, and a substantial proportion of victims will develop PTSD. Lifetime prevalence of PTSD among trauma victims is estimated at 24%, and lifetime prevalence of PTSD in the general population is estimated at 9%, with over a third of these cases having chronic PTSD (3.4%; Breslau, Davis, Andreski, & Peterson, 1991). If one adds subthreshold cases, then the combined current prevalence increases to 15% (Davidson, Hughes, Blazer, & George, 1991). Women appear to be more likely than men to develop PTSD following trauma (10.4% vs. 5%; Kessler, Sonnega, Bromet, Hughes, & Nelson, 1995).

The magnitude of the problem of PTSD among women in general and rape victims in particular can be extrapolated from Resnick, Kilpatrick, Dansky, Saunders, and Best's (1993) excellent study of a representative sample of women in the United States. If, as found by Resnick et al., 12.4% of the estimated 12 million American women who have experienced a completed rape develop chronic PTSD, there are *right now* about 1.5 million adult female rape victims who suffer from this often devastating disorder. Furthermore, if, as Resnick et al. suggested, about 6.7% of adult American women who have experienced any form of trauma are currently suffering from PTSD, then at present about 6.5 million women in the United States fall into that category. The problem of PTSD following assault is monumental and growing, as more women are attacked every hour. It is incumbent on health care professionals to provide effective and efficient treatment for these women to alleviate their suffering. This book is intended to provide the knowledge that will enable professionals to participate in this endeavor.

Various psychosocial treatments for PTSD, including group psychotherapy, individual psychodynamic therapy, and cognitive-behavioral therapy, have been developed over the past decade. Of these, cognitive-behavioral treatments have been the most widely studied, and several well-controlled investigations have shown such techniques to be effective. Despite these advances in psychosocial treatments for PTSD, information about these programs has not been widely disseminated among the mental health professionals who are the front-line helpers for trauma victims. We hope that this book will help disseminate information on effective treatment programs.

This book has two aims. The first is to present a picture of PTSD and related problems that is grounded in the research literature. To this end, we review the literature on posttrauma disturbances and on the relative efficacy of various treatments in overcoming these disturbances. We also outline a theoretical account for why some victims develop PTSD and others do not, and we suggest that victims who develop certain beliefs are more likely to develop PTSD than victims who do not develop such beliefs. Specifically, we suggest that two major beliefs underlie PTSD: first, that the world is an utterly dangerous place and that people in general are untrustworthy; and, second, that the victims themselves are unworthy and inadequate people because they were assaulted (or otherwise traumatized), or because they fail to recover and have persistent symptoms. Because the interventions that we teach in this book are directly derived from this theory and are designed to correct the dysfunctional cognitions of clients with PTSD, we strongly believe that our theoretical exposition serves as a valuable introduction to the second aim of the book.

The second aim of the book is to provide a detailed guide to conducting effective treatment programs for clients who suffer from trauma-related psychological problems. Throughout the book, we focus mainly on women who have been sexually assaulted and as a result have developed chronic symptoms of PTSD that have disrupted their daily functioning and cause them persistent psychological anguish. Thus, most of our examples demonstrating how to implement cognitive-behavioral techniques are drawn from our experience in treating rape victims. However, it is important to keep in mind that the procedures outlined here have been as successful in ameliorating posttrauma disturbances of women who have been sexually abused in childhood and of adult female victims of nonsexual assault (e.g., aggravated assault and robbery). Victims of other types of trauma, such as natural disasters and car accidents, have also been helped by cognitive-behavioral treatment. In addition, many of the cognitive-behavioral techniques described here have been useful in the treatment of many other anxiety disorders.

We have also deliberately decided not to outline a step-by-step guide for a single treatment program, because we believe that clients may vary in the specifics of their problems and dysfunctional beliefs, and thus therapists may best serve their clients by designing individualized programs that can vary in emphasis and in particular combinations of interventions. Accordingly, the book presents different cognitive-behavioral techniques that have been studied and proven effective with women sufferers of PTSD following assault.

The book is divided into two sections. Section I contains a review of what we know about PTSD prevalence, diagnosis, and treatment efficacy. In Chapter 1, a rape victim and her father give a personal account of postrape sequelae. In Chapter 2, we discuss the formal diagnostic criteria of PTSD according to the DSM-IV, as well as the prevalence of this disorder in different trauma populations. In Chapter 3, we discuss other psychological disturbances that often occur after traumatic experiences, and relevant treatment strategies for these. In Chapter 4, we review the studies of the efficacy of psychosocial and pharmacological treatments of PTSD. Finally, in Chapter 5, we present psychological theories of trauma and suggest an integrated theory for the development of chronic PTSD. This theory serves as the basis for our cognitive-behavioral treatments, and it explains the mechanisms involved in successful implementation of cognitive-behavioral techniques.

Section II of the book delineates how to conduct cognitive-behavioral interventions for PTSD. In Chapter 6, we introduce a menu of effective techniques and outline suggested treatment programs. In Chapter 7, we present our methods of assessing PTSD and related problems, and describe how to collect the information that will guide the therapist in constructing a treatment program. Chapter 8 instructs the therapist in how to present the treatment program, how to convey to the client the rationale for the treatment, and how to plan the treatment. Chapters 8 to 14 outline the various cognitive-behavioral interventions used in a comprehensive treatment program for PTSD. They are breathing training and other relaxation training techniques, *in vivo* (real-life) exposure, imaginal exposure (reliving of the trauma), cognitive restructuring, thought stopping, guided self-dialogue, covert modeling, and role playing. In Chapter 15, we discuss problems and complications in implementing these techniques, discuss how to terminate treatment, and present a full case illustration.

Throughout the book, we present examples from our own clinical experience. Most of these are aggregates of several clients and thus do not represent any one distinct person. In addition, names and details about the trauma have been greatly altered to prevent any identification and to protect privacy.

Again, this book is addressed to all mental health professionals who have chosen the difficult but rewarding path of trying to help women overcome the devastating experience of sexual assault and the psychological difficulties that often follow this experience. It is primarily intended to guide clinical psychologists, psychiatrists, social workers, and rape crisis counselors who daily confront the challenge of helping rape (and other trauma) victims.

EDNA B. FOA
BARBARA OLASOV ROTHBAUM

Contents

I

WHAT DO WE KNOW ABOUT PTSD FOLLOWING ASSAULT?

1

The Clinical Picture: A Rape Victim and Her Father Tell Their Stories

In this chapter, the father of a rape victim describes his own reactions to his daughter's rape. In addition, his daughter describes the rape and her reactions. Between them, they present a clear picture of Posttraumatic Stress Disorder (PTSD) following sexual assault. Although this book focuses on treating the rape survivor through individual therapy, this chapter allows the reader to understand the impact on people close to the victim as well. Names in the account that follows have been changed, and the story is told with the permission of all family members.

The Father's Reaction to Learning of the Rape

My nightmare began when the mother of my daughter's best friend came to my office. It didn't take her long to tell me that Sarah, who was currently a senior in high school, had been raped 2 years before. It happened when she had been babysitting the daughters of neighbors whom she accompanied on a family vacation to the beach. My shock was overwhelming. I muddled through my remaining meetings, wanting to exit the office as quickly as possible. I was scared, numb, and mildly disoriented when I picked up my wife at home a short while later. We drove to a nearby parking lot, and I told her that Sarah had been raped. I began an odyssey that afternoon — one that has led, some 8 months later, to my sitting at the word processor writing this story.

All of a sudden, Sarah's changed behavior during the past 2 years made sense. She had always been an active child, strong-willed, but thoughtful and kind. Two years earlier, however, she had become belligerent, aggressive, emotionally demanding, and bitterly hostile at the least provocation with both me and my wife. In addition, she began refusing to go to school, and the hours between 7 A.M. and 8:15 A.M. (the latter being the time the school bus left) became a "war zone" in our household. We probed and questioned. I spoke with several of her friends, asking if they were aware of anything that would account for her behavior change. We learned nothing. Sarah refused adamantly to discuss any problems, and her outbursts following such questioning made the inquiries painful experiences. Her patterns at school paralleled those at home. We were told by teachers that she was argumentative, hostile, and talkative in her classes; insensitive to the class-room needs of her peers; and particularly insensitive to the teachers. Of note were the conflicts Sarah had with the gym faculty. She refused to participate in gym, refused to wear the required garb, frequently reported that her equipment had been stolen from her locker, and promptly "lost" whatever new gym equipment we purchased. It seemed to us that she was deliberately taking herself out of the academic mainstream. We had no clue of any antecedent cause. Surprisingly, she passed all her academic subjects that year.

Sarah's Disclosure to Her Family

Toward the end of my 11th-grade year, my brother Billy and I were coming home from the end-of-the-year church banquet for the youth group. We dropped off one of his friends, now one of my friends, and we started back home. Having seen all those slides of the past year's mission project brought back sudden memo-ries. I just felt so close to him that I told him everything. All he said during that time was "Yeh." He was upset, I could tell. He was angry, but not at me. I knew that. He was angry at the life I had. When we got home, we hugged and I made him promise not to tell anyone, especially Mom and Dad. He kept that promise as long as possible and as long as I needed him to keep it. Well, one of the girls that I had told at the previous summer's mission project told her mother, and she couldn't keep it silent any longer. She made an appointment with my dad 1 or 2 days after my brother Billy's college graduation. Well, then everything in my perfectly planned life fell apart, and my mom found out, and then my older brother found out. Then I realized that everyone knew. That Monday night I had to tell my family everything. That was no picnic for me, but the only good thing was that Billy was right there beside me during the whole time. He was on my side. I am really glad I told him before everybody else found out, because I don't think he and I would be as close as we are right now. That summer was very hard for me, because the only thing I thought they thought about me was that I was unclean, and of course raped. Well. I got help and love.

The Father's Response to Sarah's Disclosure

Sarah read us a diary entry she had written shortly after the rape occurred. The entry described in detail the horrible scenario that had taken place (see below).

Portions of the narrative indicated that she had been suicidal during the 10th grade. She stated that she had written these notes so that if she took her life, we would know why. She had a plan. To this day I am convinced that several of her friends—one at school and one at church—saved her life. We found out later that she had confided in both during the first year, and that they were very supportive and sympathetic. She cried while reading her diary. All I could feel was an intense rage. My oldest son expressed the same emotion. Thankfully, Billy and his mother were able to be attentive to Sarah.

Sarah's Description of the Rape

It was in the summer when I was 16. I was babysitting that summer and was having a pretty good time until Wednesday of that week, and then my life was shattered and all hell broke loose. On Wednesday I decided to go for a walk and get away from things because I needed some peace and quiet. I was staying at a beach house a couple of hours from home. I was with my next-door neighbors and their two daughters that night. I went out of my bedroom door and went down to the beach to collect my thoughts. I didn't have much time to do so. All of a sudden a man approached me from out of the blue. My back was to him, and I didn't realize anyone was there until I felt someone's eyes, and I flipped around unaware of any danger. And immediately I had to squint my eyes, because the outside light of the beach house was in my eyes. He could see me, but I could only make out a figure of a man. From what I can remember, he was wearing all black and had a scent of cheap cologne. I have not smelled it since, and I hope I will never have to. . . . Anyway, I didn't realize I was in any danger until he came closer to me, and I could feel his eyes staring straight at me. I was only 16 and I lived in the suburbs, and I thought I didn't need to feel any danger. And in a way I trusted him. Now I trust no one unless I know them well enough to my satisfaction.

He came closer to me, and I could feel his breath. He was taller than me, but then everyone was tall to me. All I saw was black until I looked around and saw, for the first time, a long knife in his left hand. It sparkled in the light, and, again, I could only make out a manly figure. I never saw his face because he was wearing a ski mask, but I could feel his eyes, and that was enough for me. I am so glad I didn't see his face, or my nightmares would probably be worse and more vivid than they are now. He pulled me out of the light and pushed me back toward some bushes. He told me I could either run and he would kill me, or I could stay and we could have a lot of fun. I still remember his voice. I can't describe it, but it is permanently in my mind. I didn't answer. He held the knife up to my throat and looked at me. Then he pushed me down to the ground on my back and ripped off my shorts and underpants. It took him a little time to get ready himself. Then he forced himself down on me. He was very heavy and strong. I felt that, so I didn't struggle, and I think that was smart. He did have a knife and who knows what else. Then I felt the pain from the lower end of my body, and then that's when I knew what this horrible man was doing to me. He was raping me. Not only raping up my insides, but my trust, my honesty, my cleanliness, my pride, my sleep, my friends, my family, my happiness—and, most of all, my life. I just lay there not doing anything, but thinking, "What am I going to tell my family?" I don't recall how long this went on, but I do recall the pain and the powerlessness. Then a wet feeling. Then he got up and said, "Thanks." That's all he said, and he left and went on his way to rape another woman, or home to his wife and kids, or back to a house out on the street. I don't know and don't care at all.

After he left, I just sat there and tried to think up some sort of reasonable solution of what to do. So I gathered my clothes and headed back to the house. Not as I had before, when I had no violent thoughts in my mind. I have never really walked the same way since. Now I always walk with distrust of the situation and myself. I got back in the house safely, and immediately went to the shower. Now I was sobbing lightly, but not wanting to let the people upstairs hear me. They were eating dinner and having a good time, while I was being ripped apart. When I got in the shower, the first thing I grabbed for was the soap. I washed every part of my body, and now I was crying. Now I was scared of everything I had trusted before tonight. Finally, after washing myself very thoroughly as best I could, I got out. I didn't want to, because I still was not clean and I wanted to stay in there until I was. But I got out, dried off, and headed to bed. I did not sleep for at least 1 month. The most I got was 30-minute spurts, and then I was wide awake waiting for him to come back and do it all over again. Well, I managed to get through the week; I don't know how. That will always amaze me. But I did go home and started my period, so that was some sort of comfort to me.

The Father's Continuing Reactions

I left town shortly after learning of Sarah's rape. I was afraid that if I stayed in the house, I might say something to Sarah that would aggravate the crisis. Frankly, I was not able to think of Sarah, my sons, or my wife—I had to get away and think of what I wanted to do next. I began to feel that I had nothing in common with others. The trauma severed my felt connection with people— my family, my intimate friends, my graduate students, and my colleagues. I became a stranger.

I returned home several days later. I began to realize, for the first time, the extent of my anger and rage. I wanted to kill the man who had hurt Sarah, and I feel now that at that point I could have done so with relish. I also became aware of feeling an intense sort of pain for Sarah, as I started thinking about her agony and torment over the past 2 years. Then an overwhelming feeling of helplessness came over me, as I realized that I was powerless to make the crisis go away. This pervasive feeling of helplessness would last for many months, until I began to see healing in my daughter, and began to feel that I could contribute to her healing process. All along, my own experience of pain and healing has been inextricably bound to Sarah's healing process.

Setting limits for Sarah in our household began to take on fearful connotations. Equivocation characterized my expectations of her behavior, because I was never certain whether my limits would inhibit the healing process. For example, she stopped attending school that year, and I didn't know whether to push her to go to school or not. We decided to let her decide what to do about school. Her sleep cycle was reversed. She couldn't sleep at night, so she slept most of the day. I was not comfortable leaving for work and knowing she was sleeping at home alone. However, there was no other alternative; my wife and I had to go to work. Finally, I learned to trust in her judgment as to what she needed.

Sarah and I also began conversing more about what had happened. She began talking to me about her insomnia, as well as her feelings of fear, pain, and despair about ever getting over the rape. In addition, she began to let me comfort her. I began to experience some hope that maybe recovery for both of us could be achieved. I increasingly trusted her to continue the struggle toward recovery, and I started feeling less and less that I had to do it all, had to make everything "OK." My wife and I then began actively dealing with the personal wreckage that had been inflicted on our marriage, home, and family. The rapist had raped our entire family and affected its destiny for over 2½ years!

At last, Sarah gave me permission to tell her story. She read what I had written before she went to bed one night. Later, I asked her what she thought about it. She said, "Thanks," and reached out for my neck. We had one of the best and longest hugs we have shared in over 2½ years.

Authors' Conclusion

The next chapter describes the traumatic reactions to rape in epidemiological and diagnostic terms. We then briefly review what is currently known about the treatment for PTSD following rape and other traumas, and present our theoretical framework. Section II is the heart of the book, in which we describe our programs for treating the trauma of rape.

2

Diagnosis and Prevalence of PTSD Following Assault

PTSD affects from 9% to 15% of the general population (Breslau, Davis, Andreski, & Peterson, 1991; Davidson, Hughes, Blazer, & George, 1991), and close to 50% of women who have been raped (Rothbaum, Foa, Riggs, Murdock, & Walsh, 1992). Because PTSD is such a prevalent and debilitating disorder, one of the top priorities for mental health professionals around the world is to develop effective and efficient treatments for it. In this chapter, we discuss the diagnosis and prevalence of the disorder following assault.

PTSD According to the DSM-IV

Human reactions to trauma have been described for more than a century under various labels, including "hysteria" (Putnam, 1881), "nervous shock" (Page, 1885), "traumatophobia" (Rado, 1942), and "war neurosis" (Grinker & Spiegel, 1943). In 1980, persistent posttrauma symptoms were introduced in the third edition of the *Diagnostic and Statistical Manual of Mental Disorders* (DSM-III) as an anxiety disorder called Posttraumatic Stress Disorder (PTSD; American Psychiatric Association [APA], 1980). The DSM-III-R (APA, 1987) described PTSD as an anxiety disorder precipitated by an event that falls outside usual human experience and characterized by symptoms of reexperiencing (e.g., nightmares, flashbacks), avoidance and numbing (e.g., avoidance of reminders, psychogenic amnesia), and arousal (e.g., difficulty sleeping, exaggerated startle) that persist longer than 1 month after the trauma. The DSM-IV has retained the symptoms described in the DSM-III-R, but has modified the trauma criterion to include characteristics of the traumatic event and the individual's perception of threat rather than the rarity of the event. The revised symptom duration criterion includes the subtypes of "acute" and "chronic" to describe the course of the reaction (see Table 2.1 for the DSM-IV PTSD cri-

TABLE 2.1. DSM-IV Diagnostic Criteria for PTSD

A. The person has been exposed to a traumatic event in which both of the following were present:
  (1) the person experienced, witnessed, or was confronted with an event or events that involved actual or threatened death or serious injury, or a threat to the physical integrity of self or others
  (2) the person's response involved intense fear, helplessness, or horror. **Note**: In children, this may be expressed instead by disorganized or agitated behavior.
B. The traumatic event is persistently reexperienced in one (or more) of the following ways:
  (1) recurrent and intrusive distressing recollections of the event, including images, thoughts, or perceptions. **Note**: In young children, repetitive play may occur in which themes or aspects of the trauma are expressed.
  (2) recurrent distressing dreams of the event. **Note**: In children, there may be frightening dreams without recognizable content.
  (3) acting or feeling as if the traumatic event were recurring (includes a sense of reliving the experience, illusions, hallucinations, and dissociative flashback episodes, including those that occur upon awakening or when intoxicated). **Note**: In young children, trauma-specific reenactment may occur.
  (4) intense psychological distress at exposure to internal or external cues that symbolize or resemble an aspect of the traumatic event
  (5) physiological reactivity on exposure to internal or external cues that symbolize or resemble an aspect of the traumatic event
C. Persistent avoidance of stimuli associated with the trauma and numbing of general responsiveness (not present before the trauma), as indicated by three (or more) of the following:
  (1) efforts to avoid thoughts, feelings, or conversations associated with the trauma
  (2) efforts to avoid activities, places, or people that arouse recollections of the trauma
  (3) inability to recall an important aspect of the trauma
  (4) markedly diminished interest or participation in significant activities
  (5) feeling of detachment or estrangement from others
  (6) restricted range of affect (e.g., unable to have loving feelings)
  (7) sense of a foreshortened future (e.g., does not expect to have a career, marriage, children, or a normal life span)
D. Persistent symptoms of increased arousal (not present before the trauma), as indicated by two (or more) of the following:
  (1) difficulty falling or staying asleep
  (2) irritability or outbursts of anger
  (3) difficulty concentrating
  (4) hypervigilance
  (5) exaggerated startle response
E. Duration of the disturbance (symptoms in Criteria B, C, and D) is more than 1 month.
F. The disturbance causes clinically significant distress or impairment in social, occupational, or other important areas of functioning.
Specify if:
  Acute: if duration of symptoms is less than 3 months
  Chronic: if duration of symptoms is 3 months or more
Specify if:
  With Delayed Onset: if onset of symptoms is at least 6 months after the stressor

Note. Reprinted with permission from the *Diagnostic and Statistical Manual of Mental Disorders, Fourth Edition* (pp. 427–429). Copyright 1994 American Psychiatric Association.

teria). We discuss both acute and chronic PTSD in this chapter; we also look at the new DSM-IV category of Acute Stress Disorder.

The impetus for formalizing the persistent posttrauma syndrome as a psychiatric disorder in the DSM-III was the large number of Vietnam combat veterans who manifested the symptoms listed in Table 2.1. But the same symptom constellation was observed in victims of traumas other than war, including accidents (Burstein et al., 1988; Muse, 1986); natural disasters, such as volcanos, fires, tornados, floods, and mudslides (Bravo, Rubio-Stipec, Canino, Woodbury, & Ribera, 1990; Green et al., 1990; Shore, Tatum, & Vollmer, 1986; Smith, Robins, Pryzbeck, Goldring, & Solomon, 1986; McFarlane, 1988a, 1988b); and disasters such as the nuclear accident at Three Mile Island as well as dam and skywalk collapses (Baum, Gatchel, & Schaeffer, 1983; Bromet & Schulberg, 1986; Green et al., 1990, 1991; Wilkinson, 1983); and rape (Kilpatrick, Saunders, Veronen, Best, & Von, 1987a; Rothbaum et al., 1992). The duration of PTSD symptoms varies across individuals: Some experience traumatic events with apparently no long-lasting adverse effects, whereas other victims seem impaired years after the occurrence of the trauma (Green et al., 1990; Kilpatrick et al., 1987a).

Validity of the Three PTSD Symptom Clusters

As described above, in the DSM-IV and its predecessors, PTSD symptoms are divided into three clusters: reexperiencing, numbing/avoidance, and arousal symptoms. These clusters were determined by clinical observations rather than by empirical research. A recent study that investigated whether elements in each of these clusters really "hang together" found partial confirmation for this division of the PTSD symptoms (Foa, Riggs, & Gershuny, 1995c). When the 17 symptoms were investigated by means of a factor analysis, three clusters (also called factors) emerged, but the symptoms in each cluster did not exactly overlap with the symptoms in the clusters of the DSM-IV. One important difference is that in the DSM-IV the avoidance symptoms (e.g., efforts to avoid thoughts about the trauma) and the numbing symptoms (e.g., restricted range of affect, feeling of detachment or estrangement from others) are lumped together into one cluster. In the Foa et al. (1995c) study, however, the numbing symptoms and the avoidance symptoms belonged to different factors. Thus, it appears that numbing and effortful avoidance may represent separate phenomena and may relate differently to other posttrauma symptoms. Later in this chapter, we discuss avoidance and numbing further in the context of examining the relationship between numbing and dissociation.

Interestingly, numbing symptoms better distinguished victims with PTSD from those without PTSD than the remaining symptoms. Very few of the victims without PTSD endorsed the numbing symptoms. In contrast, many victims who did not meet the full criteria for PTSD endorsed symptoms of intrusion, arousal, and effortful avoidance. Thus, the presence of numbing symptoms best identified individuals with PTSD. The findings that numbing symptoms distinguish victims with PTSD from those without PTSD is very interesting, because, according to the DSM-IV, a victim can receive a diagnosis of PTSD without having any numbing symptoms.

In the study on the clusters of PTSD symptoms, increased irritability/ anger belonged with the numbing factor, despite the fact that in the DSM-IV it is subsumed under the arousal symptom cluster. This suggests that angry arousal and anxious arousal may be somewhat different. Riggs et al. (1995) have suggested that anger may serve to inhibit feelings of anxiety in assault victims. Thus, like numbing symptoms, anger may serve to protect the individual from continuous anxiety when effortful avoidance fails to do so.

Another study that found numbing symptoms to be a prominent feature of PTSD was conducted by Solomon, Mikulincer, and Benbenishty (1989), who interviewed Israeli soldiers 1 year after combat and used factor analysis to ascertain the symptom clusters in this group. As in the Foa et al. (1995c) study, a psychic numbing cluster emerged, and in this study it was more prominent than other symptom clusters. The symptoms in the numbing cluster included detachment from others and from one's surroundings; numbing of responses; mental escape; and distraction. These results point again to the prominent position of dissociation in posttrauma sequelae.

Similarities and Differences between PTSD and Other Anxiety Disorders

The placement of the diagnostic category of PTSD among the anxiety disorders in the DSM reflects the recognition that anxiety is a predominant reaction to trauma. Indeed, the symptoms of PTSD overlap considerably with those of other anxiety disorders. For example, arousal symptoms such as hypervigilance, sleep disturbances, irritability, and difficulty concentrating are common to both PTSD and Generalized Anxiety Disorder (GAD). Fear and avoidance are common to PTSD, Specific Phobia, Social Phobia, and Agoraphobia. Some experts are of the opinion that flashbacks more closely resemble Panic Disorder than other anxiety disorders, and suggest that nearly all flashbacks involve panic-like features (Burstein, 1985; Mellman & Davis, 1985). However, flashbacks and nightmares remain unique to PTSD and are the more dramatic features of PTSD (McFarlane, 1988b). Moreover, patients with Panic Disorder often describe their first panic attack in terms suggesting that this experience was extremely traumatic for them; however, they rarely have nightmares or flashbacks about it. This is also true for people who have become phobic about a situation or an object after a frightening experience such as being bitten by a dog. They rarely report nightmares or flashbacks about the fearful experience. Thus, flashbacks and nightmares are unique to PTSD.

Both PTSD and Obsessive–Compulsive Disorder (OCD) are characterized by distressing intrusive cognitions, usually termed "reexperiencing" in PTSD and "obsessions" in OCD. Although the reexperiencing symptoms of PTSD differ from obsessions in OCD in content and complexity, they can be equally intrusive, vivid, and distressing. Intrusive cognitions are also present in other psychiatric conditions, such as Schizophrenia, Major Depressive Disorder and GAD. PTSD sufferers may for a while engage in compulsive behaviors. For example, rape victims with PTSD may shower excessively for some time after the rape in an attempt to reduce feelings of "dirtiness" (see Sarah's description in Chapter 1), or may check locks repeatedly to feel safer. If these compulsive symptoms become chronic and pervasive, a dual diagnosis of OCD and PTSD is warranted.

Escape/avoidance behaviors in PTSD sufferers, like many avoidance behaviors in individuals with other anxiety disorders, are driven by the strong desire of anxious individuals to avoid or escape states of high anxiety, as well as by their bias toward exaggerating the probability of threat (Foa & Kozak, 1986; Foa, Franklin, Perry, & Herbert, 1996; Foa, Steketee, & Rothbaum, 1989b). As noted above, although avoidance symptoms are common to all anxiety disorders, numbing symptoms are strongly characteristic of PTSD but are uncommon in other anxiety disorders. The state of numbness is described by PTSD sufferers as the *absence* of emotion or feelings in situations where emotional reactions are expected. However, numbness is not the absence of a reaction; the numbness is the reaction. The absence of a reaction is "nothing." When a reaction is experienced, sufferers report feeling "numb" rather than "nothing."

Unlike other anxiety disorders, the diagnosis of PTSD always requires an instigating external event, with the emphasis on major stressors such as combat, rape, severe accidents, natural disasters, captivity, and criminal assault. PTSD affects individuals with previously normal personality functioning (Breslau & Davis, 1987; Foy, Sipprelle, Rueger, & Carroll, 1984). Although symptom selection in OCD, Panic Disorder, or other anxiety disorders may at times reflect a stressor such as childbirth or a personally trying event (Foa, Steketee, & Young, 1984), most cases begin insidiously, and the specific symptoms generally are not clearly related to antecedent life events.

In summary, PTSD victims share some phenomenological features with sufferers of other anxiety disorders, including intrusive thoughts, avoidance behaviors, and hyperarousal. The features that distinguish PTSD are flashbacks, nightmares, and numbing.

The Symptom Picture of PTSD

Consistent with the diagnostic features of PTSD, experts have noted that criminal victimization produces a variety of disturbances, including anxiety, depression, intrusive thoughts and images of the assault, and sleep disturbances such as nightmares and insomnia (Calhoun, Atkeson, & Resick, 1982; Ellis, Atkeson, & Calhoun, 1981; Frank & Stewart, 1984; Kilpatrick & Veronen, 1984; Kilpatrick, Veronen, & Resick, 1979b; Nadelson, Notman, Zackson, & Gornick, 1982; Resick, 1987).

Rape victims report intrusive thoughts and images of the assault that they actively attempt to avoid (Kilpatrick & Veronen, 1984; Resick, 1987). They also report more sleep disturbance, including nightmares and insomnia (Ellis et al., 1981; Nadelson et al., 1982) and more difficulty concentrating (Nadelson et al., 1982) than nonvictimized controls. Thus, the postassault psychopathology of rape victims can be best characterized as PTSD. Indeed, 76% of rape victims in one study reported PTSD symptoms at some point within a year after the assault (Resnick, Veronen, Saunders, Kilpatrick, & Cornelison, 1989b).

Prevalence Studies

After a major trauma, the vast majority of people will experience psychological disturbance, but most will recover over time. Therefore, it is important to distinguish between a normal reaction to trauma and a chronic pathological reaction. To study the course of reaction, it is necessary to assess PTSD symptoms repeatedly, beginning soon after the trauma. Several researchers have conducted studies using such prospective methodology. Unfortunately, the course of PTSD in Vietnam veterans cannot be ascertained, because PTSD as a diagnostic entity did not exist until 1980—a considerable time after the Vietnam War. Later studies of PTSD in this population are plagued by confounding factors, such as chronic hospitalizations, substance use disorders, and other comorbid disorders. Nevertheless, for the sake of thoroughness, we also discuss the results of two retrospective studies of the prevalence of PTSD in Vietnam veterans.

Before we begin, it is useful to clarify some of the terminology used in epidemiological studies. In general, "incidence" refers to the frequency of occurrence, often considered the number of "new" cases of a disorder. "Prevalence" refers to how widespread a disorder is at a given time. For example, sampling a cross-section of the population would lead to estimates of the prevalence of PTSD present at that time. In this section, we do not focus on the distinction between prevalence and incidence; instead, we discuss prospective and retrospective studies separately.

Prevalence of PTSD among Trauma Victims in Prospective Studies

We (Rothbaum et al., 1992) conducted a prospective study on posttrauma reactions in female victims of rape and other crime. PTSD symptoms were assessed via a structured interview we developed, which is described later in this book. The PTSD symptoms assessed in the interview were reliving experiences, nightmares, flashbacks, avoidance of reminders and thoughts of the assault, impaired leisure activities, sense of detachment, blunted affect, disturbed sleep, memory and concentration difficulties, hyperalertness, increased startle response, feelings of guilt, and increased fearfulness. The results are depicted in Figure 2.1.

Rape victims ($n = 95$) were first interviewed within 2 weeks following their assault (mean = 12.64 days) and once weekly thereafter for 12 weeks. Follow-up assessments were conducted 6 and 9 months following the assault ($n = 24$). The results indicated that at the initial interview, 94% of rape victims met the symptom criteria but not the duration criteron for a PTSD diagnosis. At 1 month postassault (mean = 35 days), 65% met criteria for PTSD; this figure decreased to 52.5% by 2 months postassault and to 47% by 3 months postassault (Rothbaum et al., 1992). At 6 months postassault, 41.7% were classified as having PTSD, and at 9 months postassault, 47.1% fulfilled PTSD criteria. PTSD and related psychopathology decreased sharply between Assessments 1

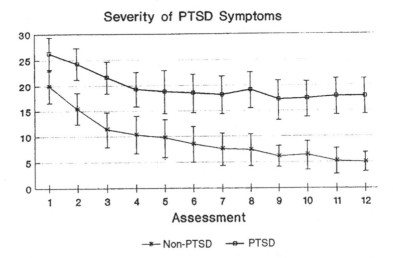

FIGURE 2.1. Severity of PTSD symptoms among rape victims over 12 weeks of assessment (Assessment 1 occurred within 2 weeks of assault). Non-PTSD, women who did not meet the criteria for PTSD at 3 months postassault; PTSD, women who did meet these criteria at 3 months postassault. From Rothbaum, Foa, Riggs, Murdock, and Walsh (1992). Copyright 1992 by Plenum Publishing Corporation. Reprinted by permission.

and 4 for all women. Women who did not meet criteria for PTSD 3 months postassault showed steady improvement over time throughout the 12 weeks of the study. However, women whose PTSD persisted throughout the 3-month study did not show as much improvement after the fourth assessment, approximately 1 month postassault. Thus, nearly all of the rape victims in this sample appeared to meet symptom criteria for PTSD immediately following the assault, but fewer than half continued to meet criteria for this disorder 3 months later.

The course of PTSD for victims of nonsexual criminal assault (simple and aggravated assault and robbery) was similar to that found for the rape victims. A majority of the crime victims reported many PTSD symptoms initially, but the incidence of PTSD decreased over time (Riggs, Rothbaum, & Foa, 1995). The results of this study are shown in Figure 2.2.

Eighty-four victims of nonsexual assault (53 women and 31 men) were prospectively examined soon after the assault (average of 18.68 days) and seen weekly for 3 months. Initially, 71% of the women and 50% of the men met symptomatic criteria for PTSD; these figures decreased to 42% of the women and 32% of the men by the fourth weekly assessment. At 3 months postassault,

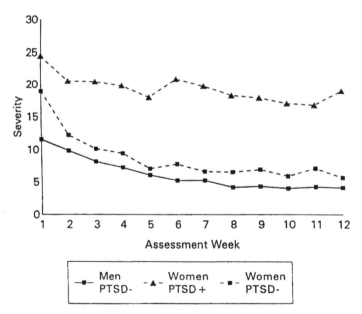

FIGURE 2.2. Severity of PTSD symptoms among victims of nonsexual assault over 12 weeks of assessment. PTSD–, subjects who did not meet criteria for PTSD at 3 months postassault; PTSD+, subjects who did meet these criteria at 3 months postassault. From Riggs, Rothbaum, and Foa (1995). Copyright 1995 by Sage Publications, Inc. Reprinted by permission.

21% of the women but none of the men evidenced the full symptom criteria for PTSD. However, many of those who did not evidence full PTSD at the final assessment did report significant PTSD symptoms, particularly reexperiencing and arousal symptoms. Examining the course of PTSD symptoms across the 12 weeks of the study indicated different patterns for those not diagnosed with PTSD at the final assessment versus those with full PTSD at that time. Victims without full PTSD at the final assessment showed a significant decline in severity of PTSD over the course of the study. However, women diagnosed with PTSD at the final assessment did not evidence a significant decline in PTSD symptom severity across time. Thus, like the rape victims, most of the nonsexual assault victims initially responded with PTSD symptoms, which decreased substantially by 3 months postassault. Although the pattern of gradual decline in PTSD incidence by 3 months postassault was the same for sexual and nonsexual assault victims, it is important to note that the rape victims were more likely to develop PTSD initially and to maintain it over time. The results of yet another prospective study comparing postassault reactions of female sexual and nonsexual assault victims conducted by Foa and colleagues yielded the same results. Rape produced more severe and more persistent reactions than nonsexual assault (Foa & Riggs, 1993), and victims with more severe initial PTSD were more likely to have persistent symptoms (Amir, Foa, & Cashman, 1996).

Evidence from other populations of trauma victims indicate that the reactions of rape and nonsexual assault victims described above are not unique to these types of trauma victims. For example, the finding that, without treatment, victims who develop PTSD early are more likely to exhibit the disorder later on also emerged from studies on firefighters who had traumatic experiences during their work. In one study (McFarlane, 1988a), 315 firefighters were assessed for PTSD at 4, 8, 11, and 29 months postdisaster. Sixty-nine percent of those who were symptomatic at 4 months postfire remained so later on, suggesting that PTSD at 4 months posttrauma is a relatively reliable predictor for the chronicity of the disorder (McFarlane, 1988a). Similar results came from another study with firefighters, in which 81% of firefighters diagnosed with PTSD at 8 months following the fire ($n = 50$) still had PTSD at 42 months postfire (McFarlane, 1988b). Thus, prospective studies suggest that by 3–4 months posttrauma, and definitely by 6–8 months posttrauma, the course of PTSD has become chronic and can no longer be expected to diminish naturally, as in a normal reaction to trauma.

Prevalence of PTSD among Trauma Victims in Retrospective Studies

Several studies have used a retrospective methodology to assess the prevalence of PTSD, and on the whole they portray a less devastating picture. Rape victims ($n = 33$) were interviewed 12–36 months postassault to assess the presence and duration of PTSD symptoms (Resnick et al., 1989). The results were remarkably similar to those reported in the Rothbaum et al. (1992) study. Seventy-six percent of the rape victims studied reported experiencing PTSD symptoms that lasted less than 1 month; 60.6% reported PTSD lasting at least 1 month; and 39.4% met criteria for PTSD at the time of inquiry, 12–36 months postassault. It is important to remember, however, that the participants in this study as well as participants in the prospective studies described earlier may not constitute representative samples, and thus a biased picture can be drawn from the results. It is entirely possible, for example, that victims who are motivated to participate in such demanding studies have more severe reactions than those who decline participation or drop out midway. It is also possible that victims who do not participate are more avoidant.

In contrast to the participants described in the studies above, who actually came into the clinic to be interviewed, Kilpatrick et al. (1987a) investigated the rate of PTSD in rape and crime victims from a community sample of 391 adult females, using a modified version of the Diagnostic Interview Schedule (DIS; Robins, Helzer, Croughan, & Ratcliff, 1981). Of those who had experienced a completed rape, 57.1% suffered from PTSD at some point following the assault, and 16.5% met PTSD criteria at the time of the inquiry (average of approximately 15 years postassault). Of aggravated assault victims, 36.8% had PTSD at some point after the assault, and 10.5% were diagnosed with PTSD at the time of the interview (average of 10.5 years postassault). Thus, again, a large number of victims initially responded to rape with PTSD symptoms, but a smaller number (a much smaller number than those emerging from prospective studies) developed a chronic disorder. Again, rape appeared to be more likely to induce PTSD than did other serious crimes not involving sexual assault.

In yet another retrospective study, lifetime and current prevalence of PTSD was investigated in a community sample of 214 adult victims of homicide in the family (called "homicide survivors"; Kilpatrick, Amick, & Resnick, 1988). Subjects were assessed for PTSD via a 30-minute telephone interview. Twenty-nine percent of criminal homicide survivors experienced PTSD at some point, with 7.0% experiencing PTSD at the time of inquiry (which was not specified). Of alcohol-related vehicular homicide survivors, 34.1% experienced PTSD at some point, with 2.2% experiencing PTSD at the time of inquiry. Thus, approximately one-third of homicide survivors evidenced an occurrence of PTSD at some point following the death, but a very small percentage developed a chronic disorder. Interestingly, the rate of current PTSD among the criminal homicide survivors was three times the rate among the vehicular homicide survivors, suggesting that trauma involving crime may be more devastating than noncriminal trauma.

The lifetime and current prevalences of trauma and PTSD were assessed in a large national sample (Resnick, Kilpatrick, Dansky, Saunders, & Best,

1993). Random dialing of telephone numbers was used to sample 4,008 women across the United States. The authors used the results of this study to estimate the number of women in the United States who had experienced different types of traumas, based on the 1989 U.S. Bureau of the Census estimate of the population of U.S. adult women (age 18 or older) of 96,056,000. In this sample, about 13% reported experiencing a completed rape; thus the authors estimated that this had occurred in approximately 12,151,084 American women. Other sexual assault was reported in 14.32% of the sample, resulting in an estimate of 13,755,219 women. Physical assault was reported by 10.28% of the women sampled; 13.37% reported the homicide of a family member; 35.58% reported any criminal victimization; and 33.31 reported experiencing a noncriminal disaster only. Overall, 68.89% of the women sampled, leading to an estimate of 66,172,978 American women, reported experiencing at least one of the traumas assessed. According to these results, two-thirds of adult American women have experienced a significant trauma.

The prevalence of lifetime and current PTSD was also assessed in the study by Resnick et al. (1993). Of the women sampled who reported experiencing a completed rape, 32% reported a history of PTSD in their lifetimes, and 12.4% indicated current PTSD at the time of questioning. Of the women sampled who reported experiencing other sexual assault, 30.8% reported a history of PTSD in their lifetimes, and 13% indicated current PTSD. Physical assault led to 38.5% lifetime PTSD and 17.8% current PTSD; the homicide of a family member or close friend led to 22.1% lifetime PTSD and 8.9% current PTSD. Any criminal victimization was associated with 25.8% lifetime PTSD and 9.7% current PTSD; any noncriminal trauma (e.g., disaster, accident) was associated with 9.4% lifetime PTSD and 3.4% current PTSD. Having experienced any of the traumas in question was associated with 17.9% lifetime PTSD and 6.7% current PTSD.

In summary, 12.3% of women who participated in the study reported having experienced PTSD at some point in their lifetimes, and 4.6% were currently experiencing PTSD at the time of the study. Women who had experienced a criminal trauma were three times as likely to have PTSD at the time of the interview. The implications of this monumental study for health in general and mental health in particular are vast, as it suggests that criminal victimization and the resultant PTSD pose a serious health problem for American women.

The prevalence of PTSD in Vietnam veterans was assessed thoroughly in the retrospective National Vietnam Veteran Readjustment Study, which used multiple measures of PTSD. The findings indicate that among theater veterans, 15.2% of the men and 8.5% of the women (nearly 500,000 people) were suffering from PTSD at the time of the interview, more than 15 years postservice (Schlenger et al., 1992). As would be expected, the lifetime prevalence of PTSD among Vietnam veterans who served in Vietnam was much higher than rates in the general population. Among nontheater veterans, 30.9% reported experiencing PTSD at some point following their service. The lifetime prevalence for female veterans was 26%. Profoundly alarming is the investigators' note that "of the 1.7 million veterans who ever experienced significant symptoms of PTSD after the Vietnam war, approximately 830,000 (49%) still experience clinically significant distress and disability from symptoms of PTSD" (Weiss et al., 1992, p. 365).

A different picture has emerged from data collected on civilians who experienced heavy shelling during wartime, although the conclusions from some of these studies rest on a small number of participants. Saigh (1988) assessed 12 undergraduate and graduate students at the American University of Beirut in 1983 and 1984, before and after a major offensive involving heavy shelling of the areas near the university. Structured interviews aimed at diagnosing PTSD retrospectively (approximately 1 year following the shelling) revealed that 9 of the 11 students interviewed (81.8%) experienced PTSD symptoms immediately following the shelling. However, the symptoms of 8 of these 9 spontaneously remitted within 1 month after the shelling; the remaining student developed chronic PTSD. These results are consistent with reports from World War II demonstrating that civilians undergoing an air raid exhibited short-lived fear reactions, but that very few developed intense persistent fear reactions (Rachman, 1989). Findings corroborating this observation were also reported from Northern Ireland (Cairns & Wilson, 1984). One reason for the apparent differences between the experiences of civilians under heavy shelling during wartime and the other types of traumatic experiences is that the former occur in more predictable and perhaps somewhat more controllable situations (e.g., people can find refuge in designated shelters). Predictable, controllable stressors in humans and in animal experiments were found to cause far less psychological and physiological injury than unpredictable, uncontrollable stress (Foa, Zinbarg, & Rothbaum, 1992).

PTSD in Traumatized Children

There are data from a prospective study to suggest that the course of PTSD in children may be similar to that in adults. The rates of PTSD in 159 children aged 5–13 were evaluated about 1 month after a fatal sniper attack on their school playground; 100 of them were also evaluated 14 months after the shooting (Nader, Pynoos, Fairbanks, & Frederick, 1990; Pynoos et al., 1987). Using the children's version of the PTSD Reaction Index completed by an interviewer, the researchers found that the rate of PTSD varied with degree of exposure. At the first interview, 77% of the children who were on the playground during the attack were classified as having severe or moderate PTSD, and 67% of children who were in the school building had PTSD. Fourteen months later, 74% of the children who were on the playground still manifested PTSD, as compared to fewer than 19% of those who were in the school. The latter did not differ from children who were not at school during the attack. Thus, nearly all of the children in the study who were on the playground during the attack and had PTSD shortly after the attack exhibited chronic PTSD 14 months later, whereas most of the children who were less exposed to the attack (i.e., were inside the school) recovered over time. Thus, the DSM-III-R and DSM-IV 1-month duration-of-symptoms criterion was an excellent predictor of chronic PTSD in the highly exposed children, but a poor predictor for the less exposed group. Perhaps an intermediate assessment would have increased the accuracy of prediction for the entire population.

Summary

A common pattern emerges from the studies reviewed above. The rape and other crime studies indicate a high incidence of PTSD initially, which decreases gradually over time; however, a certain proportion of rape victims develop chronic PTSD that can last for many years. Likewise, a significant number of Vietnam veterans continue to suffer from PTSD even two decades or more after their service. Civilians also respond with a high rate of PTSD initially, but most recover relatively quickly. Children's reactions appear to vary with their proximity to the original trauma: In the sniper attack study discussed above, most of the children in close proximity to the sniper responded with PTSD that remained chronic. However, most of the children who were not in close proximity to the sniper initially responded with PTSD which tended to dissipate over time.

Acute and Chronic PTSD

The DSM-III (APA, 1980) distinguished two subtypes of PTSD: acute, in which symptoms begin within 6 months following the trauma but have not lasted 6 months, and chronic or delayed, in which symptoms either develop more than 6 months following the trauma or last 6 months or more. The DSM-III-R (APA, 1987) eliminated these subtypes. The DSM-IV (APA, 1994) reinstated the subtypes with some modifications: acute, chronic, and with delayed onset (see Table 2.1).

Although the distinction between acute and chronic PTSD is straightforward, the identification of delayed reaction in the clinical setting is more problematic. In the only controlled comparison available, 31 Vietnam veterans with delayed-onset PTSD were compared to 32 with acute-onset PTSD (Watson, Kucala, Manifold, Vassar, & Juba, 1988). Veterans were assessed for PTSD via a structured interview based on DSM-III criteria. No significant differences between the two groups emerged. In addition, there was no evidence that delayed onset was related to the severity of the trauma, the severity of the symptoms, repression, or previous stress history. In the studies by Pynoos and his colleagues on school children following a fatal sniper attack, no cases of delayed PTSD reactions were noted; in Foa and colleagues' studies on rape victims, about 95% met PTSD symptom criteria initially, leaving little room for delayed PTSD. It seems that the DSM-III and DSM-IV category of delayed-onset PTSD has not gained much support from prospective studies. It relies heavily on clinical anecdotes of patients whose memory regarding past symptoms may not be entirely reliable by the time they enter treatment, often years after the trauma occurred.

Acute Stress Disorder: A New DSM Category

The diagnosis of PTSD cannot be assigned to a trauma victim until the required symptom constellation has persisted for at least 1 month. This requirement presents several problems in assessing the need and eligibility of a victim for treatment during the first month after the trauma. It also does not allow for a distinction between victims who manifest moderate symptom severity (which, as we have suggested earlier, is a normal reaction after severe trauma) and victims who display severe, highly disruptive reactions that render them totally dysfunctional during this first month. The research findings that severe early reactions to trauma (sometimes referred to as "acute stress syndrome") predicts chronic PTSD, combined with studies suggesting that dissociative symptoms during or immediately after the trauma are highly predictive of later PTSD (e.g., Koopman, Classen, & Spiegel, 1994), led to the introduction of a new stress disorder in the DSM-IV (APA, 1994) called Acute Stress Disorder (ASD). The diagnostic criteria for this disorder are detailed in Table 2.2.

Careful examination of these criteria immediately suggests the considerable overlap in symptoms between PTSD and ASD, with the exception that the criteria for ASD emphasize the numbing or dissociative symptoms more than do those for PTSD. The major difference between the two disorders is the duration of symptoms. As we have noted above, ASD refers to reactions occurring immediately following a stressor, but if symptoms persist beyond 1 month, a diagnosis of PTSD should be given.

The Relationship between Acute Stress Reactions and PTSD

Because Acute Stress Disorder is a newcomer to the psychiatric nosology, studies about the course, prevalence, or validity of its symptom clusters are currently

TABLE 2.2. DSM-IV Diagnostic Criteria for Acute Stress Disorder

---

A. The person has been exposed to a traumatic event in which both of the
   following were present:
   (1) the person experienced, witnessed, or was confronted with an event or
       events that involved actual or threatened death or serious injury, or a threat
       to the physical integrity of self or others
   (2) the person's response involved intense fear, helplessness, or horror
B. Either while experiencing or after experiencing the distressing event, the
   individual has three (or more) of the following dissociative symptoms:
   (1) a subjective sense of numbing, detachment, or absence of emotional
       responsiveness
   (2) a reduction in awareness of his or her surroundings (e.g., "being in a daze")
   (3) derealization
   (4) depersonalization
   (5) dissociative amnesia (i.e., inability to recall an important aspect of the
       trauma)
C. The traumatic event is persistently reexperienced in at least one of the following
   ways: recurrent images, thoughts, dreams, illusions, flashback episodes, or a
   sense of reliving the experience; or distress on exposure to reminders of the
   traumatic event.
D. Marked avoidance of stimuli that arouse recollections of the trauma (e.g.,
   thoughts, feelings, conversations, activities, places, people).
E. Marked symptoms of anxiety or increased arousal (e.g., difficulty sleeping,
   irritability, poor concentration, hypervigilance, exaggerated startle response,
   motor restlessness).
F. The disturbance causes clinically significant distress or impairment in social,
   occupational, or other important areas of functioning or impairs the individual's
   ability to pursue some necessary task, such as obtaining necessary assistance or
   mobilizing personal resources by telling family members about the traumatic
   experience.
G. The disturbance lasts for a minimum of 2 days and a maximum of 4 weeks and
   occurs within 4 weeks of the traumatic event.
H. The disturbance is not due to the direct physiological effects of a substance
   (e.g., a drug or abuse, a medication) or a general medical condition, is not
   better accounted for by Brief Psychotic Disorder, and is not merely an
   exacerbation of a preexisting Axis I or Axis II disorder.

Note. Reprinted with permission from the *Diagnostic and Statistical Manual of Mental Disorders,*
Fourth Edition (pp. 431–432). Copyright 1994 American Psychiatric Association.

unavailable. Nevertheless, studies on immediate reactions to trauma do exist, and they are definitely relevant here. Solomon and Mikulincer (1988) described a "combat stress reaction" (CSR) that is similar in concept. CSR often occurs during war (i.e., on the battlefield) and includes "restlessness, psychomotor retardation, psychological withdrawal, sympathetic activity, startle reactions, confusion, nausea, vomiting, and paranoid reactions" (Solomon & Mikulincer, 1988, p. 264). Solomon and Mikulincer (1988) also noted that "despite the extreme variability of this phenomenon, a common denominator can be identified: the soldier ceases to function militarily and/or begins to function in a bizarre manner that usually endangers himself and/or his comrades" (p. 264). In assessing the long-term problems of Israeli veterans from the 1982 Lebanon War, these researchers found that 59% of CSR cases had developed PTSD at 1 year postwar, as compared to 16% of veteran controls who had not manifested CSR. At 2 years postwar, 56% of the CSR cases and 14% of the non-CSR controls, respectively, met diagnostic criteria for PTSD. Thus, CSR appeared to be a good predictor of later development of PTSD.

As mentioned earlier, several studies have found that dissociative or numbing symptoms during or immediately after the trauma are related to the development of chronic PTSD. In a retrospective study, Bremner et al. (1992) compared the reported dissociation at the time of specific traumatic events in Vietnam veterans with and without PTSD. PTSD patients reported more dissociative symptoms during combat traumas than did those without PTSD. A similar study was conducted by Marmar et al. (1994). These researchers also retrospectively examined the emotional experiences during combat of female and male Vietnam theater veterans. Consistent with the findings of Solomon et al. (1989) and Bremner et al. (1992), dissociative experiences reported during combat were highly associated with chronic posttrauma reactions.

Several laboratory studies have explored dissociative phenomena in combat veterans. Influenced by results from animal experiments demonstrating opiate-mediated analgesia following uncontrollable electrical shock, Pitman, van der Kolk, Orr, and Greenberg (1990b) suggested that numbing symptoms in PTSD sufferers is mediated by endogenous opiates. To test this notion, they exposed veterans with and without PTSD to combat movies. Pain tolerance was used as a measure of numbing. Veterans with PTSD showed decreased pain sensitivity in response to an ice-cold water test after watching the movies. No such decrease occurred when naloxone, an opiate antagonist, was administered, suggesting an opiate-mediated stress-induced analgesia in PTSD. The non-PTSD veterans showed no decrease in pain following the movies.

A relationship between early dissociation and PTSD was also found in victims of traumas other than war. One study (Koopman et al., 1994) interviewed survivors of the Oakland/Berkeley, California, firestorm on two occasions: within the first month after the fire, and 7–9 months later. Participants were asked to describe their experiences during and immediately after the firestorm. Dissociation and anxiety were highly correlated within the first month posttrauma, and both symptom clusters followed similar recovery courses. Interestingly, dissociative symptoms were stronger predictors of chronic posttrauma reactions than symptoms of anxiety. Similarly, McFarlane (1986) reported that DSM-III-R symptoms of avoidance (most of which are numbing symptoms) predicted persistent PTSD in survivors of Australian bush fires. All these findings point again to the cardinal role of dissociation or numbing in PTSD and explain the emphasis on these symptoms in Acute Stress Disorder.

In summary, the studies reviewed above indicate that dissociative experiences during and immediately after a trauma are frequent and are strongly associated with persistent posttrauma reactions. Moreover, dissociative symptoms during or shortly after a trauma may be a stronger predictor of PTSD than anxiety symptoms. It is unclear, however, whether the tendency to dissociate has a causal relationship to the development of chronic PTSD. It is possible that both the tendency to dissociate and the vulnerability to develop chronic PTSD are mediated by other factors, such as childhood experiences

Dissociation, Numbing, and PTSD

The emphasis on dissociative symptoms in Acute Stress Disorder and the strong relationship of these symptoms to chronic PTSD, together with the cardinal role of the numbing symptoms in PTSD, call for a discussion about what the term "dissociation" means and how it is related to the phenomenon of "numbing," which we have discussed earlier at some length.

Since the inception of PTSD as a diagnostic entity, experts have focused on the fear and anxiety components of the disorder (Foa et al., 1989b; Keane, Zimering, & Caddell, 1985). More recently, trauma researchers have become interested in the phenomenon of affective and cognitive avoidance that is commonly observed following a trauma and has been referred to as "dissociation" (e.g., Spiegel, Hunt, & Dondershine, 1988), "denial" (Horowitz, 1986; van der Kolk, 1987), or "numbing" (e.g., Foa et al., 1995c; Horowitz, Wilner, Kaltreider, & Alvarez, 1980; Litz, 1992). Common to these constructs is a diminished awareness of one's emotions or thoughts, which experts have hypothesized to be motivated by self-preservation.

The phenomenon of emotional detachment gained considerable attention in the late 19th century, but it was Pierre Janet who coined the term "dissociation" to describe the lack of connection between aspects of memory or conscious awareness observed during and after extreme stress. Since Janet's early writings, many experts have used this concept to describe different psychological characteristics.

The characteristic of interest here is the association of dissociation and traumatic experiences. Spiegel and Cardeña (1991) proposed that "posttraumatic phenomenology frequently involves alterations in the relationship to the self (e.g., depersonalization and multiple personality disorder), to the world (e.g., derealization and hallucinatory phenomena) and to memory processes (e.g., psychogenic amnesia, fugue, and multiple personality disorder)" (p. 368). Thus, it seems that the construct of dissociation is largely defined by a set of symptoms that have been observed in persons who have experienced trauma. These include amnesia, emotional detachment, feelings of depersonalization, out-of-body experiences, dream-like recall of events, feelings of estrangement, flashbacks, and abreaction. Cardeña and Spiegel (1993) have suggested that posttrauma dissociative symptoms can be classified into three types of responses: (1) detachment from others and the physical environment, (2) alterations in perceptions, and (3) impairments in memory.

A second related construct, "denial," was proposed by Horowitz (1986), who noted that a common reaction to trauma is "the massive ideational denial of the event" (p. 16). An examination of the items contained in the scale that Horowitz and his colleagues developed to measure denial (i.e., the Impact of Event Scale; Horowitz, Wilner, & Alvarez, 1979) indicates that "denial" denotes attempts at cognitive and emotional avoidance, but not alteration in perception and memory impairment.

A third term, introduced in the DSM-III (APA, 1980), is "numbing," which we have discussed earlier in this chapter. This term is sometimes used interchangeably with "denial" and "avoidance" to describe the lack of affective expression in trauma victims. As noted earlier, seven symptoms make up the avoidance/numbing cluster of DSM-IV (APA, 1994). These include both effortful cognitive and behavioral avoidance of trauma reminders, memory loss, and emotional numbing (e.g., loss of interest in activities, detachment from others, restricted affect, sense of a foreshortened future).

The grouping of avoidance and numbing symptoms into one cluster suggests that the authors of the DSM-IV have conceptualized emotional numbing and effortful avoidance as equivalent concepts. However, the Foa et al. (1995c) study described earlier, as well as a review of literature on experimental paradigms that elicit PTSD-like symptoms in animals, suggests that effortful avoidance and numbing involve separate mechanisms (Foa et al., 1992). Foa and Riggs (1993) have suggested that effortful avoidance may be regulated by strategic psychological processes, whereas numbing may be mediated by biological mechanisms resembling those underlying the freezing behavior in frightened animals. They have further proposed that upon exposure to trauma-related information, victims first mobilize effortful strategies to avoid the arousal associated with the traumatic memories. When such strategies fail, a "shutting-down" of the affective system occurs; this process is expressed as numbing symptoms.

Conclusion

In this chapter, we have described the diagnosis of two disorders that are precipitated by a traumatic experience: PTSD and ASD. We have discussed studies showing that almost all victims of severe trauma (e.g., rape) will suffer from PTSD symptoms, and that these symptoms will continue for days or weeks. In the long run, after a traumatic experience, three consequences are likely to occur. First, most victims show reduction of the symptoms over time; although they may never forget the event and even will be mildly distressed when remembering it, they resume their normal lives. Other victims will develop chronic but restricted symptoms that can be diagnosed as Specific Phobia (e.g., fear and avoidance of dogs after being attacked by a dog). But about 10–15% of victims of severe traumas will develop the full symptom constellation of PTSD, which is distinguished from other anxiety disorders by flashbacks, nightmares, and (most importantly), by numbing or dissociative symptoms. A therapist who wishes to determine whether a patient suffers from PTSD or from Specific Phobia is advised to pay special attention to these symptoms, because treatment of Specific Phobia is different from treatment of PTSD. The former can be accomplished more easily, sometimes with only one session (Ost, Salkovskis, & Hellstrom, 1991), whereas PTSD treatment is more complex, as Section II of this book makes clear.

3

Other Common Responses to Assault

The diagnosis of PTSD succinctly describes many victims' reactions to assault and other traumas. However, other reactions are very common. Many of these symptoms should respond to treatment for PTSD, but some may require attention in their own right. The therapist should be aware of these other common reactions to trauma, in order to assess them, offer treatment for them when necessary, and educate clients about what is happening to them. This review is not meant to be exhaustive and does include reactions to other traumas besides assault.

Affective Reactions

Rape Trauma Syndrome

Prior to the introduction of the PTSD diagnosis in the DSM-III (APA, 1980), Burgess and Holmstrom (1974a) described a two-phase reaction to rape, consisting of an "acute" phase and a "reorganization" phase; they termed this "rape trauma syndrome." The acute phase, characterized by disorganization lasting from several hours to several weeks, included both "impact reactions" (e.g., shock, disbelief) and "somatic reactions" (e.g., physical trauma). The reorganization phase was depicted as a long-term process of active lifestyle changes (e.g., changing residences) and long-term chronic disturbances such as nightmares and fears. Currently, most researchers and authors agree that rape trauma syndrome is best characterized and discussed as PTSD.

Anxiety

The most incessant reactions documented following rape appear to be intense fears of rape-related situations and general diffuse anxiety, which have been noted up to 16 years postassault (Calhoun et al., 1982; Ellis et al., 1981; Kilpatrick, Resick, & Veronen, 1981). In one study, only 23% of victims were asymptomatic at 1 year postrape on fear measures (Veronen & Kilpatrick, 1980). Similarly, in another study, although victims' fearfulness declined somewhat over time, they remained more fearful than nonvictim controls 1 year postassault (Calhoun et al., 1982). Again, most fear reactions are currently discussed in terms of PTSD.

Depression

Although depression is also a common reaction to rape, it appears to be less persistent than anxiety (Atkeson, Calhoun, Resick, & Ellis, 1982; Frank & Stewart, 1984; Frank, Turner, & Duffy, 1979; Kilpatrick, Veronen, & Resick, 1979a). Of 34 victims, 15 were moderately to severely depressed immediately following their rape (Frank et al., 1979). Of these 15, one-half met criteria for a major depressive episode. In a larger sample of rape victims, 43% of recent victims were diagnosed with Major Depression (Frank & Stewart, 1984); however, these symptoms declined considerably by 3 months postassault. When compared to nonvictims, victims have been found to be significantly more depressed soon after the assault, with differences decreasing 3–4 months later, and no differences between groups detected up to 1 year postassault (Atkeson et al., 1982; Kilpatrick et al., 1979a).

However, some retrospective reports are inconsistent with these results. In interviews conducted 15–30 months postassault, 41% still reported episodes of depression they felt stemmed from the assault (Nadelson et al., 1982). Another study found that victims were significantly more depressed than matched nonvictims 3 years postassault (Ellis et al., 1981). Of 44 rape victims seen at a clinic specializing in treatment of postrape PTSD and fear, 59% were suffering from Major Depression (Resick & Schnicke, 1993). Rape victims reported significantly more depression than robbery victims for 18 months postvictimization (Resick, 1988). An average of 21.9 years postassault, rape victims were found to be more depressed than nonvictims (Kilpatrick, Best, Saunders, & Veronen, 1988). Comparing the likelihood for depression as function of number of assaults, they found that 8.6% of victims of one rape were experiencing depression at the time of the interview, with 46% reporting depression at some point in their lives following the rape. In contrast, 20% of the victims who had experienced more than one rape were currently suffering from depression, and 80% qualified for a diagnosis of depression at some point in their lifetimes.

Related to depression, suicidal thoughts and behavior must be assessed in assault victims. Estimates of the number of victims who have considered suicide following their assaults range from 2.9% to 50%: 2.9% within the first month postassault (Frank et al., 1979), 27% (Frank & Stewart, 1984), and 50% of those assessed between 1 and 16 years postassault (Ellis et al., 1981). In a study of sexual assault victims seeking treatment, 43% had considered suicide and 17% had made an attempt (Resick, 1988). In a large random population survey, 19% of rape victims reported making a suicide attempt, whereas 44% reported thinking about it (Kilpatrick et al., 1985). Clearly, suicidal ideation is present in a significant proportion of victims and should be discussed.

Anger

Anger has been repeatedly observed in rape victims, other crime victims, and war veterans with PTSD (Hyer et al., 1986; Kilpatrick et al., 1981; Woolfolk & Grady, 1988; Yassen & Glass, 1984). In a prospective study, 116 rape and other crime victims were compared to a matched nonvictimized control group (*n* = 50) on measures of anger and anger expression (Riggs, Dancu, Gershuny, Greenberg, & Foa, 1992). Results indicated that in general, victims were angrier than nonvictims. Certain assault variables, such as the use of a weapon and the victim's response to the attack, predicted the anger response. In addition, it was found that elevated anger predicted the development of PTSD. The authors speculated that intense anger may interfere with the modification of the traumatic memory by inhibiting fear responses that would lead to habituation, and by allowing the victim to avoid feelings of anxiety. That is, victims who are more prone to experience anger than anxiety do not have the opportunity to confront fearful situations and thus to have that fear decrease (habituate); their anxiety-provoking cues and responses remain unchanged.

Dissociative Reactions

A dissociative reaction is a disturbance in the normally integrated functions of identity, memory, or consciousness (APA, 1987). Mild forms of dissociation are common, such as driving along a familiar route and realizing that you haven't been paying attention to where you were driving (being on "automatic pilot"). The most extreme form of dissociation recognized in the DSM-III-R is Multiple Personality Disorder (MPD), which is the existence within the patient of two or more distinct personalities (APA, 1987). (MPD has since been renamed Dissociative Identity Disorder in the DSM-IV [APA, 1994], but many researchers and clinicians prefer the older term.) A continuum of pathology lies in between these two extremes.

It is commonly held that dissociation in its more extreme forms is the result of trauma (Putnam, 1985). As a coping mechanism, dissociation psychologically removes the individual from an extremely aversive event when physical escape appears impossible. Wartime dissociative phenomena, especially psychogenic amnesia and psychogenic fugue reactions, have been estimated to range from 5% to 14% of all psychiatric combat patients (Fisher, 1943; Grinker & Spiegel, 1943; Henderson & Moore, 1944; Sargent & Slater, 1940; Torrie, 1944); in some cases, a direct relationship has been found between the degree of combat-induced stress and the degree of dissociation. In a study of 100 MPD cases, 97% were found to have experienced significant childhood trauma (Putnam, Guroff, Silberman, Barban, & Post, 1986). The most commonly reported trauma was incest (68%), followed by physical abuse, physical and sexual abuse combined, extreme neglect, witnessing of violent death, other abuses, and extreme poverty. PTSD individuals scored almost as high as MPD individuals on a measure of dissociation (Bernstein & Putnam, 1986). In that sample, the PTSD sufferers scored higher than patients with Alcohol Dependence, anxiety disorders, and Schizophrenia, and higher than normals (including adolescents). In a prospective study, adult female rape and nonsexual assault victims with and without PTSD were compared for dissociation (Dancu, Rothbaum, Riggs, & Foa, 1990). Victims with PTSD scored significantly higher than victims without PTSD on measures of dissociation, intrusion, avoidance, and assault-related distress. Higher levels of dissociation were related to greater levels of postassault distress.

At this time, the causal role of dissociation in PTSD is unclear. It is possible that a tendency to dissociate predisposes traumatized individuals to develop PTSD by inhibiting the emotional processing of the traumatic material. On the other hand, individuals with PTSD may tend to dissociate as a coping response to intrusive images and fears. It has been proposed that PTSD is, in fact, a disorder that falls somewhere in between anxiety disorders and dissociative disorders (Foa et al., 1992).

Social Problems

Even 15–30 months postassault, over half of 41 rape victims interviewed in one study reported a restricted social life, only going out with friends (Nadelson et al., 1982). Social and leisure adjustment was significantly worse for victims than for controls 2 months postassault in another study, but improved afterwards so that no differences were observed (Resick, Calhoun, Atkeson, & Ellis, 1981). By 4 months postassault, most victims' social adjustment had recovered except for work functioning, which continued to be problematic 8 months postassault (Kilpatrick et al., 1979b; Resick et al., 1981). These problems in social functioning may be related to avoidance caused by victims' fears of strangers, of going out with new people, and of people walking behind them (Kilpatrick et al., 1979b).

Marital and familial problems were reported more frequently in victims than nonvictims in one study (Ellis et al., 1981), but not in another (Resick et al., 1981). Greater threat to the victim during the assault was inversely related to poorer household adjustment (Frank, Turner, & Stewart, 1980). The authors speculated that victims of more brutal assaults may be taken to be less blameworthy, and consequently may receive more support from their families.

Sexual Problems

Sexual difficulties following rape are common. One-third of victims assessed retrospectively indicated decreased sexual satisfaction, even several years postassault (Norris & Feldman-Summers, 1981). At least one-half of victims questioned retrospectively reported at least one sexual dysfunction following the rape, with fear of sex and decreased arousal or desire as the most common problems noted (Becker, Skinner, Abel, & Treacy, 1982; Nadelson et al., 1982).

Prospective studies have produced similar findings. Two weeks postassault, 61% of 116 victims assessed in one study indicated less frequent sex since the assault. By 4 weeks postassault, 43% reported a total avoidance of sex. The frequency of sex had improved by 4 months postassault and had nearly recovered to preassault levels by 1 year. However, sexual satisfaction continued to suffer even 1 year postassault, and 12% of the victims reported sexually induced flashbacks 1 year postassault (Ellis, Calhoun, & Atkeson, 1980). Compared to nonvictims, victims experienced significantly less sexual satisfaction 18 months postassault (Feldman-Summers, Gordon, & Meagher, 1979; Orlando & Koss, 1983). However, there were no differences between the two groups in frequency of sex or orgasms. In addition, no differences were found in satisfaction with masturbation or the expression of affection.

Psychophysiological Reactions

As it is for many anxiety disorders, increased arousal is one of the prominent characteristics of PTSD. The arousal cluster of symptoms in PTSD (see Chapter 2, Table 2.1) includes sleep disturbance, irritability and anger, difficulty concentrating, hypervigilance, and exaggerated startle response; in addition, the reexperiencing symptom cluster includes physiological reactivity to reminders of the traumatic event.

Psychophysiological studies of most of these symptoms of increased arousal in PTSD sufferers are scarce, despite the fact that at least two symptoms from the arousal cluster are required for a PTSD diagnosis. Laboratory documentation is lacking for sleep disturbance (Ross, Ball, Sullivan, & Caroll, 1989b), irritability, distractibility, and hypervigilance, even though they are common symptoms of PTSD. Although exaggerated startle response has been studied, the results provide equivocal evidence for increased reactivity. Physiological reactivity to reminders of the trauma has been the only symptom repeatedly tested and demonstrated in the laboratory. Almost all of the psychophysiological studies to date have been done with male combat veterans.

Startle Reactions

Psychophysiological studies of startle responses in PTSD present a mixed picture. Combat veterans with PTSD were found to have larger eyeblink startle responses to unsignaled stimuli than controls (Butler et al., 1990). Traumatized children actually demonstrated smaller eyeblinks to an unsignaled acoustic stimulus than did nontraumatized controls (Ornitz & Pynoos, 1989). The traumatized children showed less startle inhibition with brief pre-stimuli and more startle facilitation with long pre-stimuli. However, another study of combat veterans found no difference in habituation of the startle response between PTSD and control subjects (Ross et al., 1989a). Such equivocal results measuring startle reactions are probably attributable to differences in the paradigms used to study the phenomenon. Although the current state of knowledge does not yet permit us to describe the typical effect on the startle reaction following trauma, it is definitely worthy of future study.

Cardiac, Electrodermal, and Muscular Reactions to Reminders

Physiological hyperresponsivity of combat veterans with PTSD to stimuli associated with their trauma has been well documented (Blanchard, Kolb, Gerardi, Ryan, & Pallmeyer, 1986; Blanchard, Kolb, Pallmeyer, & Gerardi, 1982; Malloy, Fairbank, & Keane, 1983; Pallmeyer, Blanchard, & Kolb, 1986; Pitman, Orr, Forgue, deJong, & Claiborn, 1987; Pitman et al., 1990a). Combat veterans with PTSD were compared to different groups, including veterans without PTSD, nonveterans, and non-PTSD psychiatric patients, and were exposed to audiotaped combat sounds or videotaped combat scenes. In general, veterans with PTSD were more reactive on cardiac, electrodermal, cardiovascular, and/or muscular measures than controls in response to trauma-specific stimuli, but not to general fear stimuli.

In a typical paradigm, Blanchard et al. (1982) compared Vietnam veterans with PTSD to matched nonveteran controls on heart rate (HR), blood pressure (BP), forehead electromyographic (EMG) activity, skin resistance level (SRL), and peripheral temperature. Measures were taken during baseline, mental arithmetic (noncombat stressor), rest (return to baseline), music, and increasing intensities of combat sounds. PTSD individuals were more reactive than normal controls to auditory presentations of combat sounds, as measured by HR, systolic BP, and forehead EMG. Blanchard et al. (1986) replicated these findings with regard to HR, using a similar paradigm (i.e., comparing PTSD Vietnam combat veterans to veterans without any disorder). Differences in HR, systolic and diastolic BP, SRL, and frontal EMG activity between Vietnam combat veterans with and without PTSD during presentations of combat sounds were also found by Gerardi, Blanchard, and Kolb (1989). Similarly, Malloy et al. (1983) compared PTSD and non-PTSD Vietnam veterans to non-PTSD psychiatric inpatients, and found the PTSD subjects to show more reactive HR and skin resistance responses to videotapes of combat scenes and sounds than the comparison groups.

In a different paradigm, Vietnam veterans with and without PTSD were compared on skin conductance responses (SCRs) to stress words related to Vietnam (e.g., "kill," "Nam," "jungle"), words phonetically related to the stress words (e.g., "kin," "none," "junkyard"), and neutral words (e.g., "mix," "brief," "shop") (McNally et al., 1987). The PTSD veterans exhibited enhanced SCRs to the stress words as compared to the other target words, and in comparison to the non-PTSD group. However, in a similar paradigm, Trandel and McNally (1987) failed to replicate the McNally et al. results; they found no differences between PTSD Vietnam combat veterans and non-PTSD noncombat veterans in SCRs to any category of stimulus word.

Selective processing of threat information in people with PTSD was investigated by means of a modified Stroop procedure (Foa, Feske, Murdock, Kozak, & McCarthy, 1991a). Participants were 15 rape victims with PTSD, 13 rape victims without PTSD, and 16 nontraumatized controls. They were asked to name the color in which different words were presented. It has been demonstrated in various Stroop paradigms that the content of the word interferes with naming the color it is presented in. For example, one can name the color red faster when the word "RED" appears in red than when the word "GREEN" appears in red. In this way, the interference caused by different words can be measured. The words used in this study fell into four categories: specific threat (rape-related) words, general threat (related to physical harm and death) words, neutral words, and nonwords. Rape victims with PTSD took longer to name the color of rape-related words than they did for other types of words. Non-PTSD victims and nonvictim controls did not differ in the length of time they took to name the colors of the different word types. The authors concluded that rape victims with PTSD, but not those without PTSD, exhibited selective processing for rape-related material.

The specificity of this hyperresponsivity to traumatic material has been further demonstrated by Pitman et al. (1987). Vietnam combat veterans with PTSD were more reactive than normal combat veteran controls (i.e., they showed higher SCRs and forehead EMG activity) to imagery of their individualized combat experiences, but not to other, non-PTSD-related stressful imagery. Moreover, anxiety-disordered combat veterans without PTSD were *not* hyperresponsive to their combat imagery (Pitman et al., 1990a). It is interesting to note that the PTSD veterans were significantly more responsive (SCR, EMG, trend for HR) than their anxiety-disordered counterparts only to their individualized combat scripts, and not to standardized combat scripts, or general fear scripts.

All of the studies described above collected autonomic data after the trauma, so it is possible that people who develop PTSD had higher tonic arousal prior to the trauma and that such arousal may have predisposed them to develop the disorder. In order to explore this hypothesis, Pitman, Orr, Lowenhagen, Macklin, and Altman (1991) examined military records of inductees' HR and BP prior to combat activity and related it to their later PTSD status. They found that PTSD combat veterans were no more aroused on these measures prior to their traumatic combat events than were non-PTSD veterans. This indicates that the increased autonomic arousal is a response to the trauma, rather than an individual trait or cause for PTSD.

Chronic Increased Arousal

Several experiments have focused on tonic autonomic activity in PTSD combat veterans, with equivocal results. Veterans with PTSD have been found to have elevated tonic HR and BP (Blanchard et al., 1986; Pitman et al., 1987), whereas in other studies baseline levels were not significantly elevated in PTSD (Malloy et al., 1983; Pitman et al., 1990a). Several studies have failed to find baseline differences between PTSD Vietnam combat veterans and normal combat veteran controls (Malloy et al., 1983; Pitman et al., 1987), anxiety-disordered combat veterans without PTSD (Pitman et al., 1990a), and non-PTSD psychiatric inpatients (Malloy et al., 1983). In another two studies, the means appeared higher for PTSD, but statistical tests were not reported (Blanchard et al., 1982; Pallmeyer et al., 1986). In female rape victims with PTSD who were compared to victims without PTSD and nonvictimized controls, resting-level HR tended to be highest for the PTSD group, and number of spontaneous fluctuations lowest, but these apparent differences were not statistically significant (Kozak, Foa, & Rothbaum, 1992). Davidson and Baum (1986) found that individuals living within 5 miles of the Three Mile Island nuclear power station had elevated HR and BP as compared to controls living 80 miles away. The inconsistencies among the results suggest that elevations in basal physiological activity may not occur in all PTSD.

One hypothesis that has been put forth to account for these inconsistent findings regards the presumed phasic shifting between periods of increased arousal and periods of numbing (van der Kolk, 1987). It is possible that individuals tested during a numb phase would not appear more aroused than controls, but that those same individuals tested during an aroused phase would demonstrate increased arousal when compared to controls. This phasic shifting has not been taken into account in physiological studies of PTSD to this point; thus, it has probably resulted in methodological errors contributing to differences in findings.

Impaired Physiological Habituation

It appears that tendencies for elevated autonomic hyperreactivity in response to fear-relevant stimuli characterize victims with chronic PTSD, but not traumatized individuals without PTSD. One possible mechanism to account for this difference is an impaired capacity for physiological habituation. We (Foa et al., 1989b; see Chapter 4) hypothesized that failure to habituate to routine encounters with situations that evoke traumatic memories could account in part for the persistence of PTSD. To explore this hypothesis, we compared habituation of autonomic reactions to auditory tones in rape survivors with and without PTSD and a nonvictimized control group. On two measures of electrodermal activity (i.e., number of trials to habituation and percentage of nonhabituators in each group), the PTSD group showed less habituation than the other two groups. The PTSD group had significantly more trials to extinction than the other groups, and the percentage of nonhabituators was significantly higher for the PTSD group than for the other two groups. Overall HR acceleration to the tones was higher for the two assault groups than for the nonvictim control group. Although the PTSD and non-PTSD individuals appeared to show more trials to habituation than the nonvictims, these differences were not statistically significant. This resistance to habituation may account for the increased physiological arousal found in other studies of PTSD, particularly with male combat veterans.

Conclusion

In summary, posttrauma reactions are numerous and varied. They may include PTSD symptoms, general anxiety, depression, anger, dissociative reactions, social and sexual difficulties, and psychophysiological changes and sensitivities, among others. It is important to keep in mind that posttrauma sequelae are complicated, and not to have tunnel vision just for the symptoms of PTSD. However, very often when the PTSD is treated successfully, the other reactions dissipate as well.

4

What Do We Know about
Treatment Efficacy for PTSD?

In this chapter, we summarize the literature on psychosocial and pharmacological interventions for PTSD. We begin with a brief review of crisis interventions. We then discuss traditional therapies for PTSD, both psychosocial and
pharmacological. Next, we examine the larger literature on the efficacy of
cognitive-behavioral procedures for PTSD. We have included reports of treatments with survivors of various traumas, not just sexual assault; as we have repeatedly noted, there are many similarities in the presentation and treatment
of PTSD across traumas, and the cognitive-behavioral programs help victims
of a varieties of traumas. In our review here, we include results of studies in
which clients are either given treatment or put on a waiting list, and the efficacy of the treatment is thus determined by this comparison. We also discuss
results of studies comparing the effectiveness of different treatments, or case
reports that clearly describe the treatment and the procedures for evaluating
treatment outcome.

   Not all studies in the review are well controlled. In controlled studies, clients are randomly assigned to the various treatment groups or comparison
groups (ideally including a no-treatment control group for comparison). Well-
controlled studies also include standardized treatment delivery, objective standardized measurement of the symptoms that are targeted for treatment, assessment of these symptoms before and after treatment, and specified rules for
inclusion and exclusion of clients in the study. The better-controlled a study
is, the stronger are the conclusions that can be derived from its results. In contrast, the results of less well-controlled studies are open to varying explanations.

Interventions Shortly after the Trauma

Crisis intervention and psychotherapy groups for trauma victims are the most
common procedures used in rape crisis centers (Koss & Harvey, 1987). Based

on crisis theory (Burgess & Holmstrom, 1976), these interventions incorporate dissemination of information, active listening, and emotional support (e.g., Forman, 1980). In the same spirit, many trauma experts have emphasized the importance of immediate intervention following a trauma to prevent chronic posttrauma problems (see Bell, 1995). Many such interventions ensue from the debriefing model proposed by Mitchell and Bray (1990), which includes seven phases that are conducted in small groups within 3 days of the traumatic event. The first phase consists of explaining the purpose of the debriefing and the rules for participation, with special emphasis on confidentiality and suspension of rank (in situations where rank is an issue — e.g., the military). Other phases include interventions such as "recreating" the traumatic event by asking all participants to discuss their perspective on what occurred, to discuss their thoughts at the time of the event, to describe the worst part of the event for them, and to discuss their reactions to the event. The final phases include an educational component, in which a group leader describes common reactions to trauma in order to normalize participants' responses. The program ends with participants' providing comments or closing statements; they may stay to meet informally with each other and the team leaders.

Interventions such as the one described above have been applied to survivors of a variety of traumatic situations, including bank workers robbed at gunpoint (Manton & Talbot, 1990), emergency workers (e.g., Armstrong, O'Callahan, & Marmar, 1991), and military personnel (e.g., FitzGerald et al., 1993). However, as noted by Raphael, Meldrum, and McFarlane (1995), randomized, well-controlled studies of such programs have not yet been conducted, and thus the efficacy of such interventions is still unknown. Raphael et al. (1995) also note that the existing uncontrolled studies suggest that the debriefing either had no effect or had a deleterious effect. Despite these negative results on more objective measures, the participants and/or the authors in these studies felt that the debriefing was helpful and valuable.

Crisis intervention has also been employed in women's centers and rape crisis clinics (e.g., Burgess & Holmstrom, 1974b). In one study, Kilpatrick and Veronen (1984) evaluated a brief behavioral program for reducing postrape symptoms, but methodological flaws such as modifications in the intervention part way through the study, lack of PTSD measurement, and small sample size precluded interpretation of the findings. However, given the utility of behavioral interventions in the treatment of posttrauma reactions, as will be described later in this chapter, these techniques might prove efficacious for acute posttrauma reactions as well.

To address this issue, Foa, Hearst-Ikeda, and Perry (1995a) conducted a study of a brief prevention program (BPP) for female assault survivors. The BPP included a number of techniques found to be helpful in treating chronic PTSD, such as exposure, relaxation training, and cognitive restructuring. In this study, 10 patients participated in the BPP and were compared with 10 matched control participants, who were repeatedly assessed in an assessment control condition. Five women in each group of 10 were rape victims, and the other 5 were nonsexual assault victims. The average time since assault was 15 days. Participants were not randomly assigned because of the pilot nature of this study. Both programs were conducted over four weekly 2-hour sessions, which began within 1 month of the assault. Patients were assessed via standardized interview and self-report measures, and evaluations were conducted by evaluators who were unaware of the treatment that each participant received. All participants met symptomatic criteria for PTSD.

Results of this study showed that following the program, 7 of 10 women in the BPP condition no longer met PTSD symptom criteria, compared with only 1 in the control condition. Furthermore, subjects in the BPP group were rated by independent evaluators as showing a mean 72% reduction in severity of PTSD symptoms, versus a mean 33% reduction in the control group. Although the small sample size precludes drawing definitive conclusions as to the efficacy of the BPP, the results are encouraging, and Foa and her colleagues are now studying this intervention in a larger sample of women.

In summary, there is no evidence to date that the commonly used crisis interventions are effective, but they have not yet been rigorously tested. With female assault victims, short-term behavioral interventions may help in preventing chronic post-trauma problems. One difference between most crisis intervention programs and the BPP in the Foa et al. (1995a) study is that the former are usually instituted within days of the trauma, whereas the BPP was instituted about 2 weeks posttrauma. Perhaps trauma victims are better able to benefit from interventions that aim at enhancing trauma processing if these are not begun immediately following the trauma, when victims may still be in a state of shock.

Traditional Psychosocial Interventions

Hypnotherapy

The use of hypnosis in the treatment of trauma-related distress can be traced at least to the time of Freud (for a review, see Spiegel, 1989), who introduced the procedure to produce the abreaction and catharsis he thought were necessary to resolve a psychic conflict. Hypnosis has continued to be used in treating trauma victims, with a variety of theoretical underpinnings. Spiegel (1989) noted that hypnosis may be useful in treating PTSD for two reasons: First, hypnotic phenomena such as dissociation are common in coping with trauma as it occurs and in its sequelae; second, hypnosis may facilitate recall of traumatic events that were encoded in a dissociative state and that therefore are not available to conscious recollection.

A number of case reports (e.g., Jiranek, 1993; Kingsbury, 1988; Leung, 1994; MacHovec, 1983; Peebles, 1989; Spiegel, 1988, 1989) have attested to the usefulness of hypnosis in treating PTSD. Most, however, lack methodological precision and thus cannot provide a basis for drawing conclusions about the efficacy of hypnosis for PTSD and related pathology. However, these case studies do provide an interesting discussion of the use of hypnosis for trauma-related disturbances. The traumas described in these reports include those typically covered in PTSD studies (such as rape and combat), less typical but yet common events (such as industrial accidents), and uncommon events (such as consciousness during surgery).

Several problems can be identified in these reports, including lack of specificity about the symptoms targeted for treatment and about diagnostic methods. Only two of the reports cited above (Leung, 1994; MacHovec, 1983) detailed how hypnotherapy was conducted, and almost none employed control conditions.

In the one controlled study (Brom, Kleber, & Defres, 1989) of 112 trauma victims, hypnosis was compared with desensitization, psychodynamic psychotherapy, and a waiting-list control. The participants in this study were victims of a variety of traumas, but the majority did not directly experience the trauma; rather, they had lost a loved, close family member. All patients met symptom criteria for PTSD. All three conditions produced superior improvement to the waiting-list condition, but no differences across the three treatments were observed. Inspection of the pre- and posttreatment means indicated that mean improvement on the Revised Impact of Event Scale (RIES) was 29% for psychodynamic therapy, 34% for hypnotherapy, and 41% for desensitization, compared with about 10% in the waiting-list condition. Although the limitations of the study should be kept in mind, the results suggest that hypnotherapy, as well as desensitization and psychodynamic therapy, may somewhat alleviate posttrauma suffering.

Psychodynamic Treatments

Treatment by dynamic psychotherapy has often been advocated as a final component of crisis intervention (Burgess & Holmstrom, 1974b; Evans, 1978; Fox & Scherl, 1972). However, empirical investigations of their efficacy are scarce. Many psychodynamically oriented psychotherapies have been used with PTSD sufferers, including individual and group therapy in outpatient and inpatient settings. Often, there is no obvious thread that ties the different interventions and no systematic rationale that connects the type of therapy to PTSD; the few exceptions include Horowitz's (1976) theory of trauma.

In an attempt to account for posttrauma reactions, psychodynamic theorists (e.g., Horowitz, 1976) emphasize concepts such as denial, abreaction, catharsis, and stages of recovery from trauma in developing treatment for posttrauma difficulties. Although deriving from a different theoretical viewpoint, such treatments include components similar to those seen in the cognitive-behavioral treatments that we discuss later. For example, Horowitz's concept of "dosing" of the traumatic experience and of "encouraging expression" are quite similar to exposure techniques. The aim of Horowitz's brief psycho-dynamic therapy is the resolution of intrapsychic conflict arising from a trau-matic experience, rather than the resolution of specific symptoms such as intrusive thoughts or flashbacks.

Other psychodynamic theorists focus largely on group process (e.g., Yalom, 1995). Although the psychodynamic therapies were derived from interesting theories of trauma and its sequelae, they have not been widely tested in con-trolled outcome studies, and those studies that exist have suffered from numer-ous methodological difficulties. Nevertheless, several studies have suggested that psychodynamic treatments may be useful in the treatment of PTSD, whereas others have not found them effective.

Psychodynamic psychotherapy was not found effective in the treatment of a traumatized Vietnam veteran (Grigsby, 1987). After 19 months of no progress with psychodynamic psychotherapy, therapy by imagery was tried. In this treatment, the therapist presented a trauma-related scene and allowed the client to develop images spontaneously through associations rather than by plan. The use of the imagery technique was not planned in advance; rather, it was introduced at appropriate times in the context of a session. The client moved on to other trauma-related scenes when he was ready. Avoidance was addressed through psychodynamic techniques of dealing with transference and resistance. Ten sessions of this imagery therapy were effective in ameliorating the client's PTSD as observed by the therapist and reported by the client. Although con-strained by the limitations of a single case report and unsystematic measures, this report suggests that traditional "talking" therapy was not helpful for PTSD, whereas behaviorally oriented techniques appeared to be effective.

Using psychoanalytically oriented therapy, Bart (1975) reported that trauma victims worsened following treatment. In contrast, short-term dynamic group therapy for nine rape victims was found to be somewhat helpful (Cryer & Beutler, 1980): On the whole, fear and hostility decreased significantly from pre- to posttreatment. Still, three of the seven victims who completed the study reported only a slight change in their overall level of distress. Unfortunately, also, no control group was included, and the content of the therapy sessions was not specified.

Roth, Dye, and Lebowitz (1988) treated 13 female sexual assault victims in a group therapy based on Horowitz's (1976) model of responses to trauma, according to which the goal is to help the patient work through the trauma experience through gradually "dosing" her/himself with the reexperiencing of the trauma at manageable levels. Treatment began with a discussion of Horowitz's model, and consisted primarily of members' sharing experiences and offering support to each other. There was a control condition, but participants were not randomly assigned to these two groups; rather, 13 women who agreed to undergo assessments made up the control group, but the attrition rate in this group was so large that its usefulness was limited. The therapy group also had a high attrition rate, and only seven women were included in the final analyses. The majority of women in the therapy group were also in ongoing individual counseling prior to beginning the group, and others began such counseling during the group, adding additional variance in the experimental condition.

After eight sessions, most of the comparisons between the treatment group and the controls indicated that the two groups were not different from one another. Indeed, contrary to expectations, on one measure (the Intrusion subscale of the Impact of Event Scale [IES]) there was a greater decrease in symptoms in the control group than in the therapy group. After session 20, the therapy group showed improvement on fear, functioning, and intrusion measures; however, no control group data were collected. Improvements were maintained through a 6-month follow-up. Results over a year of group therapy showed greater improvement in the therapy participants particularly on measures of depression.

Although the long-term results of this study may initially appear encouraging, the conclusions that can be drawn from it are actually very limited. First, control and treatment groups differed with respect to the initial severity of symptoms, the former being less impaired than the latter; second, group members were not selected randomly; third, no control data were available after eight sessions; and, fourth, all subjects in the treatment group also received individual therapy. As such, the observed gains cannot be independently attributed to the group therapy.

The effects of time-limited group therapy with female and male cotherapists were reported by Perl, Westin, and Peterson (1985). Treatment consisted of eight weekly 90-minute sessions. A total of 17 clients were treated in groups of 3 or 4. The treatment focused on helping clients reach realistic solutions for specific problems, with an emphasis on "here-and-now" issues rather than psychodynamic processes. Only rape-related problems were discussed. The effects of therapy were determined via subjective evaluations of the therapists as derived from patients' self-reports. The authors reported striking improvements following therapy for participants on all symptoms (including fear, sexual problems, etc.). Unfortunately, this report is difficult to interpret because of the absence of objective measurement and lack of a control group.

Twenty-eight victims of the Beverly Hills Supper Club fire were treated with individual short-term psychodynamic psychotherapy (6–12 sessions; Lindy,

Green, Grace, & Titchener, 1983). Diagnoses included PTSD, Complicated Bereavement, Major Depressive Disorder, and Adjustment Disorder. Therapy was conducted along the following guidelines:

1) The work is best started by asking the victim to relate in detail the thoughts and feelings experienced before, during, and after the fire.
2) When the manifest content of affect-laden associations deviates from the fire and its surrounding circumstances, the therapist should link affects where appropriate back to the fire experience.
3) Where grief is present or being resisted, the therapist should encourage memories (positive and negative) of the deceased person by identifying and explaining barriers.
4) Where unconscious anticipation of something terrible happening again dominates the present, the therapist should contrast feelings of anticipation with the actual probabilities.
5) Where guilt and shame about the way one acted at the scene are evident, the therapist should help the patient distinguish rational from irrational affect.
6) Where reactive rage dominates, the therapist should interpret the underlying feelings of helplessness and loss of control. (p. 609)

Measures included the Symptom Checklist 90 (SCL-90), three target symptoms noted by the therapist, and a psychiatric evaluation form completed by an independent research interviewer. Patients who completed treatment showed more improvement than patients with interrupted treatment. Lindy et al. (1983) subsequently observed that all treated patients "improved to a subclinical level two years after the fire" (p. 602).

As mentioned above in the section on hypnotherapy, Brom et al. (1989) conducted a controlled study of Horowitz's brief psychodynamic therapy, comparing this treatment with hypnosis, desensitization, and a waiting-list control group. Although the authors found no differences among the three active treatment conditions, inspection of the means on the RIES suggested that psychodynamic therapy in this study resulted in a poorer outcome than desensitization did (29% vs. 41%, mean pre–post reduction).

Marmar, Horowitz, Weiss, Wilner, and Kaltreider (1988) examined the efficacy of a psychodynamic treatment for conjugal bereavement by randomly assigning 61 women who had lost their husbands to 12 weekly sessions of either brief dynamic therapy or mutual-help group treatment led by a nonclinician. Although death of a husband does not necessarily qualify as a DSM Criterion A trauma, many of the women in this study reported symptoms of PTSD. Follow-up evaluations were conducted by independent evaluators using an unstandardized semistructured interview and several standardized self-report measures. Treatment was manualized for the mutual-help group condition, but not for the dynamic treatment condition, which was based upon Horowitz's (1976) model of brief dynamic therapy for stress response syndromes.

Results indicated that on both interview and self-report ratings of PTSD symptoms, patients in both conditions improved slightly, but there were no differences between groups. The findings from this study suggest that both brief dynamic therapy and peer-led mutual-help groups may be slightly effective in treating symptoms arising from conjugal bereavement, but the relevance of the results for the treatment of PTSD is unclear.

Preliminary results from another psychodynamically oriented treatment is more promising. Using a quasi-experimental design, Scarvalone, Cloitre, and Difede (1995) compared interpersonal process group therapy (IPGT) with a naturally occurring waiting-list control in a sample of 43 female childhood sexual abuse survivors. The IPGT treatment protocol developed for this study was based on the treatment guidelines established by Courtois (1988) and Yalom (1995). History of abuse was the only specified inclusion criterion; this is reminiscent of the early studies on rape victims, where victimization itself was taken as a sufficient indication for treatment.

Results indicated that IPGT patients improved on a number of measures. Percentages of women meeting criteria for PTSD at pretreatment were 91% for the IPGT group and 85% for the control group; at posttreatment, only 39% of the IPGT group versus 83% of the control group met criteria for PTSD. On some measures (e.g., self-report measure of intrusion), the IPGT group showed greater symptom reduction than did the control group, whereas on others (e.g., depression, dissociation), both groups evidenced symptom reduction. Because of the lack of blind evaluators, the extent to which expectancy for improvement was responsible for these positive findings cannot be ascertained.

In summary, early studies of psychodynamic psychotherapy were heavy with methodological flaws, including lack of controls, lack of adequate assessment of outcome, and vaguely described treatments. Thus, the information about the efficacy of traditional interventions for PTSD from these studies is quite limited and is open to various interpretations. More recent studies, however, have employed more rigorous standards. With additional studies using such standards, we will be able to evaluate the efficacy of these therapies for the amelioration of PTSD.

Pharmacological Interventions[1]

Medication has been employed to alleviate distress following trauma for over 100 years. During World War II, Sargent and colleagues (e.g., Sargent & Slater,

---

[1]Special thanks go to Drs. Jonathan Davidson and Philip Ninan for their assistance with this section of the chapter.

1940) published a number of reports describing the important benefits of rapid drug-assisted abreaction, although they noted that startle responses remained a persisting problem. In this section of the chapter, we review applications of pharmacotherapy to PTSD, as well as clinical implications and decision-making processes involved in drug treatment of PTSD sufferers.

Pharmacotherapy studies for PTSD have typically used the antidepressant class of drugs. Most have been shown to provide at least some relief of PTSD symptoms, although sometimes not more so than placebos. Tricyclic anti-depressants and selective serotonin reuptake inhibitors (SSRIs) seem to be effective for PTSD, but the effects of other drugs are equivocal. The benefits of tricyclic antidepressants have been modest, but the benefits of the SSRIs have been more impressive.

We begin by reviewing the theoretical basis for using drugs in the treatment of PTSD.

Conceptual Basis for Medication Treatment in PTSD

There are two conceptual frames of reference that advocate the use of medication in PTSD. The first, described by Sargent and Slater (1940), recommends the use of medication in an abreactive context as a means to help uncover repressed or dissociated material. Presumably, this dissociated material leads to a variety of disturbing symptoms. This model, primarily derived from immediate intervention with patients suffering from acute PTSD, has also been advocated more recently for chronic PTSD by Hogben and Cornfield (1981). They noted that pharmacotherapy aids the psychotherapeutically driven recovery process by promoting more powerful abreactive affects. Thus, Hogben and Cornfield's observations suggest that this model should also be applicable to chronic PTSD.

A seemingly contrasting model, also put forward by Sargent and Slater (1940), states that chronic PTSD responds less successfully to abreactive approaches. In this view, antidepressant drugs suppress symptoms that disrupt PTSD sufferers' lives, and allow the individuals to restore their normal effective coping mechanisms. This model views medications as largely being suppressive of symptoms rather than aiding expression of affect.

At present, the virtues and pitfalls of each particular model are debatable. Important determinants include the philosophical orientation of the therapist, the preferences of the patient, the response to previous treatments, the ability or desire of the patient to tolerate distressing affects, the social support available, and the financial resources available to help the patient go through more intense, formal therapy. Empirical testing of these two treatment frameworks has not yet been undertaken.

Biological Basis for Medications in PTSD

Pharmacotherapy in PTSD is based on the neurobiological evidence that uncontrolled life-threatening trauma leaves an imprint on the opiate and other neuropeptidergic systems, the hypothalamic–pituitary–adrenal axis, and the autonomic nervous system, among others; in other words, it results in dysregulation of multiple neurochemical systems. Evidence is building to support a unique constellation of biological abnormalities in PTSD (ver Ellen & van Kammen, 1990). However, data from phenomenological, neurobiological, and treatment response studies suggest that PTSD shares components with dissociative states (Bremner et al., 1992), panic attacks (Mellman & Davis, 1985), and obsessions. Dissociative phenomena are part of the defining criteria for PTSD (e.g., flashbacks, psychogenic amnesia, feelings of detachment), as are obsessive phenomena (e.g., intrusive recollections, attempts at avoidance). There is emerging evidence for a spectrum of disorders (various affective and anxiety disorders among them) that are responsive to antidepressants (Hudson & Pope, 1990). Although various pharmacological agents have been used to treat PTSD clinically, there are only six controlled studies. All except one (which used alprazolam) have used antidepressants to treat PTSD. Tricyclic antidepressants (amitriptyline, imipramine), monoamine oxidase (MAO) inhibitors (phenelzine), and SSRIs (fluoxetine) have all been reported to be beneficial in the treatment of PTSD at some level.

KINDLING/SENSITIZATION

Repeated presentation of a subthreshold stimulus can sensitize or "kindle" limbic circuits, producing a lowered threshold of firing. Analogously, repeated experience with severely traumatic events may ultimately produce a lowered threshold for the experience of intrusive symptoms. Related to the concept of kindling is the idea that exposure to a single or repeated stimulus may "sensitize" animals to further stresses of lower intensity.

INESCAPABLE SHOCK/LEARNED HELPLESSNESS

Anisman and Sklar (1979) proposed a model of inescapable shock/learned helplessness to parallel the human experience of depression. This model actually has more in common with PTSD than with depression (Foa et al., 1992; van der Kolk, Greenberg, Boyd, & Krystal, 1985). Inescapable shock is accompanied by the initial mobilization of catecholamines (norepinephrine and dopamine), followed by their depletion. Inescapable shock, which sets up this biochemical effect, is a close animal analogue of the inescapable stress that is characteristic of the types of trauma leading to PTSD in humans. In broad terms, it has been suggested that the intrusive and avoidant symptoms of PTSD may correspond to hypersensitivity and hyposensitivity to catecholamines. Krystal et al. (1989) have related this to disturbance of the brain's "alarm center"—the locus coeruleus, a noradrenergically rich region of the brain stem. Drugs that have antiadrenergic effects and that down-regulate the locus coeruleus are effective in PTSD and prevent the development of learned helplessness in animals that have been exposed to inescapable shock. Such drugs include the MAO inhibitors and tricyclics. Conversely, noradrenergic alpha$_2$ antagonist drugs, such as yohimbine, stimulate the locus coeruleus and also induce symptoms of PTSD in combat veterans with the diagnosis (Charney, Deutch, Krystal, Southwick, & Davis, 1993). Particular symptoms reflective of locus coeruleus overactivity may include intrusive, autonomic, and hyperarousal symptoms.

SEROTONERGIC MECHANISMS

There is growing evidence that the neurotransmitter serotonin is important in PTSD. Conditioned avoidance behavior, characteristic of the avoidance cluster of PTSD symptoms in the DSM (i.e., phobic avoidance of trauma or its reminders), is mediated serotonergically by pathways arising in the dorsal raphe and projecting to the amygdala. In this regard, it is important to recognize that serotonin antagonists, such as trazodone and mianserin, can reverse conditioned avoidance responses. Their role in PTSD remains understudied. An adaptive pathway (i.e., one that may strengthen coping responses in the face of stress), also arises in the median dorsal raphe and innervates the hippocampus. Other evidence in favor of serotonergic involvement includes the close connection between serotonin and impulse control, the lack of which is often present in PTSD. SSRI drugs, such as fluoxetine, are effective in the strengthening of impulse control and affect modulation. In addition, the regulatory effect of serotonin on sleep suggests its further relevance to PTSD. Finally, as discussed below, drugs with a marked serotonergic effect are clinically effective in PTSD.

The Efficacy of Medication with PTSD

TRICYCLIC DRUGS

The tricyclic antidepressants imipramine, amitriptyline, and desipramine have all been studied in PTSD in double-blind, placebo-controlled conditions (J. B. Frank et al., 1988; Reist et al., 1989; Davidson et al., 1990). The studies by J. B. Frank et al. (1988) and Davidson et al. (1990) revealed positive drug effects for imipramine and amitriptyline, respectively, whereas Reist et al. (1989) did not find such differences. The two positive outcome studies employed an 8-week treatment period and used doses up to 300 mg per day. Plasma levels in these studies were equivalent to those found for the same drugs in patients with Major Depression. However, at this point we do not know whether any relationship exists between the plasma levels of tricyclics and their therapeutic effect in PTSD. The negative study by Reist et al. found no difference between desipramine and placebo in a 4-week crossover trial, employing doses no higher than 200 mg per day. It is likely that the study design, the inadequacy of the doses, and the short treatment duration were important determinants of the lack of drug efficacy. Another explanation for the inconsistency between the studies is that a purely catecholaminergic drug such as desipramine may be less effective than a serotonergic compound. The two positive studies indicated that the tricyclics' effects on PTSD were unlikely to be attributable to antidepressant effects of the drugs, since treatment efficacy diminished as depression severity increased. In addition, good relief of PTSD symptoms occurred in the absence of depression.

MAO INHIBITORS

Studies by J. B. Frank et al. (1988) and Shestatsky, Greenberg, and Lerer (1988) assessed phenelzine and placebo in combat veterans with chronic PTSD. In the first study, phenelzine produced a stronger clinical effect on intrusive and avoidance symptoms of PTSD than did placebo. In the negative outcome study by Shestatsky et al., an effect was found for time; that is, improvement continued on into the second phase of the crossover study, regardless of whether the first treatment was the active drug or the placebo. However, the 4-week crossover design and the use of a low maximum dose may have hindered the effects of phenelzine. Phenelzine has limitations, including poor tolerance of side effects and potential dangers when combined with certain foods and other medications. As a result, it is usually not recommended as a first-line treatment, but may be useful in more resistant cases.

SELECTIVE SEROTONIN REUPTAKE INHIBITORS

Open studies have suggested fluoxetine to be effective for both combat veterans and sexual assault victims with PTSD. The efficacy of fluoxetine (60 mg per day, given for up to 5 weeks) has been also established in a double-blind trial (van der Kolk et al., 1994). The drug was more effective than a placebo in reducing PTSD symptoms. In van der Kolk et al.'s (1994) study with fluoxetine, the reduction in symptoms as measured by the Clinician-Administered PTSD Scale (CAPS) was 25.4% compared to 12.6% for placebo. The reduction in PTSD symptoms in the subgroup of nonveteran patients (i.e., patients from a general hospital trauma clinic, an indeterminate number of whom were rape victims) was 41.1%, compared to 20.3% for placebo. The reduction in PTSD symptoms with fluoxetine is comparable to the reduction in symptoms with phenelzine, which was 46.3% on the IES (J. B. Frank et al., 1988), but greater than that with a tricyclic antidepressant, which was 25% on the IES (J. B. Frank et al., 1988) and 21.4% on the same scale in another study (Davidson et al., 1990).

In an open trial, sertraline was effective with 19 male Vietnam veterans (mean age = 44.3 years) with PTSD and depression (Kline, Dow, Brown, & Matloff, 1993). The daily dose of sertraline averaged 98.5 mg (range = 50–150 mg) over a minimum of 3 months. Sixty-three percent of veterans were designated as positive responders on measures of PTSD, depression, anxiety, and global functioning.

There are no controlled studies looking at pharmacological treatments of PTSD in female rape victims exclusively. Fewer than 50% of the subjects in van der Kolk et al.'s (1994) study of fluoxetine were female rape victims. The vast majority of patients reported in the pharmacological literature have been war veterans who have had chronic PTSD for several years or decades, and whose cases are complicated by a lifetime history of Substance Abuse or Dependence. There is a clear need for pharmacological studies of PTSD in rape victims.

With the wide availability of SSRIs, their selective beneficial effects in OCD, and their improved side effects and safety profile compared to tricyclic antidepressants and MAO inhibitors, they are the first-choice medications among antidepressants and the most promising for PTSD. Among the SSRIs, though fluoxetine has been the medication used most extensively because of its longer availability, sertraline has some advantages. Sertraline is better tolerated than fluoxetine, with a reduced likelihood of side effects; has pharmacokinetic advantages; results in a metabolite that is clinically inactive; and does not significantly affect the cytochrome P450 IID6 liver enzyme system (von Moltke, Greenblatt, Harmatz, & Shader, 1994). Side effects reported in 1,568 patients on sertraline and 1,378 patients on fluoxetine indicated less restlessness/anxiety and insomnia (common symptoms of PTSD) with sertraline than with fluoxetine (Rickels & Schweizer, 1990). Thus, patients are more likely to tolerate the higher doses required to receive potentially greater benefits on sertraline.

A 12-week open clinical trial of sertraline (mean dose = 105 mg) in the treatment of adult female rape victims with chronic PTSD was recently conducted (Rothbaum, Ninan, & Thomas, 1996). The five completers were, on average, 39.75 years old and had been assaulted 15.12 years earlier. Sertraline reduced PTSD and related symptoms in these rape victims. The mean CAPS Total Frequency score decreased by 53%, and the CAPS Total Intensity score decreased by 52%. These preliminary results are encouraging and support the need for systematic assessment of sertraline in this population.

BENZODIAZEPINES

Two studies explored the effects of alprazolam on PTSD. One revealed positive effects in an open study, and the other failed to find differences between a placebo and the active drug in a double-blind trial. In the latter study, there was a statistically, but not clinically, significant improvement in anxiety symptoms.

OTHER DRUGS

Several reports suggest the efficacy of anticonvulsants, such as carbamazepine and beta-blockers, although to date no controlled studies have been conducted. Of particular interest is a study by Famularo, Kinscherff, and Fenton (1988) because it involved children with acute PTSD, whereas all other studies were conducted on adults with chronic PTSD.

The alpha$_2$ agonist drug clonidine, which suppresses activity in the locus coeruleus, seems to be effective in combat veterans with PTSD (Kolb, Burris, & Griffiths, 1987) and in Cambodian refugees living in the United States (Kinzie & Leung, 1989). Over a longer period, some improvement in nightmares and startle reactions was noted with an imipramine–clonidine combination, but little improvement in avoidant behavior was found.

The anticonvulsant drug valproic acid has been tested in 16 Vietnam veterans with chronic PTSD (Fesler, 1991). Ten of the 16 showed some improvement in hyperarousal, and the drug was well tolerated.

How to Implement Pharmacotherapy for PTSD

A number of studies have indicated that many individuals with PTSD retain their symptoms for a long time, even when skillful treatment has been delivered. In many instances the treatment goal is helping patients to adjust to PTSD symptoms, master them, and integrate them into their lives, rather than to eliminate all symptoms. Only some patients achieve entire remission of symptoms. Among other variables, the response to treatment will depend upon premorbid variables; the nature and duration of the trauma; availability of supports before, during, and after the trauma; and comorbidity. Clinical experience suggests that the acute use of abreactive and sedative drugs (e.g., barbiturates and benzodiazepines) may be helpful as a brief, time-limited form of treatment.

In general, antidepressants, anticonvulsants, or mood stabilizers should be considered only when the PTSD symptoms have persisted for several weeks and the disorder has assumed a more chronic course. However, we do not yet know the best point in time for intervention. It seems that a minimum of 5–8 weeks of tricyclic or SSRI therapy is required for the drug effects to begin to emerge, in contrast to the more nonspecific effects of placebos. However, significant drug effects of phenelzine relative to a placebo may emerge as early as 3–4 weeks. This is not to say that treatment has achieved its full effects at this time.

It is probable that several months of an antidepressant may lead to further improvement. In support of this, studies by Bleich, Siegel, Garb, and Lerer (1986) and Kinzie and Leung (1989) both noted a gradual but persistent improvement with amitriptyline and with an imipramine–clonidine combination, respectively. Since chronic PTSD may be associated with persistent structural changes, it is quite possible that some individuals require years of, or even lifelong, pharmacotherapy. One important observation is that startle responses can persist even following 1 year's treatment with a tricyclic drug or with an imipramine–clonidine combination (Birkhimer, DeVane, & Muniz, 1985; Kinzie & Leung, 1989). Clinical experience suggests that some combat veterans with chronic PTSD may require lifelong pharmacotherapy, and that attempts at drug withdrawal or dose reduction may lead to symptom relapse even 20–40 years following exposure to combat.

However, anecdotal reports from the Rothbaum et al. (1996) study using sertraline with PTSD rape victims indicated that some of the participants were able to deal better with their assault once they were on medication, and that they were later able to discontinue the medication successfully. They reported being able to talk about the trauma more and to work on it in ongoing therapy while they were on the drug. Perhaps the medication lessened the intensity of their PTSD symptoms, thus freeing them up to work on processing the trauma. Once the trauma was adequately processed, they no longer required the medication.

Vargas and Davidson (1993) have suggested that discontinuation of drug treatment is governed by the following considerations: degree of symptom remission, the cost of relapse, the progress that has been made in psychotherapy, the presence of drug side effects, and the freedom from ongoing stressors.

Summary and Conclusions Regarding Pharmacotherapy

The studies reviewed above suggest that antidepressant drugs of three different classes have therapeutic effects in PTSD that are significantly greater than the nonspecific effects emanating from placebos. It should be noted that placebos seem to be relatively ineffective in chronic PTSD, in that studies show a low placebo response rate of approximately 20%. This contrasts with the higher placebo response rates found in Major Depression and Panic Disorder. Antidepressant drugs do appear to reduce the intrusive, avoidance, and hyperarousal symptoms of PTSD. In one study, the presence of more severe depression rendered less likely the possibility of a good therapeutic response to amitriptyline. Perhaps patients with more severe symptoms may require combinations of different pharmacotherapeutic agents, and/or combinations of multiple drugs with psychosocial treatment. However, the use of multiple-drug therapy should be approached in a sequential, targeted way. Most forms of pharmacotherapy leave patients with significant symptoms.

We look forward to the design and implementation of studies in PTSD in which pharmacotherapy, psychotherapy (especially cognitive-behavioral approaches—see below), and their combinations are compared. It is important that medication trials be conducted in populations other than male combat veterans. More recently there have been some studies in female sexual assault victims, but no controlled study has examined pharmacotherapy exclusively in women PTSD sufferers in general or sexual assault survivors in particular. In addition, the use of medications with other trauma populations (e.g., victims of disaster, accident, chronic childhood abuse, torture) still remains largely unstudied.

Cognitive-Behavioral Interventions

Introduction

The most vigorously studied psychosocial treatments for PTSD are the cognitive-behavioral interventions. These include a variety of treatment programs, including exposure procedures, cognitive therapy procedures, anxiety management training (AMT) programs, and their combinations. Arising from an experimental background, cognitive-behavioral interventions have typically been tested with repeated assessment of target symptoms, comparison groups, and well-delineated and replicable procedures.

One set of cognitive-behavioral approaches employed with PTSD sufferers consists of exposure techniques, which involve patients' confrontation with feared situations. It is designed to activate the trauma memories in order to modify pathological aspects of these memories. Obviously, the use of exposure techniques requires that a patient remember at least some details of the trauma and is aware of some of the stimuli that activate the trauma memory. To date, it seems that programs focusing on exposure have gained the most evidence for their efficacy, their efficiency, and the ease with which clients can learn how to use them.

Despite the likely superiority of programs that include exposure techniques for ameliorating PTSD and related problems, another approach, AMT, has also been helpful with PTSD. However, AMT programs are more complex to administer, require much more training to master, and put many more intellectual demands on clients than do programs that focus on exposure. In the case of AMT, the focus is not on fear activation as much as on the management of fear, generally by teaching patients skills to control their anxiety. In PTSD, both specific fears and general chronic arousal are among the defining characteristics; therefore, both exposure and AMT have been used.

Both exposure in imagination and exposure *in vivo* to trauma-related events appear to be therapeutic. The exposure treatment that has been developed by Foa and her colleagues typically incorporates imaginal exposure, in which the patient recalls the traumatic memories in the therapist's office. A rape victim, for example, is asked to go back in her mind to the time of the rape and to relive it in her imagination. She is asked to close her eyes and to describe it out loud in the present tense, as if it were happening now. Very often, this narrative is tape-recorded (audiotaped), and the tape is sent home with the patient so that she may practice imaginal exposure at home, usually daily, between therapy sessions. This treatment is described in detail in Chapter 10. Although this reliving is often painful for the patient initially, it quickly becomes less painful as exposure is repeated. The idea behind this type of treatment is that the trauma needs to be emotionally processed, or digested, so that it can become less painful. The process is similar to the grief process: The death of a loved one is extremely painful, but when that pain is expressed (say, through crying), it gradually becomes less. Eventually, the survivor can think about the loved one without crying, although the loss will always be sad. Also, as discussed in Chapter 5, many victims with PTSD mistakenly view the process of remembering their trauma as dangerous, and therefore devote much effort to avoiding thinking or processing the trauma. Imaginal reliving serves to disconfirm this mistaken belief and thus helps reduce the PTSD symptoms associated with this belief.

Other forms of exposure involve actually confronting realistically safe situations, places, or objects that are reminders of the trauma (called *in vivo*, or real-life, exposure); the confrontation is repeated until the reminders no longer elicit such strong emotions. Some therapists have patients write repeatedly about the trauma as a form of exposure (e.g., Resick & Schnicke, 1993). In systematic desensitization (SD), patients are taught how to relax and are then presented with reminders of the trauma gradually, in order from the least disturbing to the most disturbing. If they become very anxious or upset, they relax themselves and then go back to the material for exposure, until they can encounter all memories or situations without becoming upset.

AMT techniques, including skills such as cognitive restructuring and relaxation, have also been effective with PTSD sufferers. Stress inoculation training (SIT) is the AMT program that has received the most attention. SIT typically consists of education and training of coping skills. These skills include deep muscle relaxation and other relaxation skills, breathing control, role playing, covert modeling, cognitive restructuring, thought stopping, and guided self-dialogue. The idea is that PTSD sufferers experience a great deal of anxiety in their lives because they are frequently reminded of the trauma. Very often, when they become anxious, this is a cue for them to feel they are in danger and thus to become even more scared. SIT aims to teach skills to help decrease this anxiety in many different situations — that is, to help "take the edge off." SIT techniques are described in detail in Chapters 8, 11, 12, 13, and 14. The efficacy of SIT has been supported in a few reports; as noted above, however, it is less efficient than exposure, is more intellectually demanding for patients, and requires more training for therapists.

The Efficacy of Exposure Treatments

Several forms of exposure treatments have been developed for anxiety disorders, all involving the common feature of having patients confront their fears. These techniques vary on the dimensions of exposure type (imaginal vs. *in vivo*), exposure length (short vs. long), and arousal level during exposure (low vs. high). Thus, different exposure methods vary with regard to their place on these dimensions, with SD, for example, at the extreme of imaginal, brief, and minimally arousing exposure, and *in vivo* exposure at the other extreme on each dimension. (For more details, see Foa, Rothbaum, & Kozak, 1989a).

The efficacy of exposure treatment for PTSD was first demonstrated in several case reports on war veterans (e.g., Fairbank, Gross, & Keane, 1983; Johnson, Gilmore, & Shenoy, 1982; Keane & Kaloupek, 1982). Both flooding in imagination (e.g., Keane, Fairbank, Caddell, & Zimering, 1989) and flooding *in vivo* to trauma-related events (Johnson et al., 1982) appeared to be therapeutic. Most of these treatments, however, included additional techniques, such as anger control or relaxation training. Thus, the contribution of exposure therapy to the overall improvement is unclear.

SYSTEMATIC DESENSITIZATION

Some of the earliest studies of behavioral treatments for PTSD adopted the SD technique pioneered by Wolpe (1958) (e.g., E. Frank et al., 1988; Schindler, 1980; Wolff, 1977). In this technique the therapist pairs short imaginal exposure to feared stimuli with relaxation in a graded, hierarchical fashion, starting with the least distressing scenario. Although participants in these studies showed improvement in posttrauma symptoms, methodological problems plagued each of these studies, rendering the results inconclusive. For example, most of the SD publications consisted of case reports that did not utilize adequate single-case designs, or of uncontrolled group studies. An exception was the Brom et al. (1989) study, described in detail earlier in the sections on hypnotherapy and psychodynamic therapy. In this study, patients in the SD condition showed a mean improvement of 41% on the RIES; this was higher than the improvement rates for the other treatments examined, although the difference did not reach statistical significance.

In most of the SD studies, neither standardized measurements of PTSD nor blind independent evaluations were used, further hindering interpretation of the results. Also, these reports did not include sufficient details about the treatment. Finally, some of the participants in the studies were recent assault victims, at least some of whom would be expected to recover naturally via the passage of time alone (Foa et al., 1995a; Rothbaum et al., 1992); this may have exaggerated treatment effects.

The successful outcome of SD has been demonstrated in two studies with war veterans using psychophysiological measures (i.e., EMG and HR) (Bowen & Lambert, 1986; Peniston, 1986). The treatment was effective compared to a no-treatment control group, but required a large number of sessions over an extended period of time. The magnitude of the effects of this treatment on the PTSD symptoms and on general functioning cannot be ascertained, however, because the severity of PTSD and related psychopathology were not assessed.

Several uncontrolled studies demonstrated that SD was effective with rape victims in reducing fear, anxiety, depression, and social maladjustment (Frank & Stewart, 1983, 1984; Turner, 1979). In comparison to the treatments of war veterans described above, these treatments involved fewer sessions, but it was impossible to judge the degree of efficacy on PTSD symptoms because they were not directly assessed. Moreover, in the absence of a control group, the positive effects of the treatment on anxiety and depression are difficult to interpret. As noted above, an important limitation of these studies is that many of the participants were recent victims, and some of the observed improvement after treatment may have reflected the natural reduction of symptoms over the first several months following assault. Support for this interpretation comes from a report on the use of SD with several women suffering from chronic assault-related anxiety: SD alone was not successful in reducing these symptoms (Becker & Abel, 1981).

In summary, several studies have examined the effects of SD with a variety of trauma victims, and most have shown some beneficial results. However, methodological problems (the lack of adequate control conditions and/or the absence of PTSD diagnoses and measures) in some of the studies limit the conclusions that can be drawn from them.

PROLONGED IMAGINAL AND *IN VIVO* EXPOSURE

With the empirical finding that relaxation during confrontation with feared material was not necessary, and with evidence for the inferiority of SD to flooding for most anxiety disorders (e.g., Agoraphobia; Marks, Boulougouris, & Marset, 1971), the use of SD for PTSD and other anxiety disorders was largely abandoned. In its place, researchers and clinicians have used a variety of imaginal and *in vivo* exposure techniques, which promote the experience of anxiety during confrontation with the feared situation or image.

As noted earlier, exposure treatments with PTSD involve repeated reliving of the trauma, with the aim of facilitating the processing of the trauma, which is thought to be impaired in victims with chronic PTSD (Foa & Meadows, 1997; Foa, Rothbaum, & Molnar, 1995e; Foa et al., 1989b). Following promising results from a number of uncontrolled studies (e.g., Johnson et al., 1982; Keane & Kaloupek, 1982; Schindler, 1980), several controlled studies have suggested that both imaginal and *in vivo* exposure are effective for PTSD. As in the SD studies, participants in these studies were primarily veterans and assault victims, although exposure treatments are increasingly being utilized with other populations as well.

As discussed in more detail in Chapter 5, both imaginal and *in vivo* exposure treatments emerged from conditioning theory and were especially influenced by Mowrer's two-factor theory (Mowrer, 1960). Accordingly, extinction or habituation of fear is thought to occur when the fearful individual confronts feared situations, thoughts, feelings, and memories without encountering the feared aversive consequences. This explanation was criticized by many cognitive-behavioral theorists for being too mechanistic and narrow in scope. Foa and Kozak (1986) responded to this criticism by developing emotional processing theory to explain fear reduction during exposure. Again, this theory is discussed at length in Chapter 5. To summarize, Foa and Kozak suggested that exposure corrects erroneous stimulus–stimulus and stimulus–response associations (i.e., deconditioning), as well as mistaken evaluations. This process of correction, they suggested, requires the activation of the fear structure via the introduction of feared stimuli, and the presentation of corrective information that is incompatible with the pathological elements of the fear structure. In connection with PTSD, exposure promotes symptom reduction by allowing patients to realize that, contrary to their mistaken ideas, (1) being in objectively safe situations that remind them of the trauma is not dangerous; (2) remembering the trauma is not equivalent to experiencing it again; (3) anxiety does not remain indefinitely in the presence of feared situations or memories, but decreases even without avoidance or escape; and (4) experiencing anxiety/PTSD symptoms does not lead to loss of control (Foa & Jaycox, in press).

Several controlled studies have examined the efficacy of exposure treatment for PTSD. Some studies have examined the efficacy of exposure therapy relative to other treatments or to a waiting-list condition. Other studies have either evaluated the efficacy of a given exposure program itself or compared the efficacy of specific exposure procedures.

Cooper and Clum (1989) studied imaginal flooding as an adjunct to standard psychosocial and pharmacological treatment in veterans with combat-related PTSD. Twenty-six veterans with PTSD began the study, 16 completed the treatment, and results from 14 were reported. In addition to diagnostic interviews, other measures were used; these included self-monitoring of reexperiencing and of sleep, questionnaires, and a behavioral avoidance test. Most participants were randomly assigned to either standard treatment alone or standard treatment plus imaginal flooding. The flooding treatment adjunct was fairly flexible with regard to number and timing of sessions (between 6 and 14 sessions, up to 9 of which included flooding), but otherwise was fairly well standardized. The standard treatment consisted of individual and group treatments that were also described well. There was no description of treatment adherence ratings. The results indicated that the addition of imaginal flooding to standard therapy was beneficial: It augmented improvement of some symptoms, such as nightmares (96% reduction with flooding vs. 15% with standard treatment alone) and anxiety during the behavioral avoidance test (33% reduction with flooding vs. 18% *increase* with standard treatment alone). Although the outcome was not determined by an independent evaluator, these results do suggest that adding an exposure component to standard Department of Veterans Affairs (VA) hospital outpatient treatment leads to greater reduction in PTSD and associated symptoms.

Keane et al. (1989) studied implosive therapy, or flooding, for Vietnam veterans with PTSD. In this study, 24 patients were randomly assigned either to a treatment program (14–16 sessions) or to a waiting-list control group. Treatment included relaxation training, practice in nontraumatic imagery, and flooding (imaginal exposure) to the traumatic memories. The major pitfall of the Keane et al. study is the lack of blind independent evaluators; treatment efficacy was evaluated by the therapists themselves. Treatment appeared to reduce fear (40% reduction in the flooding group vs. 33% increase in controls) and depression (39% and 0% reduction, respectively), as well as some symptoms of PTSD. However, it cannot be determined conclusively whether this improvement represented a true treatment effect or was a result of therapist and patient expectancies. Despite these limitations, the Keane et al. study does support the use of imaginal exposure in treating at least the reexperiencing symptoms of PTSD.

In another evaluation of exposure treatment in veterans with PTSD, Boudewyns and colleagues (Boudewyns & Hyer, 1990; Boudewyns, Hyer, Woods, Harrison, & McCranie, 1990) published two reports on studies conducted with Vietnam veterans on a special inpatient unit of a VA hospital. In these studies, patients who were participating in a large ongoing study were randomly assigned to either direct therapeutic exposure or a control condition of traditional individual counseling. The direct exposure consisted of 10 to 12 sessions of implosive therapy (either imaginal or *in vivo*) lasting 50 minutes each, conducted over a 10-week period. Both groups also participated in the standard inpatient milieu program on the special PTSD unit at the hospital. Whereas the treatment condition was clearly defined, the control condition appears to have been very flexible, and therapists were not given specific instructions regarding what to include in these sessions. Another drawback is that no blind assessments were conducted. Both reports showed that clients who received direct therapeutic exposure evidenced some superiority over those in the control condition on a general measure of psychological functioning based on self-report. Because improvement was defined by change on this general measure of psychological functioning, rather than on a specific measure of PTSD, the efficacy of direct exposure for PTSD cannot be determined from these reports.

In another comparison of exposure with other treatments, we (Foa, Rothbaum, Riggs, & Murdock, 1991b) randomly assigned female victims of sexual assault to one of three treatment conditions: prolonged exposure (PE, including both imaginal and *in vivo* exposure), SIT, or supportive counseling. These were compared to a waiting-list control condition. Treatment targets were symptoms of PTSD, and a PTSD diagnosis was required, although there was no minimum threshold of symptom severity. Symptoms were assessed at pretreatment, posttreatment, and follow-up evaluations by means of psychometrically sound interviews and self-report measures; the interviews were conducted by trained clinicians who were blind to treatment conditions. All treatments included nine 90-minute sessions, conducted over 5 weeks according to detailed manuals. The same therapists conducted all three treatments to avoid therapist confound, and were supervised throughout the study. Thus, with the exception of the absence of a required minimum severity threshold and details regarding ongoing interrater reliability assessments, this study fulfills all of the "gold standard" criteria mentioned at the beginning of this chapter.

Findings of this study indicated that immediately following treatment, both SIT and PE patients improved on all three clusters of PTSD symptoms. Patients receiving supportive counseling or the waiting-list control improved on the arousal symptoms of PTSD, but not on the avoidance or reexperiencing symptoms. At follow-up, PE appeared the most successful; the means in this condition were lower on all measures of psychopathology then those in the other conditions. Also, 55% of women receiving PE no longer met the diagnosis of PTSD, relative to 50% receiving SIT and 45% receiving supportive counseling.

A second study compared PE, SIT, the combination of SIT and PE, and a waiting-list control group (described in Foa & Meadows, 1997). This study was similar to the Foa et al. (1991b) study with regard to meeting the "gold standard" criteria. Treatment targets and inclusion–exclusion criteria were clearly defined and measured adequately and independently. Treatment was again conducted according to manuals, with therapists trained in each condition and regularly supervised. Sessions were audiotaped or videotaped, and treatment integrity was rated by raters not involved in the study.

In this study, subjects receiving all three active treatments showed significant improvement in PTSD symptoms and depressive symptoms at posttest, and the waiting-list control subjects did not improve. These treatment effects were maintained at a 6-month follow-up. An examination of patients who achieved good end-state functioning (defined as 50% improvement in PTSD symptoms, a Beck Depression Inventory score of 7 or less, and a State Anxiety score on the State–Trait Anxiety Inventory of 35 or less) showed that 21% of patients receiving SIT, 46% of patients receiving PE, and 32% of patients receiving the combination treatment achieved this goal at posttreatment (Foa & Meadows, 1997). At the 6-month follow-up, 75% of PE patients, 68% of SIT patients, and 50% of SIT/PE patients lost the PTSD diagnosis, whereas all waiting-list patients retained the diagnosis. The differences among the three active treatment groups were not statistically significant, but on measures of overall improvement of psychopathology, the PE group showed some superiority.

Two additional studies also provided support for the efficacy of exposure treatment for PTSD, in samples that were heterogeneous with regard to their traumas. Richards, Lovell, and Marks (1994) treated 14 participants with either four sessions of imaginal exposure followed by four sessions of *in vivo* exposure, or vice versa. All participants had PTSD. Overall, patients in both treatment conditions improved considerably. The authors noted that the percentage of symptom reduction (65–80%) seen in this study is much higher than those of most treatment studies for other anxiety disorders. Also, at posttreatment and at a 1-year follow-up, no patients met criteria for PTSD. The only notable difference between the two exposure types was in the area of phobic avoidance, on which *in vivo* exposure appeared to be more effective, regardless of the order in which it was presented. Although the Richards et al. study did not include a control group with which to compare the exposure conditions, or blind evaluations with which to judge outcome, it further supports the use of exposure for PTSD and supplies information regarding the separate effects of the two exposure modalities, imaginal and *in vivo*.

Thompson, Charlton, Kerry, Lee, and Turner (1995) conducted an open trial of eight weekly sessions of imaginal and *in vivo* exposure treatment with 23 traumatized individuals with PTSD. Treatment was well described, but no blind evaluation was conducted; thus, expectancy effects cannot be ruled out.

With these limitations in mind, the results of Thompson et al.'s (1995) uncontrolled study suggest that exposure was efficacious. Participants improved on a variety of measures at posttreatment, with reductions of 42% on the IES, 61% on a measure of general health (the General Health Questionnaire), 38% on a general symptom checklist (the SCL-90), and 35% on the CAPS; all these improvements were statistically significant.

The results from the studies discussed above consistently support the efficacy of imaginal and *in vivo* exposure for the treatment of PTSD. These results are even more impressive, given the methodological precision of some of these studies in comparison with the previously reviewed ones. There are some suggestions that the efficacy of these treatments is greater in nonveteran populations than in veterans.

EYE MOVEMENT DESENSITIZATION AND REPROCESSING

A new technique, eye movement desensitization and reprocessing (EMDR; Shapiro, 1995), is a form of exposure (desensitization) accompanied by saccadic eye movements. Briefly, the technique involves the patient's imagining a scene from the trauma, focusing on the accompanying cognition and arousal, while the therapist waves two fingers across the client's visual field and instructs the client to track the fingers. The sequence is repeated until anxiety decreases, at which point the patient is instructed to generate a more adaptive thought and to associate it with the scene while moving his or her eyes. After each sequence, patients indicate their subjective units of discomfort (SUDs) level and their degree of belief in a positive cognition (validity-of-cognition rating).

EMDR has been the focus of considerable controversy since its introduction for a number of reasons, including claims by its originator as to its remarkable success in only a single session (Shapiro, 1989). (For a full exposition of this controversy, see Tolin, Montgomery, Kleinknecht, & Lohr, 1995). A number of case studies (e.g., Kleinknecht & Morgan, 1992; Lipke & Botkin, 1992; Wolpe & Abrams, 1991) have reported positive findings (for a comprehensive review, see Lohr, Kleinknecht, Tolin, & Barrett, 1995). These reports suffer from the lack of control typical of most case reports, as well as from the use of inappropriate statistical analyses and lack of standardized measures or blind evaluations.

Several studies have compared EMDR either with alternative treatments or with variations of the EMDR technique for PTSD in either controlled or semicontrolled designs. In the first study, Shapiro (1989) randomly assigned trauma victims to either one session of EMDR or an exposure control condition (i.e., EMDR without the eye movements). This study lacked specification of the inclusion–exclusion criteria, diagnostic assessment, standardized measures or blind evaluations, and a clearly defined target of treatment. Shapiro, the originator of EMDR, was the sole therapist and thus might have introduced an expectancy bias for improvement. Thus, although results showed that clients who received EMDR reported lower SUDs ratings after the one session of EMDR than did clients in the exposure control condition, methodological flaws make this finding difficult to interpret. Also, the relevance of the SUDs reduction to improvement in PTSD is unclear.

In a second study, two 90-minute EMDR sessions were compared to an exposure control (EMDR without the eye movements) as an adjunct to standard milieu treatment for veterans with PTSD; a third group of patients received standard milieu treatment alone (Boudewyns, Stwertka, Hyer, Albrecht, & Sperr, 1993). The target of treatment was PTSD, which was assessed via diagnostic interviews as well as by standardized self-report measures and physiological data. Participants were randomly assigned to the three conditions, and several adequate measures were used to determined outcome, although no blind evaluations were included.

As in the Shapiro (1989) study, SUDs ratings to traumatic stimuli were lower in the EMDR group, and therapists rated more patients as responders in the EMDR than in the exposure control group. However, the three groups did not differ on standardized self-report measures, interviews of PTSD, or on physiological responses; none improved. Thus, EMDR was superior to other conditions on the unstandardized in-session measures (SUDs), but none of the treatments were effective on standardized assessment. This negative result, even for the exposure control condition, contrasts with the proven efficacy of exposure treatments discussed earlier. As noted by Boudewyns et al., these negative results may be attributable to insufficient number of sessions or to the difficulties in treating service-connected veterans.

Jensen (1994) randomly assigned 74 veterans with PTSD to either three sessions of EMDR conducted over 10 days or to a control condition of standard VA services. On the PTSD severity measure, the groups did not differ from one another; neither improved. SUDS ratings decreased in the EMDR group but not in controls.

The role of the eye movements is puzzling to researchers, and thus Renfry and Spates (1994) tackled this issue in a study with 23 trauma victims who received either standard EMDR or one of two variations: an EMDR analogue in which eye movements were induced by a flashing light rather than a waving finger (automated eye movement), and an analogue in which a light blinked only in the center of the visual field (visual attention). Assessment included standardized PTSD and related measures, SUDs ratings, and physiological data; blind evaluations were again not conducted. After treatment, only 5 of the 23 participants met criteria for PTSD, but none of the treatments produced superior outcome. The groups did not differ on physiological measures, SUDs, or the validity-of-cognition rating, and no analyses on PTSD severity were reported.

Using a sample of 36 victims of heterogeneous traumas, Vaughan et al. (1994) conducted a more rigorous test of EMDR, comparing the procedure with imagery habituation training, a procedure involving repeated presentation of traumatic stimuli in the form of a spoken scenario, and applied muscle relaxation training (Ost, 1987), an AMT procedure. Treatments consisted of three to five sessions conducted over 2–3 weeks. Assessment included several standardized measures, including two independent interviews. The authors concluded that all three groups showed equal improvement on the independent assessors' rating of PTSD.

Silver, Brooks, and Obenchain (1995) compared standard milieu treatment with milieu treatment plus EMDR, biofeedback, or group relaxation training in a sample of 100 veterans with PTSD. The study was uncontrolled in that no standardized measures were used, clients were not randomly assigned to treatment conditions, and no blind evaluations were included. Results indicated that EMDR led to greater reduction of symptoms than did the control and the biofeedback conditions. Because of the many methodological flaws noted above, these results cannot be interpreted.

Wilson, Becker, and Tinker (1995) compared EMDR to a delayed-treatment condition in a mixed sample of "traumatized" individuals (only 30% of the target events met the DSM-IV definition of a trauma), about half of whom were said to have PTSD. Outcome was assessed via self-report measures, and clients were randomly assigned to the two conditions. Because a PTSD diagnosis was not required, the extent to which participants suffered from trauma-related symptoms is unclear. Overall, patients in the EMDR group reported decreases in presenting complaints and in anxiety at posttreatment, as well as increases in positive cognitions, whereas the waiting-list group reported no improvement. Since the results are based solely on self-report data, they may reflect effects of expectancy for improvement rather than effects of EMDR. Moreover, the generalizability of these results to individuals with PTSD is unknown.

A well-controlled study on the efficacy of EMDR was conducted by Rothbaum (1997), who randomly assigned 21 female victims of rape to either EMDR or a waiting-list control condition. Measures consisted of standardized self-report and interview instruments, with the interviews conducted by a blind evaluator. Treatment consisted of four weekly sessions conducted by a well-trained clinician, and treatment adherence was monitored and deemed acceptable by an independent evaluator designated by EMDR's originator. EMDR led to improvement on PTSD symptoms as assessed via interview (57% reduction in symptom severity) and via the RIES (74% reduction), and gains were maintained at a 3-month follow-up. These reductions were significantly different from the results for the control group, who evidenced no change in symptoms. Thus, this study suggests that a brief course of EMDR can effectively reduce symptoms of PTSD, but are eye movements necessary?

In a study addressing the role of eye movements, Pitman et al. (1996) compared EMDR with and without the eye movement component in a crossover design with 17 male veterans diagnosed with PTSD. Patients were randomly assigned to the two conditions. Measures included standardized self-report and independent interviews. Treatment was provided according to a manual, by therapists who had completed advanced training in seminars developed by the originator of EMDR. Adherence to treatment was rated by an independent assessor, who judged that treatment was delivered adequately in most cases.

The results of this methodologically rigorous study indicated that both treatments effected modest improvement in symptoms as measured by the RIES, but not by the independent assessment. In contrast to expectations, on the RIES there was slightly more improvement in the eyes-fixed condition than in EMDR. Thus, this study suggests that the eye movements, which constitute the primary component of EMDR other than exposure and nonspecific factors, do not explain the outcome.

In summary, the picture emerging from the studies reviewed here is mixed. In general, the studies of EMDR indicate reduction in subjective anxiety during the therapy session, but the efficacy of this treatment with PTSD has been demonstrated only in the Rothbaum (1995) study. Some studies have found improvement with EMDR, but methodological flaws render most (though not all) of these findings uninterpretable. The test of the efficacy of this much-discussed treatment awaits adequately controlled studies.

The Efficacy of AMT Programs

AMT (e.g., Suinn, 1974) is grounded in the assumption that pathological anxiety is rooted in skills deficits; accordingly, the goal of AMT is to equip clients with a set of procedures to handle anxiety. These include relaxation training, positive self-statements, breathing retraining, biofeedback, social skills training, and distraction techniques. Unlike exposure therapy (Foa & Kozak, 1986) and standard cognitive therapy (Beck, Emery, & Greenberg, 1985), which are designed to modify the dysfunctional components underlying pathological anxiety, the aim of AMT is to furnish the clients with ways to manage anxiety when it occurs. Foa et al. (1995a) have noted that one of the most commonly used sets of AMT procedures for PTSD is SIT (Kilpatrick & Veronen, 1984). This treatment program, originally developed by Meichenbaum (1974b) for anxious individuals, incorporates a number of educational and skills components such as relaxation, thought stopping, and guided self-dialogue. Although other AMT techniques have been suggested for use with trauma victims, such as biofeedback (e.g., Blanchard & Abel, 1976; Hickling, Sison, & Vanderploeg, 1986), we focus here on SIT because it has been more widely studied with trauma victims.

The benefit of SIT for female rape victims was examined in two uncontrolled studies (Kilpatrick, Veronen, & Resick, 1982; Veronen & Kilpatrick, 1982), with promising results. Although these studies were not controlled, they are among the first attempts at systematically examining treatment efficacy for rape victims, and thus are significant for their leading role in the research on treatment for rape victims. In the Kilpatrick et al. (1982) study, clients were permitted to choose among three treatments that were offered to them; the authors felt that this policy seemed more ethical than random assignment, given that being a rape victim involves a sense of helplessness and loss of control. The treatments of choice were SIT, SD, and a peer counseling condition; no client chose the SD treatment, 70% chose SIT, and the remaining 30% chose peer counseling.

Both these reports focused on postrape sequelae of fear, intrusions, and avoidance, rather than the full syndrome of PTSD, which was quite new at that time. Thus, although standardized measures were used in these studies, the instruments assessed some PTSD symptoms (i.e., via the IES) and general fear/anxiety rather than the entire range of PTSD symptoms. Additional outcome measures were personalized target fears and situations, which were derived in collaboration with each victim. Inclusion criteria included the presence of fear, anxiety, and avoidance related to the rape.

The results indicated that SIT was effective in reducing rape-related fear, anxiety, and avoidance, as well as general tension and depression, and that most of these gains were maintained at a 3-month follow-up. Although the lack of a control group precludes definitive conclusions about the efficacy of SIT in this study, the results suggest that SIT can effectively reduce rape-related psychopathology.

Following these encouraging results, a more controlled study was conducted to examine the efficacy of SIT for postrape psychological disturbances (Resick, Jordan, Girelli, Hutter, & Marhoefer-Dvorak, 1988). Rape victims were assigned to four conditions: SIT, assertion training, supportive psychotherapy, and a naturally occurring waiting-list. Treatment assignment was based upon openings in the next available treatment. Inclusion criteria were described only as having been raped at least 3 months prior to study participation, as having no incest history or severe competing psychopathology, and as having problems with rape-related fear and anxiety. Several self-report measures were included, such as the RIES; a structured interview was also used at the initial evaluation. At posttreatment, all three treatments produced improvement in fear and anxiety, whereas patients on the waiting list did not show such improvement. Improvement, however, was modest. On the RIES, SIT produced 27% reduction, compared to an increase of 14% in the waiting-list controls. On fear measures, reduction was 8% and 1.5%, respectively; on depression, both groups evidenced a reduction of 7%.

Other studies examining the efficacy of SIT have been reviewed in detail in the section on exposure therapy, and thus are only summarized briefly here.

Foa et al. (1991b) treated female assault victims in one of three treatment conditions: PE, SIT, or supportive counseling. These were compared to a waiting-list control condition. At posttreatment, both SIT and PE patients improved on all three clusters of PTSD symptoms. At follow-up, however, PE appeared to show somewhat superior outcome. On an independent evaluation of total PTSD severity, there was a 60% mean reduction for PE, versus 49% for SIT and 36% for supportive counseling. A second study (see Foa & Meadows, 1997) compared PE, SIT, the combination of SIT and PE, and a waiting-list control group. At posttreatment, mean PTSD severity as judged by an independent evaluation was decreased by 66% in PE and 52% in SIT. At follow-up (mean of 10 months), PE led to an average of 66% reduction, and SIT to 48%.

In summary, the efficacy of SIT for reducing PTSD and related symptoms has been supported by controlled studies. However, all of these studies were conducted with female assault victims, and thus the efficacy of SIT for other trauma populations is still unknown. Compared with the several studies on PE both with veterans and with female assault victims, there are only two well-controlled studies on SIT, both from the same research group. Thus, a firm conclusion as to the efficacy of SIT awaits further studies by other groups with other groups of PTSD sufferers.

The Efficacy of Combined Treatment Programs

Because both SIT and PE demonstrated positive results, it has been hypothesized that combining these programs may augment treatment benefit. It is thought that such combined programs may provide the means for clients to manage their stress and anxiety, and at the same time to learn how to overcome their fears of confronting trauma reminders. The efficacy of two such programs for women with assault-related PTSD has been studied.

The first of these studies (see Foa & Meadows, 1997) has been discussed in previous sections, but it is mentioned again briefly here. This study compared the efficacy of PE, SIT, their combination, and a waiting-list control. In contrast to the expectation that the combined therapy would be superior to either SIT or PE alone, all three groups produced similar improvement on overall PTSD severity. At both posttreatment and follow-up, the combined treatment produced a mean of 53% reduction in PTSD symptom severity. Because the combined treatment was delivered in the same number and length of sessions, clients who received this treatment did not get as much imaginal exposure as the PE group, nor did they receive as much SIT as the SIT group. This might explain the failure of the combined program to show more benefit than the single-component treatments.

The second combined treatment approach, cognitive processing therapy (CPT), was developed by Resick and Schnicke (1992). Drawn from cognitive and information-processing models, CPT was designed specifically for rape victims. Whereas CPT includes exposure and cognitive components, they differ somewhat from those described in previous sections. In CPT, exposure consists of describing the rape in writing and then reading this account, rather than imagining and reliving the traumatic event. Cognitive restructuring is adapted from other treatments for anxiety disorders. In contrast to earlier attempts to use cognitive therapy for rape victims (e.g., E. Frank et al., 1988), CPT focuses on five primary themes that have been identified by trauma experts (McCann & Pearlman, 1990) as being particularly relevant to rape: safety, trust, power, esteem, and intimacy. Nineteen rape victims were treated with group CPT, and their results were compared with those for a naturally occurring waiting-list control group. Treatment was focused on reduction of PTSD. Assessment included standardized self-report measures of PTSD symptoms, such as the PTSD Symptom Scale — Self-Report (Foa, Riggs, Dancu, & Rothbaum, 1993a). However, because of changes in measures over the duration of the study, not all participants completed the same assessment.

Overall, women who received CPT improved significantly, compared with those in the waiting-list group. On the SCL-90-R PTSD scale, the mean symptom reduction for the CPT subjects was 40%, versus 1.5% for the waiting-list controls. Thus, the results suggest that CPT may be an effective treatment for PTSD in rape victims. Since CPT was not compared to other treatments or dismantled, it is unclear which components were active; nor do we know whether these components act differently within CPT than they do on their own. In an updated report of this study, Resick and Schnicke (1992) examined a larger sample of 54 female rape victims. Clients in this study included the sample from the previous study, plus additional clients. Initially, 96% of the patients met criteria for PTSD; following CPT, about 88% lost their diagnosis. A decrease in depressive symptoms was noted as well.

A modified version of Foa and Meadows (1997) SIT/PE program was adopted by Blanchard and Hickling (personal communication, 1996) to treat 10 motor vehicle accident victims. The modification consisted of the addition of pleasurable-activity scheduling and discussion of existential issues. The results of this study indicated that the 9–12 sessions of combined treatment reduced PTSD symptoms by 68% on the CAPS. Thus, treatment was effective in reducing symptoms of PTSD in victims of vehicular accidents, but it is unclear which aspect of treatment was most active.

In summary, the studies to date have not supported the use of combination treatments over PE or SIT alone. However, taking into account the possible explanations for these findings noted earlier (i.e., the reduced time allotted to each treatment component in multicomponent programs), Foa and her colleagues are testing a simplified version of the PE/SIT treatment, comparing PE alone with a treatment that combines PE with cognitive restructuring. Also, Resick and her colleagues are comparing PE and CPT to a waiting-list control condition. Preliminary results of this study indicate that the two techniques are both quite effective but do not differ from one another.

The Efficacy of Cognitive-Behavioral Treatments: Summary and Conclusions

Overall, the largest number of controlled studies have been conducted on cognitive-behavioral treatments. These studies demonstrate that both PE and SIT are effective in reducing symptoms of PTSD. CPT has shown promising initial findings, but it awaits more rigorously controlled studies before its efficacy can be determined. Resick and her colleagues are currently conducting such a study, but the efficacy of CPT needs to be investigated also in other settings. The vast majority of the studies examining EMDR have serious methodological flaws, and the results are mixed. Thus, the efficacy of this treatment cannot yet be estimated.

Contrary to clinical intuition, there is no evidence indicating the superiority of programs that combine different cognitive-behavioral techniques. Perhaps the combination programs that have been examined have not been the most suitable and have shortchanged the individual components by allotting only limited time to each. Also, SIT includes several techniques, some of which (e.g., thought stopping) have not been found to be effective with other anxiety disorders, such as OCD (Stern & Marks, 1973).

Because our findings indicate that the combination of SIT and PE did not produce a better outcome than each one separately, we do not recommend that the therapist adopt this program routinely with each client. However, since the program of SIT alone has proven quite helpful, we describe each of the techniques involved in this program in Section II. At this point, we do not actually know which and how many of the various SIT techniques are responsible for the effectiveness of the program, and it will be extremely costly to conduct research that will study the separate effects of each of the SIT components.

It is important to note that one of SIT's techniques, cognitive restructuring, is a promising candidate for enhancing the efficacy of PE. Indeed, a combination of PE and cognitive restructuring was found to be superior to either technique alone for other anxiety disorders (Butler, Fennell, Robson, & Gelder, 1991; Mattick, Peters, & Clarke, 1989). Because of the proven efficacy of cognitive restructuring with other anxiety disorders and its promise for PTSD, we devote an entire chapter (Chapter 11) to carefully delineating how to apply this procedure for PTSD following assault.

Given the current state of the art, in which SIT alone and PE alone perform as well as combined programs, PE might be considered the treatment of choice for PTSD for three reasons. First, there are more studies attesting to the efficacy of PE in a variety of trauma populations than there are for SIT and CPT. Second, PE is fairly simple to implement, and thus this treatment can be more readily disseminated to clinicians who are not experts in cognitive-behavioral therapy. In contrast, SIT and CPT include more components and more complex techniques, and thus require more training. Third, SIT and CPT place more intellectual demands on clients, and many find it difficult to follow. However, as we discuss at length in Section II of the book, it is important to remember that exposure therapy may not be suitable for all trauma victims, and that in some cases the technique may need to be modified to be effective. For a review of such indications, see Jaycox and Foa (1996). In particular, problems have been noted with exposure techniques in Vietnam veteran populations, including negative posttrauma appraisal accompanied by shame, guilt, anger, and increase in alcohol and drug use (Pitman, Orr, Lowenhagen, Macklin, & Altman, 1991). This report suggests that PTSD sufferers whose traumatic memories are about being perpetrators rather than victims may not benefit from, and perhaps may even deteriorate as a result of, such treatment. But this limitation is irrelevant to the goal of this book, which is to teach therapists how to help victims. Also, some PTSD sufferers may reject treatment that includes exposure because of the temporary increase in distress (Rothbaum & Foa, 1992b). Stress management techniques cause less anxiety in sessions; however, they may not be as helpful as exposure in the long term and are more complicated to deliver.

As noted earlier, nonbehavioral treatments have not been the subject of well-controlled studies to the extent that cognitive-behavioral treatments have. However, this is not to say that they cannot prove effective as well. Let us hope that the recently emerging literature on these treatments will clarify their efficacy for treating PTSD.

5

Theoretical Bases for PTSD and Its Treatment

As we have discussed in Chapter 4, controlled studies of cognitive-behavioral treatments have demonstrated that PE procedures and SIT are effective with PTSD symptoms. In this chapter, we first briefly discuss how the psychopathology of chronic PTSD has been conceived of by the two major cognitive-behavioral theoretical approaches. We then outline a third approach, emotional processing theory, which incorporates principles of the two within an information-processing framework. We conclude the chapter by considering how emotional processing theory guides the therapeutic procedures that have been found to ameliorate PTSD, and how it accounts for their efficacy.

Theoretical Underpinnings of Cognitive-Behavioral Therapies for Anxiety Disorders

Two major theoretical traditions influenced the development of cognitive-behavior therapies for anxiety disorders, including PTSD. The first was learning theory, which encompasses both classical and operant conditioning principles. Exposure therapies have their roots in this theoretical tradition. The second tradition was that of cognitive theories, which emphasize the influence of evaluative processes or of core assumptions and beliefs as mediating the development and maintenance of pathological anxiety. Beck and colleagues' cognitive therapy, and other cognitive approaches, stem from this line of thought.

Learning Theory

The learning theory that was most influential in the development of behavioral treatment techniques for anxiety reduction was Mowrer's (1960) two-factor theory. In this theory, fear acquisition occurs through classical conditioning, in which a neutral stimulus (the conditioned stimulus, or CS) is paired with an aversive stimulus (the unconditioned stimulus, or UCS), so that the CS comes to elicit a conditioned response (CR) of fear. This process was invoked to explain some of the symptoms of PTSD (e.g., Foa et al., 1989b; Keane et al., 1985; Kilpatrick et al., 1985), in which previously neutral stimuli that were present during the trauma come to elicit anxiety themselves. In addition, through generalization and second-order conditioning, stimuli associated with both the feared and neutral stimuli that were present during the trauma also come to evoke fear. For instance, words, thoughts, and images acquire the capacity to cause anxiety.

Subsequently, through the process of operant conditioning, avoidance behavior is established. That is, an individual learns to reduce trauma-related anxiety though avoidance of, or escape from, the CS. Escape and avoidance behaviors become established through the process of negative reinforcement—that is, through their predicted capacity to terminate the aversive fear state. Because avoidance obstructs the realization that the CS has ceased to be followed by the UCS, fear is maintained.

It follows from Mowrer's two-stage theory that successful treatment should include confrontation with the CS in the absence of the UCS, until the CR (anxiety) is extinguished. As noted above, learning theory provided the original impetus for the development of exposure techniques, which have become the treatment of choice for Specific Phobia (e.g., Ost et al., 1991) and OCD (e.g., Foa & Kozak, 1996). Moreover, early on, the major mechanism invoked to explain the efficacy of exposure therapy was "extinction" (Stampfl & Levis, 1967)—that is, a decrease in the CR (anxiety) in the absence of the UCS. One difficulty with this conceptualization in phobic anxiety is that outside the laboratory it is difficult if not impossible to distinguish between a UCS and a CS, as well as between an unconditioned response (UCR) and a CR. To circumvent this difficulty, researchers have resorted to the concept of "habituation," which is represented by decreased responding to a stimulus, to describe the process of fear reduction observed during exposure treatment (e.g., Watts, 1979). Other difficulties in invoking automatic processes to explain phobias and their treatment have been discussed by Rachman (1980).

Cognitive Theories

Even during the period when Mowrer's theory was influential, discontent with nonmediational accounts of anxiety stimulated the development of cognitive approaches. Theories about cognitive mechanisms in the development and maintenance of PTSD have come from two different disciplines within psychology. In clinical psychology, cognitive theory about the psychopathology of depression has been extended to explain pathological anxiety, including trauma-related anxiety and PTSD. In personality and social psychology, the focus has been on the cognitive "schemas" or structures of meaning that are most disrupted following victimization. We discuss each of these developments in turn.

Cognitive therapy (Beck, 1976; Beck, Rush, Shaw, & Emery, 1979; Ellis, 1977) was first developed for the treatment of depression, but was later extended to the treatment of anxiety disorders (e.g., Beck et al., 1985). This therapy is founded on the assumption that it is not events themselves, but rather one's interpretations of events, that are responsible for the evocation of emotional reactions. Accordingly, an event can be interpreted in different ways and consequently can evoke different emotions. An example is a woman's hearing a noise at the window in the middle of the night. If she thinks that the noise is made by a burglar, she will immediately become anxious. However, if she thinks it is just the wind, she will be perhaps slightly annoyed to be awakened, but will not be anxious.

Cognitive therapy further assumes that each emotion is associated with a particular class of thoughts. In anxiety, the characteristic thoughts revolve around the perception of danger. The thoughts that produce anger involve the perception that other people have behaved in a wrong or unfair way. The thoughts that produce guilt involve the perceptions that one has behaved oneself in a wrong or unfair way. The thoughts that produce sadness involve the perception of fundamental loss.

In everyday life, people experience a wide range of events that evoke negative emotions. However, sometimes the emotional responses are more intense and/or more prolonged than would be expected, interrupting an individual's daily functioning. These exaggerated emotional responses are thought to originate from distorted or dysfunctional interpretations. Cognitive therapy aims to make people aware of these dysfunctional thoughts, and to correct them. It is assumed that the corrected cognitions will produce normal rather than dysfunctional emotional responses.

The originators of cognitive theory for anxiety disorders gave little attention to PTSD. They did suggest, however, that people with traumatic neuroses do not discriminate between safe and unsafe signals, and that their thinking is dominated by the concept of danger. They also suggest that traumatic fear can be maintained through a sense of incompetence to handle stressful events (Beck et al., 1985).

Personality and Social Psychology Theories

In contrast to the general nature of the learning theory and cognitive therapy approaches to posttrauma pathology, more specific hypotheses about cognitive factors that mediate posttrauma emotional responses have been advanced by scholars employing personality and social psychology theories (e.g., Epstein, 1991; Janoff-Bulman, 1992; McCann & Pearlman, 1990). Only a brief discussion of these theories is given here; a more extended explication of their ideas is presented in Foa and Jaycox (in press). To explain the psychological effects of traumatic experiences, these theories invoke the concept of "schemas" — that is, core assumptions or beliefs that guide the perception and interpretation of incoming information. Common to these theories is the supposition that the processing of a traumatic experience requires modification in existing beliefs. It is thought that such modification is accomplished through two mechanisms derived from Piaget's (1954) model of cognitive development: assimilation and accommodation.

Epstein (1991) suggested that four core beliefs change after a traumatic experience: the beliefs that the world is benign, that the world is meaningful, that the self is worthy, and that people are trustworthy. Influenced by Epstein's concepts, Janoff-Bulman (1992) noted that these core assumptions are incompatible with a traumatic experience. Therefore, the victim must struggle either to assimilate the traumatic experience into the old set of assumptions, or (more often) to change the assumptions so that they can accommodate the traumatic experience.

After an extensive review of the literature on adaptation to trauma, McCann and Pearlman (1990) proposed seven fundamental psychological needs: frame of reference, safety, dependence on trust of self and others, power, esteem, intimacy, and independence. (Frame of reference is similar to Epstein's and Janoff-Bulman's notion of a meaningful world.) McCann and Pearlman further suggested that trauma causes disruptions in any or all of these need areas, which then lead to troublesome emotions and thoughts or images.

The conceptualizations that come from personality and social psychology have not concerned themselves with specific clinical issues surrounding factors involved in the production of psychopathology following a traumatic experience. After all, as noted by Foa and Riggs (1993), not all trauma victims develop posttrauma psychopathology (i.e., PTSD), and traumas vary in their likelihood of producing PTSD.

Another approach that invokes schema theory concepts but does attempt to explain posttrauma psychopathology was advanced by Horowitz (1986). Drawing on both psychoanalytic and information-processing concepts, Horowitz suggested that people have a basic need to match trauma-related information with their "inner models based on old information" (p. 92). The process of recovery entails the repetitive "revision of both [sources of information] until they agree" (p. 92), which Horowitz referred to as the "completion tendency," and which explains the reexperiencing symptoms observed in individuals with PTSD. Horowitz further noted that if the trauma information is incongruent with existing inner models, then "alterations of inner working models and plans for adaptive actions are accomplished" (p. 96). It seems, then, that the persistent incongruity between the traumatic experience and internal mental structures is central to posttrauma psychopathology.

In all the schema-based theories about the psychological effects of trauma reviewed above, a basic difficulty arises: All seem to hypothesize that pretrauma information models or schemas contain information that the world is positive, and that difficulties arise because the trauma violates this inner knowledge. This assumption may be true for the few people who have not experienced major stressors prior to the index trauma. Epidemiological studies, however, inform us that most people have experienced major negative events, including extremely traumatic experiences (Resnick et al., 1993), before the occurrence of the index trauma. How would a new trauma violate preexisting schemas in individuals with histories of multiple traumas? Such individuals, according to Horowitz's view, should experience a match between their inner models of the world and the trauma information, such that their models need not undergo alterations; consequently, they should show fast recovery. Research findings, however, do not support this prediction. The experience of multiple traumas increases, rather than decreases, the probability of chronic PTSD (Burgess & Holmstrom, 1978; Resick, 1987).

Emotional Processing Theory

Foa and her colleagues (Foa & Riggs, 1993; Foa et al., 1989b, 1992) have advanced a theoretical approach called "emotional processing theory," which integrates learning, cognitive, and personality theories of PTSD, and has been developed to explain why some individuals recover satisfactorily from a traumatic experience while others develop chronic disturbances. The starting point of the theory is the observation that emotional experiences can often be relived well after the original emotional events have occurred, and that this reliving involves the reexperiencing of the emotion itself, as well as details of the original event and the thoughts associated with that event. This phenomenon is clearly exemplified by the common experience of recurring grief following the loss of a loved one. The memories of the lost person coincide with sadness as felt at the time of the loss. Likewise, a rape victim, when remembering the rape, is likely to experience the feelings of dread and helplessness she originally felt during the rape long after the rape's occurrence. This phenomenon can be construed as emotional reexperiencing.

Usually, the frequency and the intensity of emotional reexperiencing decrease over time. Thus, a rape victim will for a while experience intense fear when reminded of the rape. With the passage of time, this fear tends to lessen, although perhaps it never entirely disappears. Likewise, the mother of a child who has died will in time be able to recall memories of her child without feeling overwhelmed with grief. Empirical studies concur with this clinical observation. Two studies examined the process of recovery in women who had been assaulted within 10 days prior to the first assessment (Foa & Riggs, 1995; Rothbaum et al., 1992). On average, assault victims demonstrated some decline in psychological disturbances over time.

Rachman (1980), in his classic paper on emotional processing, emphasized the significance of processes underlying the decline of emotional reexperiencing. For when these normal processes are impaired, psychopathology emerges. According to Rachman, the index of unsuccessful emotional processing is "the persistence or return of intrusive signs of emotional activities such as obsessions, nightmares, pressure of talk, phobias, inappropriate expressions of emotions" (1980, p. 51). The symptoms that Rachman describes as signs of inadequate emotional processing overlap considerably with the symptom criteria of PTSD described earlier, and thus we can view the presence of PTSD as reflecting impairment in emotional processing of a traumatic experience. As noted in Chapter 2, not all individuals who experience a given trauma develop chronic PTSD. Empirical data suggest that assault victims who exhibit more severe symptoms immediately after the trauma evidence difficulties in processing later on, whereas those who react less severely show more successful emotional processing over time (Foa & Riggs, 1995; Rothbaum et al., 1992). Thus, individuals seem to differ from the beginning in how strongly they are affected by a similar trauma, and their initial reaction influences their later psychopathology. We propose that the identification of factors differentiating victims with chronic PTSD from those without PTSD would help elucidate the mechanisms that hinder or facilitate successful emotional processing. Moreover, as we discuss later in this chapter, emotional processing theory takes the position that the essence of successful treatment of PTSD is the promotion of emotional processing; thus, the identification of the factors that facilitate or hinder such processing should aid in the development of more effective treatment techniques.

Representation of the Trauma as a Cognitive Structure

The concept of "emotional processing," which is thought to mediate recovery, requires elaboration. We start with the hypothesis that a traumatic event is represented differently in the memory of a victim who remains disturbed than it is in the memory of a victim who recovers. Indeed, several researchers have suggested that chronic disorders reflect pathological cognitive structures (Williams, Watts, MacLeod, & Mathews, 1988). How can such cognitive structures be conceptualized?

To explain pathological anxiety, Foa and Kozak (1985, 1986) adopted Lang's (1979) bioinformational theory of emotion, in which fear is viewed as a cognitive structure that serves as a program for escaping danger. Accordingly, fear is represented as a network in memory that includes three kinds of information: information about the feared stimulus; information about verbal, physiological, and overt behavioral responses; and interpretive information about the meaning of the stimulus and response elements of the structure. Foa and Kozak (1986) reasoned that if a fear structure is indeed a program to escape danger, then it must involve information that stimuli and/or responses are dangerous. In a subsequent exposition of emotional processing theory, Foa and Kozak (1991) took the position that it is essentially this meaning information that distinguishes the fear structure from other information structures.

The Structure of Pathological Fear

Most people experience fear in some circumstances; this implies the "running" of a "program" for fear. Normal fear occurs with the perception of real threat and disappears when the danger is removed. When does fear become pathological? Foa and Kozak (1986) have suggested that several characteristics distinguish a pathological fear structure from a normal one.

First, fear becomes pathological when it is disruptively intense. In other words, a pathological fear structure involves excessive response elements (such as representations of avoidance and physiological activity), and these responses are resistant to modification, as in the case of phobic anxiety and PTSD symptoms. Second, this structure includes unrealistic elements. This implies that stimulus–stimulus associations do not accurately represent the world. Third, associations between harmless stimuli and escape or avoidance responses are also evident in a pathological fear structure.

Furthermore, several types of erroneous evaluations or interpretations are typically evidenced in the fear structures of individuals who exhibit pathological anxiety. First, there is a reluctance to engage in fear-provoking experiences because of an individual's evaluation that anxiety will persist until escape is realized. Second, the fear stimuli and/or responses are estimated to have an unrealistically high potential for causing psychological harm (e.g., going crazy, losing control) or physical harm (e.g., dying, being ill). Third, the anticipated consequences have a relatively high negative valence; that is, they are extremely aversive for the individual.

As noted by Foa and Kozak (1986), not all elements of an emotional structure are accessible via introspection. Although individuals may be aware of some aspects of their fear, their knowledge is surely imperfect. Just as a person may be unaware of some response information in a fear structure (e.g., information that underlies increased blood pressure), so also may the person be unaware of the meaning of those responses.

Fear Structures and PTSD

We suggest that, like the other anxiety disorders, PTSD can be construed as reflecting a fear memory that contains erroneous associations and evaluations, whereas a normal trauma memory reflects associations and evaluations that better match reality. To illustrate the difference between normal and pathological memory structures, we present two schematic models derived from the case of a rape victim who presented to our clinic with severe chronic PTSD, and was successfully treated with cognitive-behavioral techniques.

NORMAL TRAUMA MEMORY STRUCTURE

As discussed above, like any fear structure, a trauma memory structure contains three information elements: stimulus elements, response elements, and meaning elements.

Figure 5.1 illustrates a schematic model of a normal trauma memory. The ovals in this model represent stimulus elements (e.g., "man" and "gun"), and those that are related to each other are connected by lines. The rectangles represent meaning structures, such as the self as confused, afraid, or incompetent, or the world as uncontrollable or dangerous. Finally, the diamonds represent response elements—that is, the individual's responses during the trauma (e.g., "scream" and "freeze"). The model illustrates realistic associations between stimulus representations such as "gun" and "shoot," and the meaning element of "danger." Guns and shooting are indeed potentially dangerous. On the other hand, characteristics of the rapist himself, such as "man," "bald," and "tall," are not associated with danger. The absence of such associations reflects the

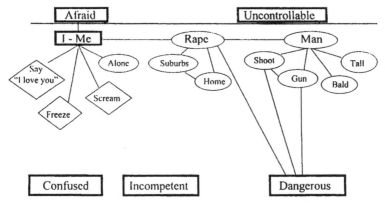

FIGURE 5.1. Schematic model of normal rape memory.

correct perception that the rapist was a unique person, and that baldness and maleness are not dangerous in and of themselves. Thus, the connections between stimulus elements and meaning elements are realistic and appropriate. A person with such a memory structure will not develop the notion that the world has become an entirely dangerous place because she was raped.

With respect to the response elements, the trauma memory includes representations of details of the rape itself and of the responses of the victim during the assault, such as "afraid" scream" and "freeze." These include also the memory that she yielded to the rapist's command to say, "I love you." These response elements, however, are not associated with negative meaning about herself (i.e., "I am a confused, incompetent person"). Thus, being raped has not altered the victim's view of herself.

PATHOLOGICAL TRAUMA MEMORY STRUCTURE

A schematic model of a pathological trauma memory structure is presented in Figure 5.2. The realistic associations are represented by solid lines, whereas the erroneous associations are represented by dashed lines. Several characteristics of this memory structure are illustrated in the model. First, like any pathological fear structure, this structure involves excessive response elements such as avoidance, escape, and physiological activity. These are represented in the diamond that denotes "PTSD symptoms." Second, in addition to the realistic associations that are present in Figure 5.1, this structure includes erroneous stimulus–stimulus associations that do not accurately represent the world, such as an association between "gun" and "bald man." That is, it indicates that because the woman was raped at gunpoint by a bald man, bald men have be-

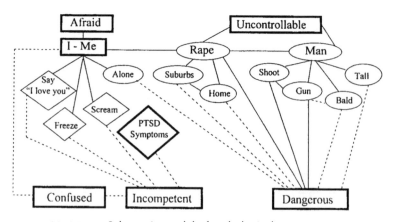

FIGURE 5.2. Schematic model of pathological rape memory.

come strongly associated with guns. In reality, however, bald men are not more likely to carry guns or to rape than men with a full head of hair. Third, the structure also includes erroneous associations between harmless stimuli, such as "bald," "home," and "suburbs," and the meaning "dangerous." Being raped at home once in the suburbs does not tangibly increase the chance of encountering violence in that environment. Fourth, the structure includes erroneous associations between harmless stimuli and escape or avoidance responses. For example, because the victim was raped by a bald man, she tends to run away from such men. In reality, however, running away from bald men is not likely to enhance her safety. These erroneous associations are depicted on the right side of the model.

The left side of the schematic model depicts the erroneous associations between response elements and the meaning "incompetent." The victim's memory that she indeed told the rapist "I love you," and the fact that she froze, are interpreted as signs of inadequacy and incompetence. The signs of emotional disturbance, such as PTSD symptoms, are also interpreted by the victim to mean that she is incompetent.

The erroneous connections found on the right side of Figure 5.2 are also typical of the fear structure of simple phobics, except that, as we have suggested (Foa et al., 1989b), the number of stimulus elements in the structure underlying PTSD is assumed to be particularly large; this is thought to lead to the perception of the world as extremely dangerous. As can be inferred from the erroneous associations depicted on the left side of the model, we suggest that in addition to the erroneous associations that lead to the perception of the world as extremely dangerous, in a pathological trauma memory structure there are erroneous associations that lead to the evaluation of oneself as incompetent. As we discuss at the end of this chapter, it is the goal of effective treatment to correct the pathological elements of the trauma memory structure that have been specified above, and thereby to lessen the trauma-related disturbances.

Why Do Some Victims Recover and Others Fail to Process the Trauma?

Foa and Riggs (1993) have suggested that three factors influence the development of chronic PTSD (i.e., the failure to process the trauma successfully): the victim's schemas about the world and the self prior to the index trauma, and pretrauma records of specific events; the victim's memory records of the trauma itself (what was recorded during the trauma); and the victim's memory records of posttrauma experiences. They have further suggested that the three factors are interconnected, such that the pretrauma schemas and records influence what will be recorded during the trauma and how these records will be interpreted; the pretrauma schemas and trauma records will both influence how posttrauma experiences will be interpreted; and the interpretations of posttrauma experiences will in turn influence the schemas about world and self, as well as modify the memory record of the trauma itself.

Figure 5.3 depicts a schematic model of these interrelationships. External events are symbolized by the solid rectangles, and their representations in memory are depicted by dashed-line rectangles. The model suggests that, first, pretrauma records, via their impact on self and world schemas, exert influence on the representations of the traumatic event; second, in the same way, memory records of the traumatic event exert influence on the representations of posttrauma events; and third, pretrauma records affect posttrauma records, again via their impact on self and world schemas. Thus, all three factors work in concert to determine whether a traumatized individual will recover or will develop chronic disturbances. We now proceed to discuss the effects of each factor.

PRETRAUMA SCHEMAS

As discussed earlier, trauma theorists (Epstein, 1991; Horowitz, 1986; Janoff-Bulman, 1992; McCann & Pearlman, 1990) imply with various degrees of explicitness that trauma victims who previously viewed themselves as invulnerable and worthy, and perceived their world as benevolent, are more likely to develop chronic emotional disturbances than victims who did not hold such extreme positive beliefs. Such individuals, Horowitz (1986) would predict, will need to invest considerable energy to match their inner models with incoming trauma information. Janoff-Bulman (1992) asserts that the individual's positive assumptions are shattered by the traumatic experience and cause emotional disturbances. However, as noted above, these conceptions are

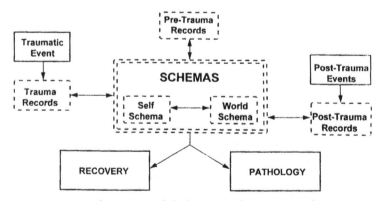

FIGURE 5.3. Schematic model of emotional processing of trauma.

incongruent with empirical studies indicating that multiple traumatic experiences and pretrauma psychological disturbances increase the likelihood of PTSD (Burgess & Holmstrom, 1978; Resick, 1987; Rothbaum et al., 1992). Presumably, individuals with such a history do not perceive themselves as competent and the world as safe. Rather, they are more likely to perceive the world as extremely dangerous and themselves as extremely incompetent. To reconcile these seeming contradictions, we suggest that it is not the holding of positive assumptions that renders an individual less adept at processing a traumatic event, but rather the holding of an extreme, rigid view. Accordingly, individuals who previously experienced multiple traumas also hold rigid extreme views, but those views are negative rather than positive.

Hence, there may be two quite distinct and even opposite ways in which pretrauma information structures can interfere with emotional processing. First, emotional processing may be impeded when the trauma violates existing knowledge of oneself as extremely competent and of the world as extremely safe. A rape experience for a woman who, prior to the trauma, perceived herself to be particularly invulnerable and strong may be highly disruptive to her self-image. For example, a confident college student who believed that she could handle any difficult situation, including protecting herself from possible assault, may blame herself for being raped because she thinks she should have been able to avoid it, and may thus begin to view herself as utterly incompetent. The same difficulty arises from holding extremely positive views about the safety of the world. For example, the victim of an industrial accident who believed that the safety measures taken by his company were flawless, would have difficulty assimilating the experience of being seriously injured in an equipment explosion. With his trust in the flawlessness of his company shattered, he would have difficulty determining which situations are dangerous and which are safe; consequently, the entire world would become dangerous for him.

The second way in which emotional processing may be impeded is when the trauma primes existing knowledge of oneself as extremely incompetent and of the world as extremely dangerous. With regard to self-view, for a woman who already held an extremely negative view of herself prior to the index trauma, this trauma is taken as conclusive proof that her self-perception is correct. In the instance of a rape victim, two lines of reasoning can reinforce her negative self-view. First, the brutal and impersonal way in which she was treated by the rapist can be seen by her as confirmation that she is an unworthy person. Second, the fact that she could not foresee the rape or prevent it may be interpreted as a sign of general incompetence. These lines of reasoning may be particularly common in women with a history of childhood sexual abuse or other prior traumatization. Thus, the index trauma reinforces the previous belief that the world is untrustworthy and entirely dangerous.

In contrast to the difficulty inherent in holding extreme views, trauma victims whose previous life experiences have equipped them with rules of interpretation that allow finer discriminations of degree of "dangerousness" and "self-competence" will be better able to process the trauma as a unique and unusual event—one that should not substantially alter their evaluations of themselves or of the world. For these victims, with more moderate and more realistic evaluations, "guns" and "rape" will continue to be associated with danger. But "bald men" and "suburbs" will be interpreted as relatively safe, even if a victim has been raped by a bald man in the suburbs.

TRAUMA MEMORY RECORDS

The second factor that may interfere with emotional processing is what is recorded "on-line" during the traumatic events. During the trauma, a memory of the trauma is constructed "on-line." This memory includes representations of stimulus elements (e.g., "bald man," "gun"), response elements (e.g., "scream," "freeze"), and meaning elements (e.g., "dangerous," "incompetent"). As noted earlier, we (Foa et al., 1989b) have suggested that trauma memories may be distinguished from other fear structures by containing a particularly large number of stimulus elements. Experiments in aversive conditioning suggest that presentation of an uncontrollable intense stimulus (electric shock) not only facilitates fear response to danger signals, but also breaks the previously established discrimination between safety and danger signals (see Hearst, 1969). If trauma is conceptualized as an uncontrollable aversive experience, then the trauma victim is expected to exhibit fear not only to dangerous situations but also to safe ones. The effect of an aversive stimulus on the emotions and behavior of the organism increases with its intensity (Baum, 1970). Accordingly, a trauma memory of an aggravated assault with a weapon will be expected to have a larger number of stimulus–danger associations than a trauma memory of a simple assault.

The number of stimulus–danger associations can also be affected by pretrauma schemas. As noted above, victims holding an extremely rigid view of the world would be expected to form a trauma memory with a panoply of stimulus–danger connections. It is reasonable to assume that a trauma memory with a larger number of stimulus–danger associations will require more processing efforts.

A trauma memory with a particularly large number of stimulus–danger associations will result in the perception of the world as entirely dangerous. Such a perception underlies the irrational reluctance of a war veteran to stand with his back to the door in the therapist's office, for fear he will be attacked from behind. Similarly, it may also lead a rape victim to view all men as potential rapists and to sleep with the lights on in her own home. Thus, the severity of the trauma, as well as pretrauma schemas of the world, will determine whether the victim will develop the unrealistic perception of the world as entirely dangerous.

We propose that trauma memories may also be distinguished from other fear structures by a large number of diverse response elements. First, the perception that the world is completely dangerous engenders a particularly large number of the typical physiological (e.g., HR) and behavioral (e.g., escape) response elements in a fear structure. Second, a trauma memory often includes a large repertoire of behaviors aiming at reducing the traumatic impact (e.g., numbing, pleading, screaming, attempts to assist others), and those are also encoded during the trauma and represented in the trauma memory. Victims who develop chronic PTSD seem to interpret their emotional responses and behavior during the rape in a way that gives them an enduring negative view of themselves, which interferes with recovery. For example, a war veteran may interpret his behavior during combat as reflecting personal incompetence because he moved away from the spot that was hit by a grenade, killing his best friend. A rape victim who becomes sexually aroused at some point during the rape may interpret this physical reaction as a sign of being a despicable human being, and her failure to prevent the rape as a sign of personal incompetence. A particularly distressing response is dissociation or numbing during the traumatic event, which is again taken as a sign of incompetence or poor coping ability (e.g., "Other people would have struggled and prevented it," "I can't trust my body," "I can't trust myself," "In stressful situations I fall apart"). Thus, the actual large numbers of responses during the trauma, in concert with rigid pretrauma schemas about the self, may result in a large number of response–self–incompetence associations, and thus will determine whether the victim will develop a view of the self as totally inept.

POSTTRAUMA REACTIONS OF SELF AND OTHERS

The third factor that can impede emotional processing is what gets recorded in memory *after* the trauma. This includes records of interactions with others, as well as records of posttrauma disturbances and difficulties in resuming daily functioning. We suggest that emotional processing of the trauma will be impeded when there is a tendency to interpret the reactions of others as negative and thus as further indications that the world is unsafe, or to interpret initial emotional difficulties (e.g., PTSD symptoms) as further signs of incompetence. The tendency to generate such dysfunctional interpretations can be traced to pretrauma schemas as well as what was recorded "on-line" during the trauma (i.e, what actually happened). As noted earlier, a pretrauma schema of the self as incompetent is likely to lead to a rapid interpretation of initial PTSD symptoms as further signs of incompetence. In addition, traumas involving violence produce PTSD in three to four times as many victims as nonviolent traumas do (Resnick et al., 1993). It stands to reason that being assaulted by another human being will produce a bias to interpret others as untrustworthy, and their reactions as negative. Also, more violent traumas result in more intense symptoms, which are more likely to lead to the interpretation that the victim is inept.

Let us first illustrate the way in which negative interpretations of the initial symptoms of PTSD can be destructive. A female prison officer who before the trauma perceived herself as exceptionally emotionally stable, and thought that she could master any stressful situation, viewed her initial distress symptoms as a sign that she was going insane. Naturally, if she thinks that intrusive recollections or flashbacks of the trauma signal a danger of going crazy, she will be likely to try to push the intrusions out of her mind. Paradoxically, however, such attempts at thought suppression are likely to increase the frequency of the intrusions (see Wegner, 1994), and hence to strengthen her belief that she is going crazy. This results in a vicious circle that maintains the symptoms. Similarly, the belief "Other people would have got better by now; only weak people can't recover" can also feed into this vicious circle. Another example concerns numbing and detachment from others, which can be interpreted as a sign that one will never experience normal feelings again or as a sign of poor functioning (e.g., "How can I not love my children/husband?", "I have died emotionally," "I'll never recover").

As noted earlier, the reactions of others can contribute to an increased sense of danger and incompetence. Some people do not respond to victims in a supportive way. Others care a great deal but don't want to discuss the trauma with the victims because of the distress it generates in themselves, and because of their concern that such conversations will also exacerbate the victims' distress. The victims can misinterpret these responses as signs that other people do not care about them, or that others blame them for not having prevented the trauma or for overreacting. Indeed, empirical studies indicate that negative social interactions (e.g., blaming or disbelieving victims) have strong negative effects on victims' adjustment, whereas positive reactions from others have little impact on adjustment (Davis, Brickman, & Baker, 1991; Ullman, 1995). This asymmetry may be attributable to a general negative interpretation of other people's reactions, and this bias strengthens the vicious circle that serves to reinforce the victims' perceptions of the world as an unsafe place and of themselves as ineffectual copers.

In summary, the victims' persistent symptoms, the disruption in their daily functioning, and the negative reactions of others are all remembered. And they are interpreted as confirming the victims' evaluation of themselves as incompetent, and of the world as extremely dangerous.

INTERRELATIONSHIPS AMONG FACTORS

From the discussion to this point, it is clear that the three factors—pretrauma schemas, the trauma memory, and posttrauma experiences—are interrelated through a myriad of vicious circles (see Figure 5.3). As noted earlier, pretrauma schemas influence perceptions of the traumatic event; the traumatic event influences posttrauma experiences; and pretrauma schemas and records affect posttrauma experiences both directly and through their influence on the trauma memory. Thus, all three factors that are involved in the formation of chronic PTSD work in concert to reinforce the two negative schemas that we hypothesize to underlie chronic psychopathology: The world is completely dangerous, and the self is totally inept.

The cognitive processes that determine whether a victim will recover or develop chronic pathology are summarized in Figures 5.4 and 5.5. Thus far, we have considered the self schema and the world schema separately. But, as depicted in Figures 5.3, 5.4, and 5.5 in the central rectangle that contains current world and self schemas, the two are interrelated, forming an additional set of vicious circles that also contribute to the maintenance of the posttrauma psychopathology. For example, the perception of the world as a dangerous place reinforces a victim's belief of self-incompetence: If the world is indeed utterly dangerous, then there is no way for the victim to protect herself (i.e., the victim is incompetent). Similarly, the belief of self-incompetence reinforces the view that the world is dangerous. These perceptions will in turn produce or exacerbate PTSD symptoms, such as phobic anxiety (reexperiencing), numbing, avoidance, and general arousal.

The foregoing discussion of the mechanisms underlying the formation of chronic PTSD suggests that successful treatment can be construed as promoting emotional processing, and therefore involves the correction of the two main erroneous cognitions: "The world is extremely dangerous" and "I am extremely incompetent." Cognitive-behavioral techniques are examples of such treatment. Indeed, Foa and Kozak (1985, 1986) have proposed that successful therapy

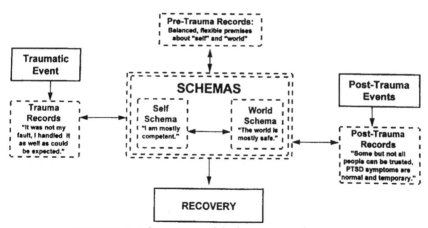

FIGURE 5.4. Schematic model of processes of recovery.

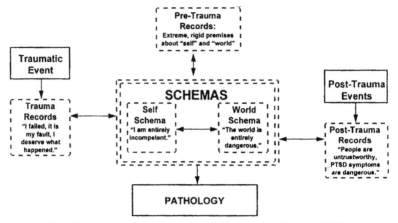

FIGURE 5.5. Schematic model of processes underlying PTSD.

involves correcting the pathological elements of the fear structure, and that this corrective process is the essence of emotional processing. It follows, then, that the therapeutic process can be viewed as involving the same mechanisms that underlie natural recovery from trauma.

How Do Cognitive-Behavioral Techniques Ameliorate PTSD?

Clearly, cognitive-behavioral techniques are helpful in reducing PTSD symptoms in many victims, and especially in women who have been the victims of sexual assault. Now that we have proposed a theory for understanding the psychological disturbances that underlie PTSD, we conclude this chapter by presenting an account of how cognitive-behavioral interventions correct these disturbances.

Emotional processing theory (Foa & Kozak, 1986) proposes that successful therapy involves correcting the pathological elements of the fear structure, and that this corrective process is the essence of emotional processing. Foa and Jaycox (in press) suggest that successful therapy can be viewed as involving the same processes that underlie natural recovery from trauma, which were considered earlier. In discussing the processes involved in successful treatment for anxiety, Foa and Kozak (1986) have suggested that, regardless of the type of therapeutic intervention used, two conditions are required for fear reduction. First, the fear structure must be activated via the introduction of fear-relevant information. If the fear structure is not activated (i.e., fear is not evoked), the structure will not be available for modification. Second, new information must be provided that includes elements incompatible with the existing pathological elements, so that the latter can be corrected.

Mechanisms of Change in Trauma Reliving and *In Vivo* Exposure

As noted in Chapter 4, exposure procedures consist of confronting the patient with trauma-related information, thus activating the trauma memory (i.e., eliciting the trauma-related fear). This activation constitutes an opportunity for corrective information to be integrated, and thus to modify the pathological elements of the trauma memory. Foa and Kozak (1986) have suggested that fear reduction (habituation) within and across exposure sessions, as well as changes in threat appraisals, are indicators that meaning changes in the fear structure have taken place. Several studies lend support to the proposition that activating the pathological fear structure facilitates treatment efficacy (see Foa & Kozak, 1986; Kozak, Foa, & Steketee, 1988). Of particular relevance to PTSD is a study demonstrating that fear activation during treatment promotes successful outcome (Foa, Riggs, Massie, & Yarczower, 1995d).

Several mechanisms are thought to be involved in the specific changes relevant to improvement of PTSD. First, repeated imaginal reliving of the trauma is thought to promote habituation and thus to reduce anxiety previously associated with the trauma memory, as well as to correct the erroneous idea that anxiety stays forever unless avoidance or escape is realized. Second, the process of deliberately confronting the feared memory blocks negative reinforcement connected with the fear reduction following cognitive avoidance of trauma-related thoughts and feelings. Third, reliving of the trauma in a therapeutic, supportive setting incorporates safety information into the trauma memory, thereby helping the patient to realize that remembering the trauma is not dangerous. Fourth, focusing on the trauma memory for a prolonged period helps the patient to differentiate the trauma event from other, nontraumatic events, and thus enables the patient to consider the trauma as a specific occurrence rather than as a representation of a dangerous world and of an incompetent self. Fifth, the process of imaginal reliving helps change the meaning of PTSD symptoms from signs of personal incompetence to signs of mastery and courage. That is, during trauma reliving the patient experiences many of the PTSD symptoms and comes to realize that this does not result in losing control or "going crazy." In this manner, the dysfunctional schema of self-incompetence is corrected and replaced by a sense of control and personal competence. Sixth, prolonged, repeated reliving of the traumatic event affords the opportunity for focusing on details central to negative evaluations of themselves and modify those evaluations. For example, a 36-year-old patient who was raped at age 18 by four men with a weapon erroneously held to the belief that she could have prevented the rape. It was only through focusing on the details of the event that she spontaneously realized, "There was no way in the world that I could have escaped those guys."

In addition to the six mechanisms suggested above, Foa and Riggs (1993) have suggested that the fear structures of traumatic memories are more disorganized than those of nontraumatic memories. A disorganized memory, they have proposed, is particularly resistant to modification. The repeated trauma reliving generates a more organized memory record, which can be more readily integrated with existing schemas. Support for this contention comes from a study analyzing victims' narratives of their traumas during exposure (Foa, Molnar, & Cashman, 1995b). Signs of disorganization (such as unfinished thoughts and repetitions) decreased from the first to the last narrative, and this decrease was correlated with improvement.

Many of the mechanisms discussed above also operate in *in vivo* exposure. However, the mechanism most salient during *in vivo* exposure is the correction of erroneous probability estimates of danger. For instance, a trauma victim may come to fear a certain time of day, physical characteristic of an assailant, and part of the city because they are related to the trauma, even when they are objectively safe. Repeated confrontation with such harmless situations will prompt a more realistic appraisal.

It is apparent from the foregoing exposition that although exposure procedures do not involve formal discussions of the patients' beliefs about the world and themselves, they are thought to affect cognitive changes in two ways. First, repeated exposure promotes the realization that the trauma was a distinct event rather than a prototype of the world as a whole, and this realization serves to increase discrimination between danger and safety signals. Second, the successful processing of the trauma leads to a reduction in PTSD symptoms. This symptom reduction promotes positive self-perception.

Mechanisms of Change in Cognitive Restructuring

In contrast to exposure therapy, cognitive restructuring formally addresses negative automatic thoughts and the dysfunctional beliefs about oneself and the world that these thoughts reflect by invoking a technique called the "Socratic method" (Beck et al., 1985; Clark, 1986). This technique involves discourse in which the patient, after having identified the thoughts and beliefs underlying fear, examines whether or not these accurately reflect reality, and replaces mistaken thoughts or beliefs with more realistic, helpful ideas. Thus, cognitive restructuring, like exposure techniques, aims at reducing symptoms via correcting the erroneous elements of the pathological trauma structure underlying PTSD.

One possible advantage of cognitive restructuring over exposure is that in addition to addressing the thoughts and beliefs underlying fear, it is equally adept to deal with those underlying anger, guilt, and shame. Although these emotions are often processed through imaginal and *in vivo* exposure, they can be targeted more directly via cognitive restructuring.

Mechanisms of Change in AMT Techniques

Although the direct goal of AMT is to teach patients techniques to manage their anxiety, the successful acquisition of such techniques can have indirect effects on schemas of self and of the world. The experience of oneself as being able to control the anxiety fosters a more positive self-image; in turn, the perception of oneself as a successful coper can reduce the negative valence of potential future threats. Victims who perceive themselves as "adequate copers" will expect to be better able to avert potential dangers in the world. Finally, the increased perception of control over anxiety may allow a victim to tolerate the trauma memories for longer periods of time, thus fostering self-directed exposure and the resulting increased organization of trauma memory.

Considerations for Specific Trauma Populations

VETERANS

A number of issues are unique to veterans as a group. First, almost all studies of veterans and treatments of this population are conducted through the VA system, where secondary-gain considerations such as benefits may mitigate against recovery. Second, many veterans who have more resources have access to private treatment, and thus have not been represented in the studies described in Chapter 4. Third, a clear difference between veterans and many other types of trauma victims is the level of perpetration versus victimization experienced by the clients. Although guilt and shame are common reactions among many trauma victims (e.g., rape victims frequently blame themselves for not having been successful in deterring the rapist, or for "giving in"), the cause for guilt and shame in veterans may be more closely linked to their behavior in causing others harm. Thus, whereas it is appropriate to challenge the guilt associated with being raped, such challenge may not be a suitable goal in the treatment of a veteran who killed civilians during wartime.

SEXUAL ASSAULT VICTIMS

Unlike veterans who have returned to peace zones, sexual assault victims must face the reality that their traumas may recur unpredictably. Thus, addressing daily safety issues becomes an important part of the treatment of sexual assault victims, and therapists need to assess the clients' ability to discriminate dangerous from safe situations and to introduce discrimination training when necessary. A related issue arises in developing *in vivo* exposure exercises. To do this, a therapist and patient generate a list of situations the patient avoids, and the patient is given assignments to confront these situations. However, in some cases, a woman may be fearful of situations that remind her of the trauma, but are in fact unsafe (such as walking alone at night in deserted areas). Such situations should obviously not be included in exposure practices, and training that focuses on differentiating PTSD-related avoidance from realistic precautions is particularly salient in this population.

It appears that the effects of exposure on PTSD symptoms in the studies on female assault victims are more impressive than those found in Vietnam veteran studies (see Chapter 4). But no study has found that a treatment being tested, whether it is medication or psychological therapy, is completely successful for Vietnam veterans with PTSD. At this point in time, Vietnam veterans' problems appear to be so chronic and complex that a combination of treatment approaches is probably warranted.

II

HOW TO CONDUCT EFFECTIVE TREATMENT OF PTSD

6

An Overview of Cognitive-Behavioral Techniques and Programs for PTSD

An Overview of Treatment Planning Options

In Chapters 4 and 5, we have reviewed the literature on treatment efficacy for PTSD and have described a theoretical model for its etiology and treatment. In this section we show you, the therapist, how to apply the cognitive-behavioral techniques found to be most effective in treating PTSD sufferers, especially rape trauma victims. These techniques range from prolonged exposure (PE) procedures to the components of stress inoculation training (SIT). The different techniques are presented with step-by-step guidance for using them with clients. They can be used within three different treatment programs that use a progressively larger number of techniques, as shown in Table 6.1. These three programs are (1) the PE program, (2) the PE/cognitive restructuring program, and (3) the PE/SIT program.

As we have suggested at the end of Chapter 4, a program of PE alone can be considered the treatment of choice for PTSD. This program begins with breathing retraining, which is described in Chapter 8. It then focuses on exposure in reality to feared situations (*in vivo* exposure) and repeated reliving of the trauma (imaginal exposure). These techniques are described in Chapters 9 and 10, respectively, and are the foundation of PTSD treatment. The research tells us that these two exposure techniques are extremely effective. In fact, they are sometimes more effective than a program that also includes the other techniques. More is not always better. The program of PE alone is simpler and easier both for most clinicians to implement and for most clients to follow. But exposure therapy alone may not be suitable for all trauma victims.

For some clients, the major problem lies in their dysfunctional thoughts, which produce guilt and shame. We know that cognitive restructuring (one of the components of SIT) is an extremely effective technique with these clients

TABLE 6.1. Treatment Plan Options

Technique	Program 1 (PE)	Program 2 (PE/CT)	Program 3 (PE/SIT)
Imaginal exposure	×	×	×
In vivo exposure	×	×	×
Breathing retraining	×	×	×
Cognitive restructuring		×	×
Thought stopping			×
Guided self-dialogue			×
Deep muscle, cue-controlled, and differential relaxation			×
Covert modeling and role playing			×

and with individuals who suffer from other anxiety disorders. In these cases, you may want to choose the second treatment context, the PE/cognitive restructuring program. It combines exposure with breathing retraining and cognitive restructuring. Chapter 11 details the use of cognitive restructuring for PTSD.

In other cases, clients may suffer from extreme, continuous tension. They may be reluctant to engage in exposure until their level of arousal is decreased. In these cases, you may want to select the PE/SIT program. We are including the full array of SIT techniques, but these can be individualized to suit each client's needs. In addition to cognitive restructuring, these include the cognitive techniques presented in Chapter 12 (i.e., thought stopping and guided self-dialogue), as well as various forms of relaxation (Chapter 13) and covert modeling and role playing (Chapter 14). The efficacy of thought stopping, guided self-dialogue, covert modeling, and role playing alone is largely unknown. But their use in combination with cognitive restructuring and relaxation is effective in reducing PTSD.

A Typical Treatment Program

Beginning with a Thorough Evaluation

Before you can determine which combination of techniques will be suitable for a client, a thorough assessment of the client's PTSD and related symptoms needs to be conducted. Thus, assessment should be done before the first treatment session. This special pretreatment evaluation uses some of the instruments and interviews described in Chapter 7. If you have concluded at the end of the evaluation that your client could benefit from some form of cognitive-behavioral treatment, you need to decide which of the three programs described in this chapter you will start with. Remember that in most cases the PE-alone program will be effective, and it is the simplest and most straightforward program to use. Conclude the evaluation session with a brief description of the treatment program that you are planning to employ.

This interview may or may not be conducted by you as the treating therapist. If it is conducted by someone other than yourself (such as person responsible for all intakes in the clinic), then all the information gathered in this evaluation should be given to you, and you should review it before the treatment and decide whether you need additional information before choosing the treatment program. The information-gathering phase may extend beyond one session and include a general psychosocial and history assessment. We suggest that in the majority of cases, two evaluation sessions are quite sufficient.

How Long Should the Treatment Program Be?

The typical treatment program consists of nine weekly treatment sessions of 90 minutes each. However, some clients may need fewer than nine sessions, and others may require more. Every client requires special consideration, and you should use clinical judgment in deciding whether to modify the program according to the client's needs. The decision regarding the length of therapy should be based on continuous assessment of the client's symptoms during treatment, as we describe in Chapter 7. We recommend that clients who do not show substantial improvement in symptom severity (defined as 70% improvement from pretreatment) of PTSD symptoms on the PTSD Diagnostic Scale (PDS; Foa, Cashman, Jaycox, & Perry, in press) after nine sessions may be offered three additional sessions. At the end of nine sessions, you and the client should evaluate her progress in the program.[1] Together, you will decide whether she will receive the three addition sessions, terminate treatment, or focus on other issues.

We have found that clients who fail to benefit substantially from cognitive-behavioral treatments after 12 sessions do not profit from additional sessions. More of the same is not necessarily beneficial. We advise that, rather than using the same approach indefinitely, you reevaluate the client's problems and to try to ascertain why the treatment has not helped the client. Throughout this section of the book, we consider difficulties that may arise during treatment and offer suggestions for how to overcome these difficulties. Chapter 15 in particular devotes much attention to this topic.

[1]Because our emphasis throughout this section is on the treatment of female rape victims suffering from PTSD, we use feminine pronouns from this point on to refer to a patient/client. However, we ask you to keep in mind that many of the techniques described in this section have been used with PTSD sufferers of both genders, and with patients suffering from other anxiety disorders as well.

General Considerations in Treating Assault Victims

A fact to bear in mind continually when a client is a survivor of rape (or non-sexual assault) is that the client has experienced a major trauma that was caused deliberately by another person. It is not surprising, therefore, that she is likely to experience extreme fear, and that her view of the world is dominated by pessimism and distrust. After all, she has sought treatment because the assault has caused long-lasting emotional distress. Your client may be involved in pressing charges against her assailant, serving a restraining order, working closely with the police, or coping with financial difficulties because she is not able to work. She may have responsibilities for others, such as taking care of her children or other family members, at a time when she can barely take care of herself. In addition, often family members and friends do not realize how debilitating posttrauma reactions can be.

Therefore, in addition to offering the client technical guidance about how to control her PTSD symptoms, you as the therapist need to become a source of general support and encouragement. In fact, one of the primary goals of the first two sessions is to form a therapeutic alliance in which the client will feel comfortable with you as well as with the treatment program. We suggest the following guidelines for forming a constructive working relationship with your client:

- *Adopt a nonjudgmental attitude.* It is highly likely that your client has been subjected to a judgmental attitude after the trauma. Try not to be a "Monday-morning quarterback" and contemplate what you would have done in her situation. Even if she made a mistake in judgment, she did not deserve to be assaulted.

- *Display a comfortable attitude when the client describes her traumatic experience.* This doesn't mean you have to sit there stoically and listen to atrocities without reacting. Your client has probably experienced people who do not want to hear about the assault, especially the gory details. She needs to know that you can hear everything she has to tell.

- *Demonstrate knowledge and expertise about PTSD and its treatment.* Your client needs to feel that she has found an expert who will help her. Many PTSD sufferers feel as if they are going crazy, and just hearing from an expert that the reactions they are experiencing are common helps normalize their reactions.

- *Express confidence in the efficacy of the treatment program.* Your confidence will allow your client to continue in treatment and to trust you to help; it will also assist her in accomplishing the goals that frighten her. She may be skeptical about the treatment or about any treatment. She may worry that she will not be able to handle reliving the trauma and that she will "fall apart" during reliving because of the intense emotions she may have. But trauma reliving is a very potent technique, and your confidence will help her feel safe to do what she needs to do.

• *Highlight the client's personal resources and praise her for having the courage to work on her problems.* We define courage as "approaching in the face of fear—being scared and doing it anyway." Your client needs to know that you appreciate how difficult this is for her and how much she's accomplished already.

• *Normalize the client's response to the assault.* Let your client know that you do not think she's weak, or losing her mind, or exaggerating. By letting her know she's experiencing a normal reaction to trauma, you give her hope and alleviate her shame and guilt for not having recovered sooner.

Specific Considerations in Applying Cognitive-Behavioral Treatment with Assault Victims

Assault victims with PTSD are characterized by extreme cognitive and behavioral avoidance. This avoidance may interfere with the treatment program in several ways:

1. A client may be reluctant to attend sessions that focus on confrontation with the distressing images, thoughts, situations, and other cues associated with the assault. We have had clients phone and tell us that they drove to the clinic but couldn't bring themselves to get out of the car and come inside. When you detect avoidance, it is important to display empathy and express understanding of the client's reluctance to face the pain associated with the traumatic memories. At the same time, it is important to point out to her that this reluctance is one of the PTSD symptoms and at the same time the cause for the chronic psychological problems that she has been experiencing since the trauma. Remind the client of the rationale for exposure treatment (see Chapters 9 and 10). In order to make progress, it is essential to learn to face the traumatic memories. However, when all is said and done, you may have to allow more latitude in the treatment of assault survivors with PTSD than in the treatment of clients with other difficulties. We allow more cancellations and appointment changes than usual, and we will call clients who don't show for appointments and give support rather than criticism.

2. Individuals with anxiety disorders usually express concerns that are largely unrealistic and irrational. For example, individuals with Panic Disorder may fear having heart attacks resulting from a fast heartbeat, and individuals with OCD disorder may fear catching AIDS from sitting on a public toilet seat. In contrast, the fears of women who have experienced a brutal physical and emotional assault are strongly rooted in reality. It is therefore very important to assess the degree to which such a client's fears are realistic when the *in vivo*

hierarchy is constructed and *in vivo* exposure homework is assigned. The reality of a rape survivor's fear was demonstrated with one of our clients, who was murdered in her own home just hours after her therapy session. But during this process of evaluating safety, we do not categorically designate situations as either "safe" or "dangerous," since in real life one can never ascertain absolute safety. Rather, we think in terms of "an acceptable level of risk," and we instruct our clients to approach situations that someone who is neither foolhardy nor phobic would feel comfortable doing.

3. Because the PTSD symptoms are connected to a traumatic event that has actually occurred, it can be difficult to use cognitive techniques to change the client's perception of danger associated with specific events. Whereas some situations that the client avoids are clearly "safe" and demand the correction of her beliefs (e.g., wearing the running shoes she was wearing when she was attacked), other situations are more ambiguous (e.g., going to a bar late at night by herself). When the safety of the situation is uncertain, you should discuss with your client rules for determining what types of situations and behaviors are safe enough and thus should not be avoided.

Therapeutic Do's: Additional Guidelines

• *Do* be active and directive in encouraging the client to attend the sessions, comply with therapeutic instructions, learn new skills, and practice them during homework.

• *Do* be supportive and sensitive when your client confronts assault-related memories, feelings, and thoughts about her assault.

• *Do* remember that the treatment programs described in this section are time-limited. However, if a client needs further help, it is important that you help her to find appropriate resources or continue to work with her yourself.

Remember, the goal of these programs is to alleviate chronic PTSD symptoms—not to produce personality changes or to solve problems that are not directly related to the assault. Again, if a client needs further help, refer her to the proper resource or establish new goals for your continuing relationship.

Suggested Treatment Schedules

In the chapters that follow, we describe the various cognitive-behavioral techniques to ameliorate PTSD, including PE techniques and SIT procedures. Again, we have elected to describe each technique or set of techniques separately, in order to present the full scope of cognitive-behavioral techniques that have been used with female assault victims; as noted earlier, some clients may not require all of the techniques presented. Our research has demonstrated that PE alone (including trauma reliving and *in vivo* confrontation of trauma reminders) is as effective as, if not more effective than, more complicated programs. Nevertheless, all three of our programs—PE alone, PE plus cognitive restructuring, and PE plus SIT—are outlined below.

Program 1: PE Alone

Many clients, especially those with uncomplicated PTSD characterized mainly by anxiety and avoidance symptoms, may require PE techniques only. The repeated imaginal exposure and *in vivo* exposure exercises may be sufficient to reduce their suffering. This is our recommendation as a first-line approach to treatment. In this approach, each session is devoted to PE, both imaginal and *in vivo*. This program is as follows:

Session 1 is devoted in part to collecting information about the assault itself, the client's reactions to the assault, and preassault stressful experiences. Use the Assault Information and History Interview (AIHI; see Appendix) to guide you in obtaining the information you will need for designing her treatment program. (Other information will have been collected during the pretreatment assessment session; see Chapter 7.) The session also includes presenting the client with a rationale for the treatment program and introducing breathing retraining (Chapter 8). For homework, instruct the client to practice the breathing retraining on a daily basis, and give her the Breathing Retraining handout to facilitate the practice of this exercise (Chapter 8).

Overview of Session 1

A. Present the rationale for the overall program (25–30 minutes).
  1. Discuss the treatment procedures that will be used in the program.
  2. Explain that the focus of the program is on PTSD symptoms.
B. Collect information relevant to the assault, using the AIHI (45 minutes).
C. Introduce breathing retraining (10–15 minutes).
D. Assign homework (5 minutes):
  1. Practice breathing retraining for 10 minutes, three times a day.
  2. Listen to audiotape of session one time.

Session 2 presents the client with an opportunity to talk in detail about the assault and her reactions to the assault and its effects on her. Common reactions to sexual assault are discussed, using the Common Reactions to Assault Handout (see Chapter 8); this discussion should be didactic and interactive. Next, the rationale for *in vivo* exposure is presented, and you and the client together construct a hierarchy of situations that the client is avoiding.

She will begin confronting situations in *in vivo* exposure after this session. This session concludes with the identication of *in vivo* assignments for homework. The client is also encouraged to continue to use breathing retraining throughout the day when she feels anxious, and to read the Common Reactions to Assault handout daily.

Overview of Session 2

A. Review homework (5 minutes).
B. Present agenda for the session (5 minutes).
C. Use Common Reactions to Assault handout to educate client about PTSD symptoms (25 minutes).
D. Discuss the rationale for *in vivo* exposure (10 minutes).
E. Introduce subjective units of discomfort (SUDs) (5 minutes).
F. Construct *in vivo* hierarchy (20 minutes).
G. Select *in vivo* assignments for homework (5 minutes).
H. Assign homework (10 minutes):
   1. Read Common Reactions to Assault handout daily.
   2. Continue to practice breathing retraining.
   3. Review the list of avoided situations at home and add more situations.
   4. Begin *in vivo* exposure assignments.
   5. Listen to audiotape of session at least once.

Session 3 presents the rationale for prolonged imaginal exposure, and this type of exposure is conducted in session for the first time. The client is told that she will listen to the imaginal exposure part of the session daily at home. During imaginal exposure, the client is instructed to relive the trauma for approximately 60 minutes. Homework includes listening to the audiotape of the imaginal exposure and continuing with *in vivo* exposure.

Overview of Session 3

A. Review homework (10 minutes).
B. Present agenda for session (5 minutes).
C. Present rationale to client for imaginal exposure (5 minutes).
D. Conduct imaginal exposure (60 minutes).
E. Assign homework (10 minutes):
   1. Continue breathing practice.
   2. Listen to audiotape of imaginal exposure at least once a day.
   3. Continue with *in vivo* exposure exercises daily, working up the hierarchy with SUDs levels.
   4. Listen to audiotape of session at least one time.

Sessions 4–8 (or 4–11) consist of about 45 minutes of imaginal exposure, and 30–45 minutes of *in vivo* exposure and/or discussion of the *in vivo* homework assignments. As treatment advances, the client is encouraged to describe the assault in much detail during the imaginal reliving. In Session 8, the client's progress in treatment is evaluated, and a decision is made about whether to continue through Session 12 or to terminate at Session 9 (as discussed in Chapter 15). This is calculated by comparing the client's total score on the PDS at Session 8 with her score at the pretreatment assessment. If she shows 70% improvement, or does not wish to continue, therapy will end in Session 9. If she has not shown 70% improvement, continue with this format for another three sessions, and terminate therapy in Session 12.

Overview of Sessions 4–8 (or 4–11)

A. Review homework (10 minutes).
B. Present agenda for session (5 minutes).
C. Conduct imaginal exposure (45 minutes); focus on "hot spots" progressively as therapy advances.
D. Conduct *in vivo* exposure discussion/implementation (20–30 minutes).
E. Assign homework (10 minutes):
　　1. Continue breathing practice.
　　2. Listen to imaginal exposure tape daily.
　　3. Continue to perform *in vivo* exposure exercises.
　　4. Listen to audiotape of each session one time.
F. Session 8 only—administer the PDS and determine whether additional treatment is needed.

The final treatment session, whether Session 9 or 12, includes 30 minutes of imaginal exposure and a detailed review of progress in treatment. The final part of the session is devoted to discussing follow-up assessments and treatment termination.

Overview of Final Session (9 or 12)

A. Review homework (20 minutes).
B. Present agenda for session (5 minutes).
C. Conduct imaginal exposure (30 minutes).
D. Review progress in detail, and make suggestions for continued practice (30 minutes).
E. Terminate therapy; saying goodbye (5 minutes).

Program 2: PE Cognitive Restructuring

For clients with PTSD that is characterized not only by anxiety but also by guilt, shame, or debilitating anger, PE with the addition of cognitive restructuring may be the treatment of choice. Additional training on your part is required for the cognitive component, but cognitive restructuring can be useful for clients who suffer from guilt, shame, or rage. To administer PE and cognitive restructuring, we suggest the following program:

Session 1 is devoted in part to collecting information about the assault itself, the client's reactions to the assault, and preassault stressful experiences, using the AIHI (Appendix). (Again, other information will have been collected during the pretreatment assessment session.) The session also includes presenting the client with a rationale for the treatment program and introducing breathing retraining. For homework, the client is instructed to practice the breathing retraining on a daily basis, and she is given the Breathing Retraining handout to facilitate the practice of this exercise.

Overview of Session 1

A. Present the rationale for the overall program (25–30 minutes).
    1. Discuss the treatment procedures that will be used in the program.
    2. Explain that the focus of the program is on PTSD symptoms.
B. Collect information relevant to the assault, using the AIHI (45 minutes).
C. Introduce breathing retraining (10–15 minutes).
D. Assign homework (5 minutes):
    1. Practice breathing retraining for 10 minutes three times a day.
    2. Listen to audiotape of session one time.

Session 2 presents the client with an opportunity to talk in detail about the assault and her reactions to the assault and its effects on her. Normal reactions to sexual assault are discussed, using the Common Reactions to Assault handout; this discussion should be didactic and interactive. Next, the treatment program is outlined and the general rationale of exposure and cognitive restructuring is presented, and you and the client together construct a hierarchy of situations that the client is avoiding. She will begin confronting these situations after this session. The session concludes with the presentation of the Common Reactions to Assault handout to the client. She is instructed to read the handout daily. The client is also encouraged to continue to use her breathing exercises throughout the day when she feels anxious.

Overview of Session 2

A. Review homework (5 minutes).
B. Present agenda for the session (5 minutes).
C. Use Common Reactions to Assault handout to educate client about PTSD symptoms (25 minutes).
D. Discuss the rationale for PE/cognitive restructuring (10 minutes).

E. Introduce SUDs (5 minutes).
F. Construct *in vivo* hierarchy (20 minutes).
G. Select *in vivo* assignments for homework (5 minutes).
H. Assign homework (10 minutes):
1. Read Common Reactions to Assault handout daily.
2. Continue to practice breathing retraining.
3. Review the list of avoided situations at home and add more situations.
4. Begin *in vivo* exposure assignments.
5. Listen to audiotape of entire session at least once.

Session 3 involves the presentation of an extensive rationale for cognitive restructuring and a description of common cognitive distortions that cause negative automatic thoughts and dysfunctional beliefs. The client is taught how to use the Daily Diary (see Chapter 11) to record situations that trigger negative automatic thoughts and distressing feelings; she is also helped to identify the types of cognitive distortions she utilizes. For homework, the client is instructed to use the Daily Diary at least three times a day, and also to identify her cognitive distortions.

Overview of Session 3
A. Review homework (10 minutes).
B. Present agenda for the session (5 minutes).
C. Give rationale for cognitive restructuring (5 minutes).
D. Define negative automatic thoughts and dysfunctional beliefs (5 minutes).
E. Teach client to identify automatic thoughts and uncover underlying assumptions (20 minutes).
F. Describe common cognitive distortions (10 minutes).
G. Teach client to challenge thoughts and beliefs, and provide rational responses (15 minutes).
H. Review use of Daily Diary, and work through second example (10 minutes).
I. Assign homework (10 minutes):
1. Continue breathing practice.
2. Study Common Cognitive Distortions handout (see Chapter 11), and fill in more examples.
3. Use Daily Diary to monitor negative thoughts, feelings, and behaviors at least three times a day, and preferably each time a negative feeling or thought emerges.
4. Continue with *in vivo* exposure and add more situations to the list.
5. Listen to audiotape of session at least once.

Session 4 presents the rationale for prolonged imaginal and *in vivo* exposure. The client is told that the imaginal exposure part of the session will be audiotaped so that she can listen to the tape at home. Imaginal exposure is then conducted for the first time; during imaginal exposure, the client is instructed to relive the trauma for approximately 60 minutes. In addition, information from the Daily Diary is used to continue teaching her to identify negative automatic thoughts and to challenge distorted cognitions. Homework is assigned to listen to the audiotape of the imaginal exposure, start performing *in vivo* exposure exercises, and use the Daily Diary to monitor automatic thoughts, feelings, behaviors, and cognitive distortions.

Overview of Session 4

A. Review homework: cognitive restructuring (15 minutes).
B. Present agenda for session (5 minutes).
C. Present rationale to client for imaginal exposure (5 minutes).
D. Conduct imaginal exposure (60 minutes).
E. Assign homework (5 minutes):
   1. Continue breathing practice.
   2. Listen to audiotape of imaginal exposure at least once a day.
   3. Continue with *in vivo* exposure exercises daily, working up the hierarchy with SUDs levels.
   4. Continue to use the Daily Diary at least three times a day.
   5. Listen to audiotape of session at least one time.

Sessions 5–8 (or 5–11) consist of 30–45 minutes of prolonged imaginal exposure and 30–45 minutes of cognitive restructuring. As treatment advances, the client is encouraged to describe the assault in complete detail during the imaginal reliving. Also, throughout the treatment the client is instructed about how to identify and challenge her automatic thoughts and dysfunctional underlying assumptions.

If the client improves 70% or more on PTSD symptoms, or does not wish to continue with treatment, therapy will end in Session 9. If the client has not improved at least 70% on PTSD symptoms, she may be offered three additional sessions, as discussed above and in Chapter 15. If she continues her participation in the program, Session 9 involves treatment planning.

Overview of Sessions 5–8 (or 5–11)

A. Review homework (10 minutes).
B. Present agenda for session (5 minutes).
C. Conduct imaginal exposure (40–45 minutes); focus on "hot spots" progressively as therapy advances.
D. Conduct cognitive restructuring (20–25 minutes).

E. Assign homework (10 minutes).
   1. Continue breathing practice.
   2. Listen to imaginal exposure tape daily.
   3. Use Daily Diary to record and evaluate the accuracy of negative thoughts at least three times a day.
   4. Continue to perform *in vivo* exposure exercises.
   5. Listen to audiotape of session at least once after each session.
F. Session 8 only—administer the PDS and determine whether additional treatment is needed.

The final treatment session, whether Session 9 or 12, will include a detailed review of the coping skills the client has learned during treatment and an evaluation of their helpfulness. The final part of the session will be devoted to treatment termination.

Overview of Final Session (9 or 12)

A. Review homework (20 minutes).
B. Present agenda for session (5 minutes).
C. Conduct imaginal exposure (30 minutes).
D. Conduct cognitive restructuring (20–25 minutes).
E. Review progress in detail and make suggestions for continued practice (30 minutes).
F. Terminate therapy, say goodbye (5 minutes).

Program 3: PE plus SIT

For some clients, the entire array of PE and SIT procedures is recommended. However, it can be modified to meet each client's needs. For example, if a client is very aroused and feels out of control, and/or is extremely hesitant to engage in exposure, it is possible to work on reducing this arousal and increasing her sense of control through the SIT. Exposure can be added at a later date, or begun when the client feels ready for it. This treatment program proceeds as follows:

Session 1 is devoted in part to collecting information about the assault itself, the client's reactions to the assault, and preassault stressful experiences, using the AIHI (Appendix). (Again, other information will have been collected during the pretreatment assessment session.) Session 1 also includes presenting an overview of the treatment program and introducing breathing retraining. For homework, the client will be instructed to practice the breathing exercise daily, and is given the Breathing Retraining handout to facilitate the practice of this exercise. As new skills are taught, they are added to the homework assignment. For example, breathing retraining is practiced daily throughout the treatment program, while relaxation skills are practiced from Sessions 3–9.

Overview of Session 1

A. Present the rationale for the PE + SIT program (25–30 minutes).
   1. Discuss the treatment procedures that will be used in the program.
   2. Explain that the focus of the program is on PTSD symptoms.
B. Collect information relevant to the assault, using the AIHI (45 minutes).
C. Introduce breathing retraining (10–15 minutes).
D. Assign homework (5 minutes):
   1. Practice breathing retraining for 10 minutes three times a day.
   2. Listen to audiotape of session one time.

Session 2 presents the client with an opportunity to talk in detail about the assault, her reactions to it, and its effects on her. Normal reactions to sexual assault are discussed, using the Common Reactions to Assault handout; this discussion should be didactic and interactive. Next, the treatment program is outlined and the general rationale for exposure and stress inoculation training is presented, and you and the client together construct a hierarchy of situations that the client is avoiding. She will begin confronting these situations after this session. In addition, the rationale for learning SIT skills is presented for each channel of fear response:

- Physiological: breathing retraining and relaxation skills
- Cognitive: thought stopping, guided self-dialogue, and cognitive restructuring
- Behavioral: role playing and covert modeling

This session concludes with the presentation of the Common Reactions to Assault handout to the client. She is instructed to read the handout daily. The client is also encouraged to continue to use her breathing exercises throughout the day when she feels anxious.

Overview of Session 2

A. Review homework (5 minutes).
B. Present agenda for the session (5 minutes).
C. Use Common Reactions to Assault handout to educate client about PTSD symptoms (25 minutes).
D. Discuss the rationale for the treatment program (10 minutes).
E. Introduce SUDs (5 minutes).
F. Construct *in vivo* hierarchy (20 minutes).
G. Select *in vivo* assignments for homework (5 minutes).
H. Assign homework (10 minutes):
   1. Read Common Reactions to Assault handout daily.
   2. Continue to practice breathing retraining.

3. Review the list of avoided situations at home and add additional situations.
4. Begin *in vivo* exposure assignments.
5. Listen to audiotape of entire session at least once.

Session 3 involves the presentation of the rationale for learning relaxation skills. During this session you will teach the client deep muscle, cue-controlled, and differential relaxation. Finally, thought stopping is taught, and homework is assigned. Instruct the client to practice deep muscle relaxation, cue-controlled, and differential relaxation exercises twice daily. Also, the client is instructed to set aside a time each day to recall a distressing image or thought and apply the thought-stopping technique, as well as to use thought stopping each time she spontaneously experiences a distressing thought or image.

Overview of Session 3

A. Review homework (10 minutes).
B. Present agenda for the session (5 minutes).
C. Give rationale for, and teach, deep muscle relaxation (50 minutes).
D. Give rationale for, and teach, cue-controlled relaxation (10 minutes).
E. Give rationale for, and teach, differential relaxation (10 minutes).
F. Give rationale for, and teach, thought stopping (15 minutes).
G. Assign homework (10 minutes):
   1. Continue breathing practice.
   2. Practice deep muscle relaxation twice a day.
   3. Practice cue-controlled and differential relaxation twice daily.
   4. Set aside a time each day to recall a distressing image or thought and apply the thought-stopping technique; also, use thought stopping each time a distressing thought or image is spontaneously experienced.
   5. Listen to audiotape of session at least once.

Session 4 presents the rationale for prolonged imaginal and *in vivo* exposure. The client is told that the imaginal exposure part of the session will be audiotaped so that she can listen to the tape at home. Imaginal exposure is then conducted for the first time; during imaginal exposure, the client is instructed to relive the trauma for approximately 60 minutes. Homework is assigned to listen to the audiotape of the imaginal exposure and to start performing *in vivo* exposure exercises, as well as to continue practicing the SIT skills.

Overview of Session 4

A. Review homework (10 minutes).
B. Present agenda for the session (5 minutes).

C. Give rationale for imaginal and *in vivo* exposure (5 minutes).
D. Conduct imaginal exposure (60 minutes).
E. Assign homework (10 minutes):
   1. Continue breathing practice.
   2. Practice deep muscle relaxation.
   3. Practice cue-controlled and differential relaxation exercises.
   4. Practice thought stopping.
   5. Listen to audiotape of imaginal exposure.
   6. Continue with *in vivo* exposure exercises daily, working up the hierarchy with SUDs levels.

Sessions 5–8 consist of 30–45 minutes of prolonged imaginal exposure and 30–45 minutes of work on SIT skills. As treatment advances, the client is encouraged to describe the assault in more detail during the imaginal reliving. Also, the client is instructed throughout the treatment to use the SIT skills she has learned as she needs them. The specific SIT skills that are taught during sessions 5–8 are cognitive restructuring, guided self-dialogue, role play, and covert modeling, respectively.

The session structure for all of these PE/SIT sessions follows roughly the same format:

A. Review homework (5 minutes).
B. Present agenda for session (5 minutes).
C. Conduct imaginal exposure (30–45 minutes).
D. Teach SIT skill (30–45 minutes):
   1. Rationale.
   2. Demonstration.
   3. Non-assault-related application.
   4. Assault-related application.
   5. Skill review.
E. Assign homework (5 minutes):
   1. Listen to imaginal exposure tape daily.
   2. Continue to perform *in vivo* exposure exercises.
   3. Practice SIT skills learned to this point.

Overviews of Sessions 5–8 with the specific SIT skills taught in each session follow:

Overview of Session 5

A. Review homework (5 minutes).
B. Present agenda for session (5 minutes).
C. Conduct imaginal exposure (30–45 minutes).

D. Teach cognitive restructuring (30–45 minutes):
   1. Rationale.
   2. Demonstration.
   3. Non-assault-related application.
   4. Assault-related application.
   5. Skill review.
E. Assign homework (5 minutes):
   1. Listen to imaginal exposure tape daily.
   2. Continue to perform *in vivo* exposure exercises.
   3. Practice relaxation techniques, thought stopping, and cognitive restructuring.
   Handout: Common Cognitive Distortions (Chapter 11).

Overview of Session 6

A. Review homework (5 minutes).
B. Present agenda for session (5 minutes).
C. Conduct imaginal exposure (30–45 minutes).
D. Teach guided self-dialogue (30–45 minutes):
   1. Rationale.
   2. Demonstration.
   3. Non-assault-related application.
   4. Assault-related application.
   5. Skill review.
E. Assign homework (5 minutes):
   1. Listen to imaginal exposure tape daily.
   2. Continue to perform *in vivo* exposure exercises.
   3. Practice relaxation techniques, thought stopping, cognitive restructuring, and guided self-dialogue.
   Handout: Guided Self-Dialogue Examples (Chapter 12).

Overview of Session 7

A. Review homework (5 minutes).
B. Present agenda for session (5 minutes).
C. Conduct imaginal exposure (30–45 minutes).
D. Teach role play (30–45 minutes):
   1. Rationale.
   2. Demonstration.
   3. Non-assault-related application.
   4. Assault-related application.
   5. Skill review.
E. Assign homework (5 minutes):
   1. Listen to imaginal exposure tape daily.
   2. Continue to perform *in vivo* exposure exercises.

3. Practice relaxation techniques, thought stopping, cognitive restructuring, guided self-dialogue, and role play.
Handout: Assertive Behaviors (Chapter 14).

Overview of Session 8

A. Review homework (5 minutes).
B. Present agenda for session (5 minutes).
C. Conduct imaginal exposure (30–45 minutes).
D. Teach covert modeling (30–45 minutes):
   1. Rationale.
   2. Demonstration.
   3. Non-assault-related application.
   4. Assault-related application.
   5. Skill review.
E. Administer the PDS and determine whether additional treatment is
   needed.
F. Assign homework (5 minutes):
   1. Listen to imaginal exposure tape daily.
   2. Continue to perform *in vivo* exposure exercises.
   3. Practice relaxation techniques, thought stopping, cognitive restruc-
      turing, guided self-dialogue, role play, and covert modeling.
   Handout: None.

If the client improves 70% or more on PTSD symptoms, or does not wish
to continue with treatment, Session 9 includes reviewing the newly learned
skills in detail and evaluating their helpfulness. The client also spends 30 minutes reliving the trauma in imaginal exposure. The final part of Session 9 is
devoted to treatment termination.

If the client has not improved at least 70% on PTSD symptoms, she may
be offered three additional sessions. If she continues her participation in the
program, Session 9 involves treatment planning. Sessions 10 and 11 consist of
30–45 minutes of imaginal exposure and 30–45 minutes of focusing on the
SIT skills that the client has found most useful. Homework is assigned to practice the SIT skills daily and to listen to the audiotape of the imaginal exposure.
Session 12 consists of 30 minutes of imaginal exposure, a review of the helpfulness of all skills, and a detailed review of the client's progress during the
program; this is the final session of treatment. Discuss the follow-up assessments
with the client and terminate therapy.

Overview of Additional Sessions 9–11

A. Review homework (5 minutes).
B. Present agenda for session (5 minutes).

C. Conduct imaginal exposure (30–45 minutes).
D. Conduct SIT skills review (30–45 minutes).
E. Assign homework (5 minutes):
1. Listen to audiotape of imaginal exposure twice a day.
2. Listen to relaxation tape once a day.
3. Continue to conduct *in vivo* exposure exercises daily.
4. Continue to use previously learned coping skills as needed to cope with stressful situations: relaxation techniques, thought stopping, cognitive restructuring, guided self-dialogue, role play, and covert modeling.

Overview of Final Session (9 or 12)

A. Review homework (5 minutes).
B. Present agenda for session (5 minutes).
C. Conduct imaginal exposure (30–45 minutes).
D. Review the client's progress in detail, and evaluate the helpfulness of all skills (30–45 minutes).
E. Discuss continued practice (15 minutes):
1. Imaginal exposure.
2. *In vivo* exposure.
3. Continued use of SIT skills as needed to cope with stressful situations: relaxation techniques, thought stopping, cognitive restructuring, guided self-dialogue, role play, and covert modeling.
F. Terminate therapy; say goodbye (5 minutes).

7

Assessment of PTSD
and Related Problems

As it is with any clinical intervention, assessment is an integral and ongoing component of the treatment of PTSD and related problems. In this chapter, we first describe the specific goals and purposes of the accurate assessment of PTSD. Next, we discuss methods of assessment, and describe several good measures for the assessment of PTSD and related symptoms. Finally, we note some common assessment problems.

As we have mentioned in Chapter 6, most of the assessment methods and measures described in this chapter are employed during a special pretreatment evaluation session. (In a few cases, two such evaluation sessions may be needed.) The exception to this is the Assault Information and History Interview (AIHI; see Appendix), which we prefer to utilize during Session 1 of the treatment.

Goals for Assessment

Providing Differential Diagnosis

Does a client have full-blown PTSD or just partial PTSD? Is she also suffering from Major Depressive Disorder? Is she checking door locks and/or showering so excessively as to warrant a diagnosis of OCD? Is she dissociating to a clinical degree? Is she abusing or dependent on alcohol or other substances? Obviously, the diagnoses she receives will guide treatment, and certain problems may need to be addressed before others. For example, a client who is abusing alcohol or drugs probably requires treatment for her Substance Abuse or Dependence before she will be ready to deal with her assault. We do not advocate using the techniques we describe in this book with clients who have current substance use disorders. In the same vein, if a client is so depressed it is difficult for her to function, or is actively suicidal, these problems need to be controlled before the assault can be addressed.

Providing an Accurate Baseline

It is important to understand the severity of the client's problems at the time she presents for treatment. Progress in treatment, or lack of it, can be measured against this baseline. Even if the client is not doing as well as she had hoped by the end of treatment, it may be useful to compare where she is with where she used to be. It can be encouraging for her to realize that progress has been made. For example, if a client is disheartened because she still feels jumpy occasionally, it will help her to realize that before treatment this was happening daily, whereas now it occurs less than weekly.

Providing an Accurate, Ongoing Record of Response to Intervention

The goal of providing an accurate, ongoing record of treatment response is tied to the goal of providing an accurate baseline. We recommend assessment as an ongoing process throughout therapy; in this manner, it becomes clear whether and in what ways the client is responding to treatment. It is not enough to think, "Well, she looks and sounds better," or even for the client to report feeling better. It should be clear in what ways she is improving and what remains to be worked on. A comparison of ongoing assessment results to the baseline assessment will furnish answers to these questions. It is also useful to have pre-, mid-, and posttreatment assessments to compare to follow-up responses. This provides a relatively quick and objective means to "take the client's PTSD temperature."

Validating, Normalizing, and Educating

We have found it invaluable to educate our clients about PTSD—its common symptoms, and the rationale for why they have these. Understanding that their "jumpiness," for example, goes along with PTSD, is commonly experienced, and is not a sign that they are just "paranoid" helps to validate their experience and normalize their reactions. They are already likely to feel alone and incompetent; it often helps them greatly to know that what they are experiencing is normal, is shared by other survivors, and is to be expected. Frequently, our clients do not connect many of their current problems to the assault when it is clear to us that the symptoms are a result of the assault. Linking many of these problems to the assault helps them become more aware and start to feel that at least their reactions are consistent and predictable—that this is part of the syndrome. This awareness helps them to label their internal events more accurately. Think back to when you've been sick: If you were informed that a medication's side effects included stomach upset, then you were probably much less worried when you experienced stomach upset than if you thought that there was yet another thing wrong with you. It helps to know what to expect and what it's caused by.

Methods of Assessment

There are multiple methods of assessment, all of which have advantages and disadvantages. We discuss three main types: self-monitoring, clinical interviewing, and standardized measures.

Self-Monitoring

Self-monitoring involves having the client record each occurrence of a target behavior (e.g., nightmares). Most commonly, this involves indicating on a form the number of occurrences of the target behavior as well as other relevant information, including the date and time, situation, thoughts, and reactions. Reactions may be recorded as subjective units of discomfort (SUDs), rated on a 0–100 scale where 0 indicates no anxiety or discomfort and 100 indicates panic-level anxiety or discomfort. Figure 7.1 shows a partial page of a self-monitoring sheet completed in a typical manner.

The date and time are important in determining the patterns of problems—for example, higher-risk times for strong reactions. It is often the case that nighttime is more difficult for rape survivors. The situation (e.g., location, others present, activity) is also important in determining relevant factors. A client may report that it scares her to go to the grocery store; however, what actually scares her may be going to a certain store at night by herself. She may not be bothered by other stores, or by this store at other times of the day or when she is accompanied. The client's thoughts surrounding strong reactions are important and can be addressed with cognitive restructuring (see Chapter 11). Are her thoughts centered around safety concerns, embarrassment, guilt, trust, or other issues?

When you are using self-monitoring with a client, you need to explain its rationale, emphasizing the importance of accuracy. Does the self-monitoring record accurately reflects the rate and severity of problems, both for the period covered and the period before treatment began? Without accuracy, treatment effects cannot be determined or client awareness increased. The therapeutic benefits of self-monitoring should also be discussed. You should inspect the self-monitoring record and respond to it accordingly. If the client reports problems but has not completed her self-monitoring form, you need to discuss the importance of these procedures and gain the client's agreement to comply in

Self-Monitoring

Target Behavior A: Nightmares
Target Behavior B: Anger/irritability outbursts
(Examples of target behaviors include nightmares, exaggerated startle reactions, outbursts of anger, etc.)

Date & Time	Situation	Thoughts	Target Behavior	SUDs
Sun 6/17 4 AM	in bed	"Someone's trying to get me"	A	90
Sun 6/17 9 AM	Kitchen	"Stop bothering me!"	B	65
Tues 6/19 3 PM	work	"Boss is picking on me"	B	50
Wed 6/20 3 AM	bed	"Someone's trying to get me"	A	90
Fri 6/22 9 PM	husband grabbed me	pissed me off	B	85

FIGURE 7.1. Part of a typical self-monitoring sheet.

the future. Compliance should be praised. Other methods of self-monitoring include keeping a simple count of occurrences of the target behaviors (e.g., by using a pocket counter or check marks) and making duration ratings (i.e., ratings of how long strong reactions last).

One advantage of self-monitoring is that it is prospective and thus more accurate recording. It also enables related relevant information to be recorded prospectively. In addition, it increases the client's awareness of target behaviors and problematic situations, and teaches the client to think in contextual terms; thus, self-monitoring is useful as a therapeutic aid. A disadvantage is that as a measure of baseline, self-monitoring is very reactive during the period of monitoring and thus often does not reflect an accurate baseline. As an ongoing measure throughout treatment, however, self-monitoring is valuable.

Clinical Interview

No assessment is complete without a sensitive clinical interview of the client regarding all aspects of her assault, other traumatic experiences, PTSD and related symptoms, social support, reactions following the assault, coping behaviors, alcohol and drug use, and psychiatric history, as well as a general psychosocial assessment. For the collection of information related to the assault itself, the client's preassault stressful experiences, and her reactions to the assault, the AIHI (see Appendix) can be used either as a standardized clinical interview or as a guide to information that may be important to gather. As we have noted in Chapter 6 and stress again in Chapter 8, the AIHI—unlike the other methods and measures we describe in the current chapter—is recommended for use in Session 1 of treatment. There are several reasons for this. First, the AIHI provides a structured way for you and the client to build rapport and begin working together to overcome assault-related symptoms. This is especially important if the pretreatment evaluation has been conducted by someone other than yourself, as if often the case in busy mental health clinics. Second, the more you know about the client's assault experience, the more assistance you can provide in prompting the client during imaginal exposure. Furthermore, in discussing ways in which the client's life has changed during the assault, you may discover areas of avoidance that can be targeted during *in vivo* exposure. Finally, the AIHI will give you a sense of areas of particular importance to the client (such as ongoing legal action, or the fact that she occasionally sees her assailant in her neighborhood); this will allow you to prepare early in treatment for some of the issues that are likely to arise.

When we reach the part of the AIHI asking for information about the assault itself, we often find it much more natural and comfortable simply to allow a client to tell her story without a great deal of interruption. It is important to remember how difficult this retelling is for many clients and to respond accordingly—expressing sorrow that they went through this experience, thanking them for sharing it with you, and/or praising their courage for being able to tell it to you. We try to avoid discussions of their behavior at the time of the assault, as this will come up later in therapy when we have taught the clients techniques for evaluating and changing their thoughts. However, some reassuring comments may be in order, especially if the client may be feeling judged by you. Here are some examples of reassuring comments:

- "You must have done the right thing, since you are here to tell about it."
- "I'm a great believer in instincts, and sometimes our instincts tell us that the way to survive is to freeze—to lie still and not fight or run."
- "Even if you feel you did something to encourage him or are to blame, it did not give him the right to rape you. In our society, people do not have the right to hurt you unless you hurt them first and they are acting in self-defense. The punishment did not fit the crime."
- "People seek help when it is the right time for them. When it is not the right time, it will probably be a frustrating experience. When it is the right time, things can work like a charm. It wasn't the right time for you until now."

Information gathering for a general psychosocial assessment should include a history of problems, results of previous treatments, other problems, family history, and so forth. However, this information (as opposed to that covered in the AIHI) is usually obtained in the pretreatment evaluation session.

The advantages of interviewing the client to gather information, in addition to those noted above, are that a clinical interview allows flexibility in responding to information gathered, in making comments, and in conducting ongoing assessment. The disadvantages are that it is often unstructured (although the use of a structured instrument like the AIHI will help), so that information may be missed if you do not happen to ask the appropriate questions and the client does not volunteer information. It is also easy to become sidetracked by a talkative or distressed client. However, a clinical interview should always be part of the assessment package.

Standardized Measures

Currently, no single universal or even common standardized measure of PTSD exists. Several questionnaires and interviews assessing PTSD severity and diagnosis, as well as related problems, are reviewed below (please note that our listing is far from exhaustive). Standardized measures permit the valid and reliable measurement of symptom severity and change. Their disadvantages center on their retrospective nature and dependence on client self-report.

CLINICIAN-ADMINISTERED MEASURES

The Clinician-Administered PTSD Scale (CAPS; Blake et al., 1990) is a 30-item interview designed to evaluate the frequency and intensity of individual PTSD symptoms as well as associated features. It contains the 17 DSM PTSD symptoms, as well as related symptoms such as guilt, depression, and occupational and social impact. It has been shown to be sensitive to treatment outcome (van der Kolk et al., 1994) and has good psychometrics. The CAPS is probably the most widely used PTSD interview and has been used for several different populations, including war veterans and sexual assault survivors. The CAPS requires about 45 minutes to administer.

The PTSD Symptom Scale (PSS; Foa et al., 1993) is a 17-item interview assessing the presence and severity of PTSD. Items (which correspond to the 17 DSM symptom criteria for PTSD) are rated on a scale of 0 ("not at all") to 3 ("very much"), with subscores available for reexperiencing, avoidance, and arousal. Psychometrics are excellent for this instrument, and it has been shown to be sensitive to treatment outcome (Rothbaum, 1997). It has been used primarily with survivors of sexual and other criminal assault. The PSS requires about 20–30 minutes to administer.

The Structured Clinical Interview for DSM-III-R (SCID; Spitzer, Williams, & Gibbon, 1987) is a structured clinician-administered interview to diagnose the various DSM-III-R Axis I disorders (e.g., Schizophrenia). The SCID has been widely used, primarily as a screening instrument, and has good psychometric properties. It requires administrators to have special training and a clinical background, and takes about 1–2 hours to administer.

The Clinical Global Improvement Scale is a global measure of change in severity of symptoms. The scale is bipolar, with 1 = "very much improved," 7 = "very much worse," and 4 = "no change." It has been used extensively in clinical trials for a variety of psychiatric patients (National Institute of Mental Health, 1985). With only one question, it is administered quickly and is based on clinical assessment. Since it assesses progress in relative terms (i.e., improvement from baseline), it is important to have the same clinician complete it at all administrations.

SELF-REPORT MEASURES

A number of self-report measures have been developed to assess PTSD symptoms in traumatized individuals. Although many of these scales provide information about PTSD severity, none yields a PTSD diagnosis that corresponds to the full DSM criteria set, except the PDS (see below). The vast majority of these scales have been validated using one index trauma (e.g., rape, combat).

The PTSD Diagnostic Scale (PDS; Foa et al., in press)[1] independently provides PTSD severity scores and yields a PTSD diagnosis according to DSM-IV criteria. It is a 49-item self-report instrument that includes all of the DSM-IV diagnostic criteria for PTSD. A total of 230 subjects who had experienced a wide variety of traumas (e.g., accident/fire, natural disaster, sexual and nonsexual assault, combat, life-threatening illness) were administered the PTSD module of the SCID, the PDS, and scales measuring trauma-related psychopathology. The PDS demonstrated high internal consistency and test–retest reliability. The PDS-derived diagnoses had high agreement with the SCID, and good sensitivity and specificity. The good validity of the PDS was further supported by its high correlations with other measures of trauma-related psychopathology. The satisfactory psychometric properties of the PDS render it a useful tool for screening current PTSD in clinical and research settings. The PDS can be completed in approximately 10–15 minutes.

The PTSD Symptom Scale — Self-Report (PSS-SR; Foa et al., 1993) is a self-report version of the PSS and assesses the same 17 DSM symptoms of PTSD. The PSS-SR requires about 5–15 minutes to complete.

---

[1]The PDS is available from National Computer Systems (NCS), 5605 Green Circle Drive, Minnetonka, MN 55343, 1-800-627-7271.

The Impact of Event Scale (IES; Horowitz et al., 1979) is a 15-item self-report scale measuring two dimensions of PTSD: event-related intrusion and avoidance. The frequency of each item is rated as 0 ("not at all"), 1 ("rarely"), 3 ("sometimes"), or 5 ("often"). Horowitz et al. reported good psychometric properties for the IES. The IES has been found to be sensitive to therapy effects in rape victims (Foa et al., 1991b; Resick et al., 1988; Rothbaum, 1997). The IES is probably the most widely used instrument to measure PTSD symptoms and has been used in most trauma populations. Horowitz et al. (1979) consider any avoidance or intrusion score over 19, with a combined score over 38, as clinically significant. With only 15 items, the IES requires only about 5–15 minutes to complete.

The Rape Aftermath Symptom Test (RAST; Kilpatrick, 1988) is a 70-item self-report inventory of psychological symptoms and potentially fear-producing stimuli rated on a 5-point Likert scale (range = 0–280). It consists of items from the Symptom Checklist 90 — Revised and the Veronen–Kilpatrick Modified Fear Survey that were found to differentiate rape victims from nonvictims. The reported psychometrics are good. The RAST usually requires about 15–20 minutes to complete.

The State–Trait Anxiety Inventory (STAI; Spielberger, Gorsuch, & Lushene, 1970) consists of 40 items divided evenly between state anxiety and trait anxiety. The authors reported good reliability for trait anxiety; as expected, figures were lower for state anxiety. The STAI is a good measure of general anxiety and requires about 10–20 minutes to complete.

The Beck Depression Inventory (BDI; Beck, Ward, Mendelson, Mock, & Erbaugh, 1961) is a 21-item self-report questionnaire assessing numerous symptoms of depression. The authors report good psychometric properties, and the BDI has been shown to be sensitive to treatment in numerous studies. The BDI is probably the most widely used self-report measure of depression and is easy to administer and score (the score is simply the total of positive responses). It takes about 5–15 minutes to complete.

The Dissociative Experiences Scale (DES; Bernstein & Putnam, 1986) is a 28-item self-administered questionnaire that assesses dissociative symptoms. Clients indicate with a slash mark on a horizontal line how often they experience a number of examples of dissociation. The lines are measured to achieve a score for each item. DES scores of 30 or greater indicate a dissociative disorder. The DES has been shown to have good psychometric properties and to differentiate clinical groups.

Assessment Packages

Many therapists use combinations of the standardized measures listed above, as well as of the three forms of assessment we have discussed. As we have mentioned, a clinical interview is usually included in all assessments. The addition of self-monitoring and/or of various standardized measures can strengthen any assessment package.

Problems in Assessment

We end our review of assessment with a discussion of some common assessment problems.

Noncompliance

One of the most problematic aspects in any assessment or treatment is client noncompliance. If the client is noncompliant with assessment endeavors, it is highly likely that she will be noncompliant with treatment instructions. The importance of the information obtained via assessment, as well as the other advantages noted earlier (i.e., increasing awareness, etc.), should be reemphasized and discussed. Obstacles to compliance should be explored, and problem-solving to try to circumvent these obstacles should be applied. For example, if a client finds it inconvenient to carry her self-monitoring sheet with her, she can note any occurrence of the target behavior on any available piece of paper and then transfer it to the self-monitoring sheet when she gets home. As her therapist, you should be persistent but not punitive.

Reactivity

It has been demonstrated repeatedly that the self-monitoring of any behavior influences the frequency reported for that behavior. Someone attempting to quit smoking who is self-monitoring the number of cigarettes smoked will probably smoke less than before the self-monitoring began. As mentioned above, self-monitoring also increases the client's awareness of the target behavior, so more occurrences may be recorded than were previously estimated. Therefore, even asking the client to self-report the frequency of target behaviors increases her awareness of those behaviors once she leaves your office, and thus interferes with the process. No research has been conducted to determine the parameters of this interference. Retrospective self-report at pretreatment does not have the problem of reactivity, but it does suffer from the inaccuracies noted above. Reactivity often renders self-monitoring inaccurate as a baseline measure. However, this can be used therapeutically (e.g., to increase awareness, etc.), and it does not interfere with ongoing assessment.

Lack of Objective Criteria

Even when standardized measures are used to assess PTSD, the results are certainly not as accurate as measurements of someone's height or weight. Certain PTSD symptoms are easily measured and quantified (e.g., the number of nightmares, flashbacks, sleep disturbances, or outbursts of anger or irritability per week). But other symptoms are less concrete and therefore more difficult to quantify objectively, such as a sense of a foreshortened future, feelings of detachment or estrangement, and avoidance. Many of the standardized interviews to assess PTSD give parameters for measuring these symptoms, but the interviewer's experience becomes important in determining the severity of a particular client's symptoms. Where none exist, it is important for the interviewer (yourself or the person who does intake in your clinic) to establish his or her own rules and apply them consistently.

Secondary Gain

As with any disorder, there may be factors maintaining PTSD symptoms that are not readily noticeable. If someone is in the "sick role" and is receiving more attention for the affliction and/or is escaping chores or duties, the sick behavior is reinforced. We have seen many women who married men who "came to their rescue" after the assault. In such a case, much of the relationship may be built on the man's protection and nurturance of the woman. If she becomes more independent and stronger, it may threaten him and the relationship. In addition, many rape victims are scared to go out alone or at night, and their PTSD symptoms help to keep them at home and/or to keep people around them.

Shame

Most women who have been raped are extremely embarrassed about what happened to them and may be ashamed of their behavior during the assault. They often hide it from even their closest friends and family members. It is important to encourage such a client to tell you all that happened to her, so that you can help her deal with it. She will not be able to accept what happened if she cannot even tell her therapist about it. You need to provide the right atmosphere to make disclosure as easy as possible. She needs to feel that you have a nonjudgmental attitude and will accept whatever she tells you. It may be helpful to acknowledge her difficulty in disclosing and thank her for her efforts.

Defining the Target Behavior

It is sometimes difficult to determine the target behavior. Nightmares? Avoidance? Flashbacks? Depression? Ideally, all of the client's problems will be assessed in the battery of measures you choose, but together you two can determine the particular target behaviors to monitor. What are the most troubling symptoms for her? What's happening the most frequently? When you ask what kinds of problems she's currently having as a result of the assault, what are the first ones she mentions? These will be your clues. If, after careful self-monitoring, it appears you chose incorrectly, you can change the target behaviors for monitoring. However, this means that you will not have a baseline measure of the original target behaviors, and therefore will not be able to assess response to treatment as accurately for those behaviors. Do not make the mistake of switching symptoms "with the wind" because your client complains of different symptoms each week. Also, when primary symptoms are controlled better, previously minor symptoms may gain importance because their overshadowing symptoms are gone. Do not switch the target behaviors for self-monitoring to these previously minor symptoms; they will be assessed with the general measures.

Conclusion

Accurate assessment is critical to all interventions, especially those that are behaviorally oriented. The assessment process is closely tied to the therapeutic process, in that continuing evaluation of problems throughout treatment guides treatment and monitors response. It also provides feedback to the client regarding her progress and areas for continued work.

8

The Beginning of Treatment

Session 1

Session 1 begins with giving the client the rationale for the treatment techniques selected. Next information is collected about the assault itself, the client's reactions to the assault, and her preassault history. As noted in Chapters 6 and 7, the Assault Information and History Interview (AIHI; Appendix) has been developed to guide you in the collection of information that you will need to evaluate the client's difficulties and plan her treatment. It can be modified or adapted for any other type of trauma for use with other clients. We suggest that you familiarize yourself with the interview before the first session, so that you are comfortable asking questions about the assault and the client's history.

The next part of Session 1 is devoted to introducing breathing retraining. Finally, for homework, instruct the client to practice the breathing exercise daily, and give her the Breathing Retraining handout (Figure 8.1) to facilitate practice. Note that throughout treatment, the client is instructed to continue daily practice of any techniques that are used during the sessions. For example, breathing retraining is practiced daily throughout the treatment program, whereas *in vivo* exposure is practiced after being introduced during the second session.

Overview of Agenda for Session 1
1. Present the rationale for the particular treatment techniques selected.
2. Collect information, using the AIHI.
3. Introduce breathing retraining.
4. Assign homework.

Explaining the Treatment Program

Introduce the client to the treatment she will receive during the next 9–12 sessions by providing a brief rationale for the treatment program you have de-

---

Breathing Retraining

Purposes:
    Slow down breathing.
    Decrease amount of oxygen in blood.
    With practice, decrease anxiety.

Breathing Instructions:
    1. Take a normal breath in through your nose with your mouth closed.
    2. Exhale slowly with your mouth closed.
    3. On exhaling, say the word "calm" or "relax" very slowly—for example, "c-a-a-a-l-l-m-m-m" or "r-e-e-e-e-e-e-l-a-x."
    4. Count slowly to 4 and then take the next inhalation.
    5. Practice this exercise several times a day, taking 10 to 15 breaths at each practice.

FIGURE 8.1. The Breathing Retraining handout.

cided to employ with her. Below are the introductions for the three programs described in Chapter 6: prolonged exposure (PE) only, PE plus cognitive restructuring (PE/CR), and PE plus stress inoculation training (PE/SIT).

RATIONALE FOR THE PE PROGRAM

Today is our first session together. I would like to spend most of the session getting to know you by asking you some questions about your past experiences and feelings. I will also explain the goals of this program to you and talk with you about the techniques you will learn while we work together.

The treatment program is set up to last 9 sessions. We will meet once a week for 90 minutes each. Most people feel better at the end of 9 weeks. But if we both feel that you would benefit from a few more sessions, we can talk about adding 3 more sessions to practice these skills.

The two main procedures of this treatment program are called "prolonged imaginal exposure" and "*in vivo* exposure." Imaginal exposure aims to enhance your ability to process the traumatic memory by instructing you to relive the memory repeatedly during the sessions. We have found that repeated and prolonged (30–60 minutes) imaginal exposure to the traumatic memory is quite effective in reducing assault-rape-related symptoms.

In addition to reliving the trauma, you will be encouraged to approach situations that you have been avoiding since the assault because these situations remind you, directly or indirectly, of the assault—for example, sleeping with the light off, walking alone in a safe place, or going to a shopping mall. This procedure is *in vivo* exposure (*in vivo* means "in real life). It has been found to be very effective in reducing excessive fears and avoidance after an assault.

We are going to work very hard, together, during the next few months to help you get on with your life. Our work will be intensive, and you may find that you are experiencing discomfort as we discuss your reactions to the assault. I want you to know that I will be available to talk with you between sessions if you feel that you need my help in coping with your feelings. Do you have any questions that you would like to ask me about the treatment program? [Encourage the client to respond.]

What I would like to do for the rest of the session is to talk with you about some of your experiences before the assault, the assault itself, and your reactions to the assault. To do this, I am going to use a standardized interview. Some of the things we discuss may be hard to talk about and may bring up unpleasant feelings. But I will help you with these unpleasant feelings. Before the end of the session I will teach you your first relaxation strategy, called "breathing retraining." It helps you breathe in a calming way and reduces anxiety.

RATIONALE FOR THE PE/CR PROGRAM

Today is our first session together. I would like to spend most of the session getting to know you by asking you some questions about your past experiences and feelings. I will also explain the goals of this program to you and talk with you about the techniques you will learn while we work together.

The treatment program is set up to last 9 sessions. We will meet once a week for 90 minutes each. Most people feel better at the end of 9 weeks. But if we both feel that you would benefit from a few more sessions, we can talk about adding 3 sessions to practice these skills.

The three main procedures of this treatment program are called "prolonged imaginal exposure," "*in vivo* exposure," and "cognitive restructuring." Imaginal exposure aims to enhance your ability to process the traumatic memory by instructing you to relive the memory repeatedly during the sessions. We have found that repeated and lengthy imaginal exposure to the traumatic memory — that is, exposure for 30–60 minutes — is quite effective in reducing assault-rape-related symptoms.

In addition to reliving the trauma, you will be encouraged to approach situations that you have been avoiding since the assault because these situations remind you, directly or indirectly, of the assault — for example, sleeping with the light off, walking alone in a safe place, or going to a shopping mall. This procedure is *in vivo* exposure (*in vivo* means "in real life"). It has been found to be very effective in reducing excessive fears and avoidance after an assault.

The third strategy you will learn in this treatment program is cognitive restructuring. This technique aims at teaching you to evaluate how realistic your beliefs about yourself and the world are. After an assault, many assault/rape survivors conclude that the world is unpredictable and uncontrollable, and view the world as entirely dangerous. Another consequence that is common after an assault is that the survivors develop extremely negative views about themselves. They believe, for example, that the fact that they are experiencing emotional reactions to the trauma indicates that they are less adequate than other people. Do you feel this way about yourself? [Encourage the client to respond.]

Also, you may believe that you are extremely vulnerable and incapable of coping with stress. These thoughts cause enduring anxiety, avoidance, and depression, and augment PTSD symptoms. As a result, you may feel anxious much of the time and may be less effective in dealing with daily responsibilities. When you learn to detect these dysfunctional thoughts and correct them, your PTSD symptoms will decrease. Thus, prolonged exposure, both imaginal and *in vivo*, and cognitive restructuring will help you correct your beliefs and provide you with skills to evaluate realistically whether a situation is dangerous or not, and whether you are able to cope with it.

We are going to work very hard, together, during the next few months to help you get on with your life. Our work will be intensive, and you may find that you are experiencing discomfort as we discuss your reactions to the assault. I want you to know that I will be available to talk with you between sessions if you feel that you need my help in coping with your feelings. Do you have any questions that you would like to ask me about the treatment program? [Encourage the client to respond.]

What I would like to do for the rest of the session is to talk with you about some of your experiences before the assault, the assault itself, and your reactions to the assault. To do this I am going to use a standardized interview. Some of the things we discuss may be hard to talk about and may bring up unpleasant feelings. But I will help you with these unpleasant feelings. Before the end of the session I will teach you your first relaxation strategy, called "breathing retraining." It helps you breathe in a calming way and reduces anxiety.

RATIONALE FOR THE PE/SIT PROGRAM

Today is our first session together. I would like to spend most of the session getting to know you by asking you some questions about your past experiences and feelings. I will also explain the goals of this program to you and talk with you about the techniques you will learn while we work together.

The treatment program is set up to last 9 sessions. We will meet once a week for 90 minutes each. Most people feel better at the end of 9 weeks. But if we both feel that you would benefit from a few more sessions, we can talk about adding 3 more sessions to practice these skills.

There are several methods used in this treatment program. The first two are called "prolonged imaginal exposure" and "*in vivo* exposure." Imaginal exposure helps you process the traumatic memory by reliving it in your imagination during our sessions. We will need to do this again and again for 30–60 minutes at a time. We have found that this kind of repeated exposure to the traumatic memory is very effective in reducing symptoms like yours.

I will also ask you to try to do some of the things that you have been avoiding since the assault. These situations probably remind you, directly or indirectly, of the assault; for example, you may not sleep with the light off, walk alone in a safe place, or go to a shopping mall. This is *in vivo* exposure (*in vivo* means "in real life"). It can be very effective in reducing strong fears and the avoiding of situations after an assault.

Another group of strategies you will learn in this treatment program is called "stress inoculation training." This is a set of several techniques to help you control your anxiety. They include ways to relax your body, ways your thoughts can help you (cognitive techniques), role playing, and modeling. After an assault, many survivors feel that the world is unpredictable and uncontrollable. They see the world as very dangerous. Thinking like this makes it hard to live a normal life. I will help you to look at how realistic your thoughts about yourself and the world are. If necessary, I'll help you to make them more realistic.

After an assault, it is also common for survivors to feel very bad about themselves. This may apply to you, too. For example, since you are experiencing emotional reactions to the trauma, you may feel you are less adequate than you thought you were. Many survivors feel very vulnerable and feel unable to cope with stress. These thoughts can make your symptoms worse. They can cause great anxiety, avoidance, and depression. When you learn to catch these thoughts and change them, your symptoms will decrease. These techniques will give you skills to manage your anxiety, and help you come to grips with what has happened to you.

We are going to work very hard, together, during the next few months to help you get on with your life. Our work will be intensive, and you may find that you feel uncomfortable as we discuss your reactions to the assault. I want you to know that I will be happy to talk with you between sessions if you feel that you cannot cope with your feelings alone. Do you have any questions that you would like to ask me about the treatment program or the information that I have just given to you? [Encourage the client to respond.]

What I would like to do for the rest of the session is to talk with you about some of your experiences before the assault, the assault itself, and your reactions to the assault. To do this, I am going to use a standardized interview. Some of the things we discuss may be hard to talk about and may bring up unpleasant feelings. But I will help you with these unpleasant feelings. Before the end of the session I will teach you your first relaxation strategy, called "breathing retraining." It helps you breathe in a calming way and reduces anxiety.

Collecting Information on the Assault

Prior to this first treatment session, clients will have gone through a formal assessment session (see Chapter 7) that focuses on symptoms, diagnosis, and the appropriateness of treatment. In this first treatment session, information gathering turns directly to the in-depth details of the assault and the specific life changes the client has undergone since the assault. Again, we have developed the AIHI (see Appendix) to aid you in collecting this information. Discussing the ways in which the client's life has changed since the assault helps you and the client identify areas of avoidance that may be targeted for *in vivo* exposure, as described in Chapter 9. Moreover, as we will see in Chapter 10, the more details you know about the asssault, the better you will be able to prompt the client during imaginal exposure.

Asking specific and directive questions about assault-related topics is likely to elicit strong emotional responses from the client. Please assure your client (implicitly or explicitly) that this is OK, that you understand, and that you can handle her distress. If a particular topic provokes extreme discomfort for the client, use your clinical judgment to decide whether to focus on this area at greater length or to postpone the questioning until a later time. When you make this decision, it is important that you take into account the expressed needs and wishes of the client, and that you communicate your decision to her. We always tell our clients at the beginning of the information-gathering period what to expect, and ask them to let us know if they need a break. Although they rarely take a break, it is important that they know they have this control.

Breathing Retraining

Introduce the client to breathing retraining before she leaves the first session, in order to alleviate anxiety that may have been elicited by discussing the assault. The rationale for this technique can be presented as follows:

Most of us realize that our breathing affects the way that we feel. For example, when we are upset, people may tell us to take a deep breath and calm down. However, taking a deep breath often does not help. Instead, in order to calm down, we should take a normal breath and exhale slowly. For example, when our ancestors, thousands of years ago, were walking through the forest and spotted a lion, they probably gasped and held their breath. When the lion walked away, they signed in relief (exhaled). Therefore, it is *exhalation* that is associated with relaxation, not *inhalation*.

When you are suggesting a cue word for relaxation, find out if the client has a preference for a specific word. Most people find the word "calm" or "relax" helpful. We use the word "calm" in the example that follows, but it is important to use the word that the client prefers. First, model for the client how to inhale and exhale through the nose, and then ask the client to perform the exercise according to the following instructions:

Please try to take in a *normal* breath rather than a deep breath. Inhale normally through your nose. Unless we are exercising vigorously, we should always try to breathe through our noses. After you inhale normally, I'll ask you to concentrate on the exhalation and drag it out. While you are slowly exhaling, I will also ask you to say the word "calm" silently to yourself, and I will say it aloud when you practice in here. "Calm" is a good word to use, because in our culture it is already associated with nice things. If we are upset and someone helps us to "calm down," usually it is associated with comfort and support. It also sounds nice and can be dragged out to match the long, slow exhalation: "c-a-a-a-l-l-m-m-m."

In addition to concentrating on slow exhalation while saying "calm" to yourself, I want you to slow down your breathing. Very often, when people become frightened or upset, they feel as if they need more air and may therefore hyperventilate. Hyperventilation, however does not have a calming effect. In fact, it generates anxious feelings. Unless we are preparing for one of the "three F's"—that is, fight, freeze, or flee—in the face of a real danger, we often don't need as much air as we are taking in. When we hyperventilate and take in more air, it signals our bodies to prepare for one of the "three F's" and to keep it fueled with oxygen. This is similar to a runner's taking deep breaths to fuel her body with oxygen before a race and continuing to breathe deeply and quickly throughout the race. Usually when we hyperventilate, though, we are tricking our bodies. And what we really need to do is to slow down our breathing and take in *less* air. We do this by pausing between breaths to space them out more. After your slowed exhalation, literally hold your breath for a count of 4 [note: this may be adjusted if necessary] before you inhale the next breath.

Now instruct the client to take a normal breath and exhale very slowly as she says the word "calm" or "relax" to herself. Train her to pause and count to 4 before taking a second breath. Repeat the entire sequence 10 to 15 times, for 10–15 breaths. Try to watch the client's chest or abdomen, in order to follow her own natural breathing rhythms. Toward the end of the exercise, start fading away your instructions while she continues to practice. Here are the instructions to say aloud: "Take a normal breath [client inhales] . . . c-a-a-a-l-l-m-m-m [as client exhales] . . . And pause . . . 2 . . . 3 . . . 4." We usually start when it looks as though the client is ready to inhale naturally by instructing, "Take a normal breath now." This prompt is usually dropped by about the eighth repetition. We continue to say "c-a-a-a-l-l-m-m-m" as the client exhales throughout the entire exercise. "And pause . . . 2 . . . 3 . . . 4" follows; we drop the "2 . . . 3 . . . 4" by about the ninth repetition, and the "And pause" soon thereafter.

After teaching the technique, give the client the Breathing Retraining handout (Figure 8.1). You should also suggest to the client that she practice the breathing retraining at least twice per day, as well as when she is feeling particularly tense or distressed throughout the day.

If a client has asthma, she will probably not feel comfortable pausing without air in her lungs. In these cases, have the client take a normal breath, then pause for a count of 4, then exhale slowly.

Session 2

Session 2 presents the client with an opportunity to talk in detail about her reactions to the assault and its effects on her. Common reactions to sexual assault are discussed, using the Common Reactions to Assault handout (Figure 8.2); this discussion should be didactic and interactive. Next, the rationale for *in vivo* exposure is presented (this is discussed in more detail in Chapter 9).

Common Reactions to Assault

An assault is a traumatic experience that produces emotional shock and causes many emotional problems. This handout describes some of the common reactions people have after a trauma. Because everyone responds differently to traumas, you may have some of these reactions more than others. Please read it carefully, and think about any changes in your feelings, thoughts and behaviors since the assault.

Remember, many changes after a trauma are common. In fact, 95% of rape victims have severe problems 2 weeks after the rape. About half of these women feel much better within 3 months after the rape, but the other half recover more slowly, and many do not recover enough without help. Becoming more aware of the changes you've undergone since your assault is the first step toward recovery. Some of the most common problems after a trauma are described below.

• **Fear and anxiety** are common and natural responses to a dangerous situation. For many, they last long after the assault has ended. This happens when views of the world and a sense of safety have changed. You may become anxious when you remember your assault, but sometimes anxiety may come from out of the blue. **Triggers or cues** that can cause anxiety may include places, times of day, certain smells or noises, or any situation that reminds you of the assault. As you begin to pay more attention to the times you feel afraid, you can discover the triggers for your anxiety. In this way, you may learn that some of the "out-of-the-blue" anxiety is really triggered by things that remind you of your assault.

• **Reexperiencing of the trauma** is common among women who have been assaulted. For example, you may have **unwanted thoughts** of the assault, and find yourself unable to get rid of them. Some women have **flashbacks**, or very vivid images as if the assault is occurring again. **Nightmares** are also common. These symptoms occur because a traumatic experience is so shocking and so different from everyday experiences that you can't fit it into what you know about the world. So in order to understand what happened, your mind keeps bringing the memory back, as if to try to digest it and fit it in.

• **Increased arousal** is also a common response to trauma. This includes feeling jumpy, jittery, or shaky; being easily startled; and having trouble concentrating or sleeping. Continuous arousal can lead to **impatience and irritability**, especially if you're not getting enough sleep. The arousal reactions are caused by the fight-or-flight responses kicking in in your body. The fight-or-flight response is the way we protect ourselves against danger, and it occurs also in animals. When we protect ourselves from danger by fighting or running away, we need a lot more energy than usual, so our bodies pump out extra adrenaline to help us get the extra energy we need to survive.

People who have been assaulted often see the world as filled with danger, so their bodies are on constant alert, always ready to respond immediately to any attack. The problem is that increased arousal is useful in truly dangerous situations, such as if we find ourselves facing a tiger. But alertness becomes very uncomfortable when it continues for a long time even in safe situations. Another reaction to danger is to freeze, like a deer in headlights, and this reaction can also occur during an assault.

• **Avoidance** is a common way of managing trauma-related pain. The most common type is avoiding situations that remind you of the assault, such as the place where it happened. Often situations that are less directly related to the trauma are also avoided, such as going out in the evening if you were assaulted at night. Another way to reduce discomfort is trying to push away painful thoughts and feelings. This can lead to feelings of **numbness**, which make it difficult for you to have either fearful or pleasant and loving feelings. Sometimes the painful thoughts or feelings may be so intense that your mind just blocks them out altogether, and you may not remember parts of the assault.

- Many people who have been assaulted feel **angry** not only at the assailant but also with others. If you are not used to feeling angry, this may seem scary. It may be especially confusing to feel angry at those who are closest to you. Sometimes people feel angry because of feeling irritable so often. Anger can also arise from a feeling that the world is not fair.

- Trauma often leads to feelings of **guilt and shame**. Many people blame themselves for things they did or didn't do to survive. For example, some women believe that they should have fought off an assailant, and blame themselves for the assault. Others feel that if they had not fought back, they wouldn't have gotten hurt. You may feel ashamed because during the assault you were forced to do something that you would not otherwise have done. Sometimes, too, other people may blame you for being assaulted.

  Feeling guilty about the assault means that you are taking responsibility for what your assailant did. Although this may make you feel somewhat more in control, it can also lead to feelings of helplessness and depression.

- **Depression** is also a common reaction to assault. It can include feeling down, sad, hopeless or despairing. You may cry more often. You may lose interest in people and activities you used to enjoy. You may also feel that plans you had for the future don't seem to matter any more, or that life isn't worth living. These feelings can lead to thoughts of wishing you were dead, or doing something to hurt or kill yourself. Because the assault has changed so much of how you see the world and yourself, it makes sense to feel sad and to grieve for what you lost because of the assault.

- **Self-image** often becomes more negative after an assault. You may tell yourself, "If I hadn't been so weak or stupid, this wouldn't have happened to me." Many women see themselves more negatively overall after the assault ("I am a bad person and deserved this").

  It is also very common to **see others and the world more negatively**, and to feel that you can't trust anyone. If you used to think about the world as a safe place, the assault suddenly makes you think that the world is dangerous. If you had previous bad experiences, the assault convinces you that the world is dangerous and others aren't to be trusted. These negative thoughts often make women feel they have been changed completely by the assault. Relationships with others—even the ones you love most—can become tense, and it is difficult to become intimate with people as your trust decreases. In fact, you may find that the people closest to you are not supportive of you or have difficulty hearing about your assault.

- **Sexual relationships** may also suffer after a traumatic experience. Many women find it difficult to feel sexual or have sexual relationships. This is especially true for women who have been sexually assaulted, since in addition to the lack of trust, sex itself is a reminder of the assault.

Many of the reactions to trauma are connected to one another. For example, a flashback may make you feel out of control, and will therefore produce fear and arousal. Many women think that their common reactions to the trauma mean that they are "going crazy" or "losing it." These thoughts can make them even more fearful. Again, as you become aware of the changes you have gone through since the assault, and as you process these experiences during treatment, the symptoms should become less distressing.

FIGURE 8.2. Common Reactions to Assault handout.

During the latter part of Session 2, you and your client together construct a hierarchy of realistically safe situations that the client is avoiding because they remind her of the assault or scare her more than they should. This will be used in the treatment for *in vivo* exposure. (Again, see Chapter 9.)

You will end by giving the client the Common Reactions to Assault handout. Encourage her to read the handout several times, and to allow others close to her to read it as well. Also, remind the client to continue to practice her breathing exercises daily and to use them when she feels anxious.

Overview of Agenda for Session 2

1. Review homework.
2. Present agenda for the session.
3. Use the Common Reactions to Assault handout to educate client about PTSD symptoms.
4. Discuss rationale for specific treatment techniques (see Chapter 9).
5. Introduce client to SUDs (see Chapter 9).
6. Construct *in vivo* hierarchy (see Chapter 9).
7. Assign homework.

Discussion of Common Reactions to Assault

The Common Reactions to Assault handout is given here as Figure 8.2. We suggest you photocopy it and give it to your clients. (The following discussion and the handout do not follow the same format.) You may want to use the following introduction to begin the discussion about normal reactions to an assault.

An assault is an emotional shock. I know that you have been feeling very distressed since the assault. Right now, I want to discuss with you the common reactions of people who have undergone a severe trauma. Later, and in future sessions, I will discuss why some people continue to have difficulties long after the assault, and will explain how various treatment techniques will work to alleviate your distress.

There are reactions that are common to traumatic experiences. Although everyone who has been traumatized responds in a unique way, you may find that you have experienced many of these reactions.

1. The primary reactions people experience after an assault are **fear and anxiety**. Are you feeling fearful, tense, or anxious? [Encourage the client to respond.]

Sometimes your feeling of anxiety may be a result of being reminded of the assault; at other times the anxiety may feel to you as if it comes out of the blue. Do you notice that you are more fearful at certain times than others? [Encourage the client to respond.]

The feelings of anxiety and fear that you are experiencing can be understood as reactions to a dangerous and life-threatening situation. You may experience changes in your body, your feelings, and your thoughts because your view of the world and your perceptions about your safety have changed as a result of the assault. Certain **triggers and cues** may remind you of the assault and activate your fears. These triggers may be certain times of the day, certain places, men approaching you, an argument with someone you care about, a certain smell, or a noise. Have you noticed specific triggers that remind you of the assault? [Encourage the client to share her own relevant experiences.]

Typically, after an assault, fear and anxiety are experienced in three primary ways: continuing to reexperience memories of the assault; feeling aroused, easily startled, and jumpy; and shutting yourself off from others and from going places. Let's talk about these now.

2. Women who have been assaulted often **reexperience the trauma**. You may find that you are having **flashbacks** when visual pictures of the assailant's face or some other aspect of the assault suddenly pops into your mind. Are you having flashbacks? What is this experience like for you? [Encourage the client to respond.]

Sometimes a flashback may be so vivid that you might feel as if the assault is actually occurring again. These experiences are intrusive, and you probably feel that you don't have any control over what you are feeling, thinking, and experiencing during the day or at night. Sometimes these flashbacks are triggered by external events, and often they appear to come out of nowhere. You may also find that you are reexperiencing the assault through **nightmares**. Have you been having nightmares? What changes do you notice in your body when you suddenly wake up from a nightmare? [Encourage the client to respond.]

You may also reexperience the assault **emotionally or cognitively** without having a flashback or nightmare. Have you been having distressing thoughts and feelings about what happened to you? [Encourage the client to respond.]

3. You may also find that you are having trouble concentrating. This is another common experience that results from an assault. Are you having any trouble reading, following a conversation, or remembering something that someone told you? What is this like for you? [Encourage the client to share her own relevant experiences.]

It is frustrating and upsetting to be unable to concentrate, remember, and pay attention to what is going on around you. These experiences may lead to a feeling that you are not in control of your mind or a feeling that you are going crazy. It is important to remember that these reactions are temporary. Difficulties concentrating are due to intrusive and distressing feelings and memories about the assault. In an attempt to understand and digest what happened to you, your mind is constantly going over this material—bringing it back up, chewing on it, and trying to digest it.

4. Other common reactions to assault are **arousal** reactions—that is, agitation, feeling jittery, feeling **overly alert**, trembling, being **easily startled**, and having trouble concentrating or sleeping. Have you noticed that your body is experiencing any of these changes since the assault? Are there times when you feel panic? What happens

to your body? Sweating? Heart racing? Are you especially watchful and easily startled? [Encourage the client to share her own relevant experiences.]

Feeling tense and jumpy all the time may also lead to feelings of **irritability**, especially if you are not getting enough sleep. Have you been feeling irritable or angry? Do you find that you are having angry outbursts, or that you are more snappy than usual with people? [Encourage the client to respond.]

These changes in your body are the result of fear. Animals and people have several potential reactions to being startled, assaulted, or threatened. One reaction to danger is to freeze. You may have seen a cat that is being approached by a dog crouch down and be very still because it is afraid. A second possible reaction to being threatened is to run away or flee. A third reaction is to fight. Have you ever seen a cat puff up its fur, hiss, extend its claws, and swat at a threatening dog?

The fleeing or fighting responses require a burst of adrenaline to mobilize your body and help it respond adequately to a dangerous situation. As a result of the assault, you have realized that there is danger in the world and you want to be ready for it. Your body is in a constant state of preparedness and arousal, so you can feel "pumped" and ready to respond immediately to a dangerous situation.

5. You may find that you are physically, emotionally, or cognitively **avoiding** people, places, or things that remind you of the assault. This avoidance is a strategy to protect yourself from situations that you may feel have become dangerous, and thoughts and feelings that are overwhelming and distressing. Are you unable to go certain places or do certain things as a result of the assault? Have you been making efforts to avoid thoughts or feelings associated with the assault? How do you do that? What kinds of things do you find yourself doing to try to forget what happened to you? [Encourage the client to share her own relevant experiences.]

Sometimes the desire to avoid memories and feelings about the assault may be so intense that you might find that you have forgotten important aspects of what happened during the assault. Are there any memories that you cannot remember or gaps of time that you cannot account for? [Encourage the client to respond.]

Another experience you may have from avoiding painful feelings and thoughts about the assault is **emotional numbness**. Do you have times when you feel numb, empty, or detached from your environment? Have you found that you have lost interest in things that once were pleasurable to you? Do you feel detached and cut off from other people since the assault? [Encourage the client to respond.]

6. Other common reactions to assault are **sadness** and a sense of feeling down or **depressed**. You may have feelings of hopelessness and despair, frequent crying spells, and sometimes even thoughts of hurting yourself and suicide. A loss of interest in the people and activities that you once found pleasurable is often associated with an assault. Nothing may seem fun to you any more. You may also feel that life isn't worth living and that plans you had made for the future do not seem important any longer. Have you been feeling sad or depressed? Are you tearful? Are you feeling stuck or hopeless? Are you having any feelings or ideas that life is not worth living or that you would be better off dead? [Encourage the client to share her own relevant experiences.]

In connection with the discussion of depression as a common response to assault, a special assessment of suicidal (or homicidal) ideation and potential may be warrented. Clearly, an inquiry about suicidal thoughts is part of the general assessment process; yet, because assault victims with PTSD often contemplate suicide, you may want to evaluate this issue further in the context of discussing common reactions to assault. Ask the client about her thoughts, urges, feelings, fantasies, and plans she may have to harm herself. Inquire whether she has ever thought about hurting herself or planned to hurt herself in the past. If she has, ask her what she planned or what she did. Ask her if she has any intention of carrying out these plans. Does she have lethal means available to her? You may want to ask the client to sign an agreement to contact you, a hospital emergency room, or another mental health professional if she has thoughts or plans to harm herself. Just a reminder: Make sure you document that you have conducted a suicide assessment, and that the client has entered into an agreement to contact a professional if she starts feeling suicidal.

Many of our clients have expressed some homicidal ideation as well. Statements such as "If they find him, I'll kill him," or "I want to make him suffer like he made me suffer," are common reactions to assault. However, just as we take any suicidal talk seriously and assess it further, we always do the same for homicidal talk. We have never actually had an assault client who harmed her assailant, but it does happen (especially in cases of partner abuse), and you can be held accountable if it does and the client has told you of her intent. Assess whether the client has plans to harm the perpetrator, how she would do it, whether she really intends to harm him, whether she has access to weapons, and so forth. If she is actively homicidal, you may have a duty to warn the perpetrator and the proper authorities; check your state laws. Again, we're being cautious here. We now continue our suggested discussion of the common reactions to assault. The next response is anger—a prominent factor in homicidal ideation.

7. A feeling of **anger** is also a common reaction to assault. The anger is mostly directed at the assailant for causing you physical injury, for violating you, for abusing you, or for stealing something of yours. However, feelings of anger may be also stirred up in the presence of people who remind you of the assailant or strangers. Many assault survivors also feel angry at God for allowing them to be assaulted, at the police for not doing enough afterwards, at the hospital staff for treating them insensitively, at society for creating an atmosphere that allows this to happen, and/or at friends and family for not understanding. Are you feeling particularly angry or aggressive? Is this different from the way you felt before the assault? How do these feelings affect you or other people? [Encourage the client to share her own relevant experiences.]

Sometimes you may find that you are so angry that you want to hit someone or swear; if you are not used to feeling angry, you may not recognize or know how to handle these angry feelings. Many women also direct the anger toward themselves for something that they did or did not do during the assault. These feelings of anger directed at the self may lead to feelings of blame, guilt, helplessness, and depression. Many women also find that they are experiencing anger and irritability toward those people that they love the most: family members, friends, their partners, and their children. Has this been happening to you? [Encourage the client to respond.]

Sometimes you may lose your temper with the people who are most dear to you. This may be confusing, since you may not understand why you are most angry and irritable with those you care about most. Although closeness with others may feel good, it also increases the opportunity for feelings of intimacy, dependence, and vulnerability or helplessness. Having those feelings may make you feel angry and irritable because they remind you of the assault. We also may expect more from the people we love and get angry when they disappoint us.

8. During an assault, you may have been threatened and forced to participate in acts against your will. You were violated. During the assault, you may have felt as if you had no control over your feelings, your body, and your life. Sometimes the feelings of loss of control may be so intense that you may feel as if you are "going crazy" or "losing it." Have you had this experience since the assault? What is that like for you? Is there anything that you have found helpful to cope with these feelings and thoughts? [Encourage the client to share her own relevant experiences.]

9. Feelings of **guilt and shame** may be present. Guilt and shame may be related to something you did or did not do to survive the assault. It is common to second-guess your reactions and blame yourself for what you did or did not do. Are you blaming yourself for the assault? Do you feel that if you had or had not done something, you would not have been assaulted? Are there any people you are avoiding talking to or things you are avoiding doing because you feel guilty or ashamed? [Encourage the client to share her own relevant experiences.]

Many women feel ashamed after an assault if they have been forced to do something they would not do under other circumstances. Sometimes women believe that if they had fought off their assailant, or had been more passive, their assault would not have been so bad. Feeling guilty about what happened to you means that you are holding yourself responsible for your assailant's actions. These feelings of guilt can lead to feelings of helplessness, depression, and negative thoughts about yourself. Blame can also come from society, friends, family, and acquaintances, because many times people place responsibility on the person who has been hurt and victimized. Has anyone blamed you for the assault? What do you think about that? Would you blame your sister or your daughter if the same thing happened to her? [Encourage the client to respond.]

It is important for you to remember that you are not responsible for what happened to you. You did not ask to be treated badly or harmed by someone else. We believe that no matter what you did or didn't do, no one has the right to hurt you. Even if you feel you made a mistake in judgment, people make mistakes in judgment every day. In this case, the "punishment" didn't fit the "crime." The only time people have the right to hurt you is if you hurt them first and they are acting in self-defense, and that is not what happened here.

10. **Self-image** can also suffer as a result of an assault. You may tell yourself, "I am a bad person and bad things happen to me," or "If I had not been so weak or stupid, this would not have happened to me," or "I should have been tougher." Are you having any negative thoughts about yourself since the assault? What kinds of things do you find yourself saying or thinking about your feelings or the way you are coping? [Encourage the client to respond.]

11. It is not unusual to have **disruptions in relationships with other people** after an assault, and to **view the world more negatively** as well. If you thought of the world as a safe place before the assault, you may now see it as dangerous. If you had some bad experiences in your life before the assault, you may now be convinced that the world is a bad place and you cannot trust other people. These changes result in part from feeling sad, frightened, and angry. In order to cope with these negative feelings, you may withdraw from others or not participate in the activities that you once did. You may also find that the people you love the most and expect to be the most supportive are not. Has this been a problem for you? Have you noticed that you are having difficulties getting along with other people? [Encourage the client to share her own relevant experiences.]

It is common for people to experience anger, anguish, and guilt when a person they love is hurt. You may find that your friends and family members, especially your partner, may have difficulty hearing about your assault and may have serious reactions to it. It is important that you get support for what you are going through, and that you understand that some of the people around you may be going through a crisis, too. Imagine how you would feel if this had happened to your daughter. You might be so upset that someone could do this to her, so blinded by rage, that you were not as attentive to her needs as you usually are. Sometimes we need to learn to forgive others' reactions to us when they don't give us what we need. At the same time, the support of your family and friends plays an important role in your recovery. It is important to talk to people who you feel can support you and understand your feelings.

12. After an assault, it is not unusual to experience a **loss of interest in physical affection and sexual relations**. There are various reasons for this. For example, it is very common for women who are depressed and have not been assaulted to experience a loss of interest in their sexual drive. Also, loss of interest in or fear of physical and sexual relations is extremely common in women who have been assaulted. Are you experiencing any loss of interest in sexual relations? Have you experienced any frightening feelings, thoughts, or flashbacks during physical contact with anyone? [Encourage the client to respond.]

You may feel uncomfortable being emotionally and sexually intimate with someone, because this experience may bring back your feelings of vulnerability during the assault. In fact, you may have flashbacks or intensely distressing feelings when you are having sexual or physical contact.

13. Finally, as a result of this recent assault, you may be reminded of your past experiences. Once a negative experience comes to your mind, it tends to **provoke memories of other negative experiences**. This is the normal way in which your memory works. For this reason, you may find following the trauma that you may recall many negative memories about a past trauma that you had forgotten. These memories may be as disturbing to you as the memories of your more recent assault.

These negative memories may be stirred up as a result of a recent assault, and it may be difficult for you to think of any other situations or experiences that are not negative. In fact, it may be very difficult to believe that you will ever feel happy again or have pleasant experiences. But you will. In fact, you will find that it is possible for you to put these negative experiences behind you, and you will start to remember more positive memories. These positive memories will trigger more positive recollections, and eventually you will gain a more balanced view of your life. Have you suddenly remembered upsetting experiences that you had before the assault? [Encourage the client to respond.]

Some of these common reactions to an assault are connected with each other. For some people, having a flashback may increase their concern about losing control of their lives and may even intensify their fears. In other words, the responses of being assaulted often interact with one another and cause the overall response to be more intense. Of all these normal reactions to assault, fear is probably the most common and appears to be the most debilitating.

We use probe questions (e.g., "Did that happen to you?", "What are your most troubling reexperiencing problems?") during the discussion of assault reactions to stimulate discussion of a client's specific reactions. A case example of the interactive approach to use with clients is presented below.

Presenting Common Reactions to Assault: Case Example

Mary was a 40-year-old woman who worked as an administrative assistant in a private corporation. She lived with her husband and two children in the suburbs. Mary went to the grocery store at 6:00 one morning and was forced into her car by a young white male at knifepoint. He raped her in her car, parked in the lot of the grocery store. The therapist interviewed her 10 days after she had been raped.

During the initial interview, Mary reported nausea, anxiety, sleeping difficulties, flashbacks, nervousness, and loss of appetite. Mary also was unable to get into her car or go to work, and reported extreme irritability toward her children.

THERAPIST: I know that you are feeling very uncomfortable and upset right now, but I want you to know that the symptoms you are experiencing are normal reactions to a traumatic event. In fact, if I had experienced an assault similar to yours, I would also be experiencing nausea, anxiety, sleeping problems, flashbacks, nervousness, and loss of appetite. I know it does not decrease your discomfort level, but I want you to know that these are normal reactions and that over time, little by little, you will feel better. That's what I'm here for: to help you to feel better.

MARY: I feel like my life is turned upside down and I will never be the same. I can't concentrate on anything, and I am afraid that I am going to lose my job because I am afraid to get into my car and go to work—and even if I could, I'm scared I am going to lose control at work.

THERAPIST: I know that this is really a frightening feeling. Why don't we talk a little bit more about reactions to trauma? What I would like us to do, as we review each type of reaction, is to discuss what you are experiencing.

MARY: I don't think I am going to be able to sit here and be able to concentrate.

THERAPIST: That's OK. If you get to the point that you are uncomfortable or just need to chill out for a minute, we can take a little break whenever you feel the need. Just let me know. Have you noticed that you are having difficulties concentrating since the assault?

MARY: Yeah . . . I feel very spaced out and like I can't pay attention to anything.

THERAPIST: When you can't concentrate, what is happening?

MARY: I just keep having pictures of the rape go through my mind over and over. I can't get rid of them.

THERAPIST: I know it's frustrating and upsetting not to be able to concentrate, remember, and pay attention to what is going on around you. The images that pop into your head are called "flashbacks" and usually interrupt your ability to concentrate. They may make you feel extremely anxious. Can you give examples of specific situations when you have flashbacks?

MARY: Yes. Every time I look at that car, I see his face and the knife in his hand. I will never be able to drive that car again. Yesterday my husband drove me to the grocery store and I couldn't get out of his car, but I didn't want him to leave me there alone either. He says I am overreacting.

THERAPIST: Sometimes it seems that flashbacks come out of nowhere, but often they are triggered by external events or objects, such as your car, parking lots, the grocery store, and seeing someone who resembles the assailant. Another way that many people reexperience the assault is through nightmares. Have you been having any nightmares?

MARY: Most nights I can't even get to sleep. My husband thinks I am crazy because I want to sleep with the light on. I fall asleep toward morning and usually only sleep an hour or two before I wake up again, and I can't get back to sleep.

THERAPIST: Many women tell us that after an assault they need to sleep with the light on to help them feel safer. One of the things that you may wish to discuss with your husband are these normal reactions to trauma. You may want to give him this handout [Common Reactions to Assault] to read, so that he has a better understanding that what you are going through is a normal reaction to trauma. Are you experiencing any bad dreams once you fall asleep?

MARY: Yeah, but they are not about the assault. They are just violent and upsetting dreams. Usually someone is trying to get me.

THERAPIST: Many women report similar experiences after they have been assaulted. You may have nightmares about the assault that are violent in nature, but not specific to the assault. This is all a part of the reexperiencing that people who are survivors of a traumatic event go through. Have you noticed when you wake up suddenly that you are experiencing any physical problems?

MARY: Yeah, I sit up in bed and I look all around the room.

THERAPIST: Have you noticed that your body is experiencing any changes?

MARY: Do you mean like when my heart starts beating rapidly?

THERAPIST: Exactly. Are there any other sensations that you experience?

MARY: I feel very jittery, and it is a feeling of panic. It is very difficult for me to describe. It is like I am superalert. Like I'm frozen and waiting for something to happen.

THERAPIST: You described that very well. In fact, these are the types of symptoms that women often report after an assault. These are the body's reactions to feeling very anxious and fearful. Have you noticed that you are having chills and trembling, and that you sweat?

MARY: No, that's not what it's like.

THERAPIST: You may recall that in the beginning of this discussion, I mentioned that although there are common reactions to traumatic experiences, each person has a unique set of responses. These changes in your body are the results of fear. Animals and people have several potential reactions to fear. We call them the "three F's." One reaction is to freeze. You may have seen a cat that is being approached by a dog crouch down and be very still because it is afraid. A second possible reaction to being threatened is to run away, to flee. A third reaction is to fight. All these reactions involve a burst of adrenaline to mobilize your body and help it respond to a dangerous situation. Do you have any questions that you would like to ask about anything we have just discussed?

MARY: I can understand my feeling that way during the assault, but why do I keep feeling that way over and over again?

THERAPIST: As a result of the assault, you have realized that there is danger in the world, and you want to be prepared for it. Your body is in a constant state of preparedness and arousal so that you can feel "pumped" and ready to respond at any moment. Another reason you are feeling aroused or jumpy all the time is because there are triggers or reminders of the assault. We have already talked about a few—your car, parking lots, grocery stores, someone who looks like the assailant—but there are probably other triggers that are more subtle, such as someone coming up behind you, when your husband puts his arm around you, when you see a car that looks like yours, or strangers. Triggers or reminders do not have to be just external events or objects. You may experience feeling cold and chilly, and that may remind you of the way you felt during the assault. So feeling cold and chilly becomes a trigger for reactions of fear and anxiety. Are there any other experiences that you have had that reminded you of the assault?

MARY: Yes, my husband started kissing me and putting his arms around me. I froze. I saw the face of the man who raped me. I freaked out. My husband was very hurt. He didn't understand why I was afraid of him. I didn't understand why I couldn't feel comfortable with him. I used to love it when he would kiss me.

THERAPIST: What you are describing is a very typical reaction to any sexual or physical interaction with males after an assault. It sounds as if you have an intrusive image or flashback about part of the assault. Having a flashback is frightening, but so is feeling afraid of being uncomfortable with someone that you usually feel comfortable with and close to. Many women feel very confused and upset, because they know that their spouse or significant other is not going to hurt them, but nonetheless sexual or physical contact is a reminder of the assault that elicits distressing feelings, reexperiencing, and physical reactions. A natural response to these experiences is to avoid physical contact, especially with males. You may find that you are physically, emotionally, or cognitively avoiding people, places, or anything that reminds you of the assault. This avoidance is a strategy to protect yourself from situations that you may feel have become or could become dangerous, and from thoughts and feelings that are overwhelming and distressing to you. This is why you had those reactions when your husband was kissing and hugging you. You mentioned earlier that you are unable to go grocery shopping or even sit in your car. Are there any other places, people, or situations that you are avoiding because they remind you of the assault?

MARY: No, not really.

THERAPIST: Have you been able to go to work since the assault?

MARY: Well, no. But I don't think anybody would be able to go to work a week after something like this.

THERAPIST: You are probably right, and I think it is good that you have taken a few days off to rest and recuperate. Right now our jobs are to be detectives and find out how the assault is affecting you, so that we can use this information in your treatment. So let's look at different situations and see if some of them are more difficult than others for you at this time. For example, have you been able to go shopping at malls or go to a restaurant to eat since the assault?

MARY: No! Because I get very upset at the thought of having to park the car and being in a crowd of people.

THERAPIST: Does it make sense to you that these situations—being in your car, being in parking lots, or being with a crowd of people—are triggers that bring back memories of the assault?

MARY: I don't know if this has anything to do with the assault. I really never liked going out in crowds or shopping anyway.

THERAPIST: Well, it may not have been one of your favorite things to do, but before the assault, did you avoid going to these places because they made you anxious or upset?

MARY: No, I've always done my own shopping. I am a very independent person, or at least I was. Well . . . I guess I am avoiding doing some of these things.

THERAPIST: As I mentioned earlier, avoiding people, places, and situations that remind you of the assault is very common. One of the things that we are going to be working on during this program is helping you to confront upsetting memories and reminders of the trauma, so that you will be able to feel more comfortable doing the things that you did before the assault. Another strategy that people commonly use to avoid remembering or experiencing distressing feelings associated with the assault is to feel numb, empty, or cut off from their feelings. Do you ever have this experience?

MARY: Yeah, I feel distant sometimes and kind of out of it. I feel like I'm not really feeling anything.

THERAPIST: This is a very common reaction to experiencing reminders of a trauma. It is one of the ways that your mind is trying to avoid or turn off very distressing and disturbing feelings.

MARY: I feel that I am never going to be the same again. I look at my kids and I can feel loving feelings for a while, but then it just fades. I seem to spend a lot of time just staring off into space and feeling like a zombie.

THERAPIST: Another common reaction to an assault is just what you have described as "feeling like a zombie"—having difficulty feeling interested in people and things around you, alternating from feeling very distressed and upset to having no feelings at all. This program will help you develop some skills to help you manage the anxiety and fear that you are currently experiencing, as well as help you start to make sense of the trauma and your reactions to it. These strategies will help you to feel more comfortable again and able to feel that you don't have to protect yourself from others or from these bad memories. Many women experience strong feelings of sadness and depression after they have been assaulted. Are you having any of these feelings?

MARY: Well, I cry a lot, and I feel that I am never going to be the same again. The man who raped me robbed me of my life and my happiness.

THERAPIST: Feelings of grief about losing aspects of yourself and your life, loss of pleasure, low energy, sadness, and being teary are all common reactions to an assault. I know it feels bad to you, and it sounds like you haven't been feeling like your usual self. You will find that as you start feeling less anxious and fearful, you will also feel less depressed about what has happened to you. We also see that many women experience changes in the way they view themselves after they have been assaulted. In addition to all these uncomfortable emotional and physical reactions that you are having to the assault, are you aware of changes in your thinking and perception about yourself?

MARY: Yeah, I feel dirty and ugly and vulnerable. And I feel like I'm never going to get through this in one piece.

THERAPIST: Many women feel this way. They feel differently about themselves and the world after they have been assaulted. You may be thinking things about yourself that lead you to feel depressed and upset—for example, "I'm never going to get through this in one piece," or "I can't cope," or "What's wrong with me that I feel this way?" One reason that I wanted to talk with you about the usual reactions to assault is to help you understand that these reactions, although upsetting, are to be expected when someone has feared for her life and her safety and has been violated and hurt. As a result of the assault, you may now feel that the world is dangerous and that you are vulnerable, as well as feeling that you will be unable to handle what you are now feeling. The reactions to trauma are experienced in three ways that are interactive—how we feel, how we think, and what we do. We have talked about some triggers that bring back memories of the rape. When this happens, you said that you are fearful, you have flashbacks, you become jumpy and tense, your hands sweat, and your heart beats quickly. We have also talked about some physical or behavioral avoidance strategies that you use—like not leaving the house, not going to work, being unable to drive your car—to alleviate the anxiety that you feel. We haven't talked much about the cognitive channel except to discuss the flashbacks and nightmares that you are having. Are there any thoughts that you noticed that you are having as a result of the assault?

MARY: Like what?

THERAPIST: Well, you have already mentioned a few thoughts you are now having about yourself, such as "I am afraid that I can't cope," and "What is the matter with me?" These are negative statements that you are saying about yourself. We also see that people who go through traumas also develop negative or distressing thoughts about other people or about how safe they think the world is.

MARY: Oh, I see . . . well, I guess I feel like I'm going to be raped again if I go back to that grocery store parking lot.

THERAPIST: Yes. Any others?

MARY: No, just that I feel like I should be able to bounce back from this. And I'm upset with myself that I can't go to work. I can't be close to my husband. I can't even cook dinner for my children. I feel really bad about myself.

THERAPIST: I hear you saying a lot of negative things about yourself. Believing statements like those can lead to negative changes in your self-image and feelings of depression. You also mentioned that you believe that you will be raped again if you return to that parking lot. Notions that the world is no longer safe, that other people can't be trusted, and that you are vulnerable are very common in people who have experienced a trauma. Your thoughts about the safety of the world and yourself in it, as well as thoughts about yourself, are some of the things we are going to work on here.

MARY: That's good, because I feel so scared and I feel that I'm supposed to be able to handle this. My husband expects that of me, and my children depend on me to feed them and be there for them every day. I can't even get dressed and take a shower without spending the whole time thinking about it.

THERAPIST: You have just had a very frightening experience, and it sounds like you are being pretty hard on yourself right now. Maybe you feel a lot of guilt?

MARY: Guilt? I have plenty of that to go around. I feel guilty because I've been a bad mother and wife lately. I can't go to work, and things are going to be tight financially if this keeps up. I told my mother what happened, and do you know what she said to me?

THERAPIST: What did she say?

MARY: She told me that I should have been more careful, and basically made me feel that it was my fault that I was raped . . . because I went shopping early in the morning and couldn't fight off the rapist . . . and I feel bad enough about how I am doing now without all that extra responsibility and criticism. I've decided I'm never going to tell anyone again about the rape.

THERAPIST: I'm sorry about the rape, and I'm sorry you've gotten those reactions from people. That is very upsetting. It sounds like a lot of people are having trouble being supportive of your feelings at this time. I've talked with a lot of women who express feelings of responsibility for what happened, and feelings of guilt that they should have done this or should not have done that. It is painful to disclose uncomfortable feelings to other people and feel that they are blaming you or that they can't be understanding. It is important for you to get support from others, because this is a very difficult time. Sometimes people just need to be educated about what trauma survivors experience to be more empathic. But sometimes, for whatever reasons, the victim is blamed, even though it's clearly not your fault. You might want to show your mother the Common Reactions to Assault handout, or if you don't feel she can support you right now, maybe you can talk about this with her when you are feeling more comfortable yourself. However, it is important for you to know that many women have the same experiences—feeling guilty or being blamed by others for what happened to them. Before we move on, do you have any questions or comments about the reactions to trauma that we have just discussed?

MARY: Not really. I just don't want to talk to my mother about the rape any more.

THERAPIST: That is your decision, and I think it is important that you protect yourself now from additional stressors. Maybe once you have completed this program and are feeling better, you will want to talk with your mother about her reactions to you. For now, it sounds like talking with her is not helpful. It is important to find a balance between trying not to avoid talking with people because you are afraid of their reactions, because you need support right now, and confiding in people who cannot support you.

At the end of Session 2, give the client the Common Reactions to Assault handout and ask her to read it daily, sharing it with anyone she chooses to.

The latter portion of Session 2, as noted earlier, is devoted to introducing *in vivo* exposure. This is discussed in Chapter 9.

9

In Vivo Exposure: Confronting the Feared Situations

In all three treatment programs outlined in Chapter 6, we suggest that you use the technique of *in vivo* exposure. The steps for teaching *in vivo* exposure are as follows:

Overview of Steps for Teaching In Vivo *Exposure*

1. Present the rationale for *in vivo* exposure to the client.
2. Give concrete examples of habituation.
3. Introduce the subjective units of discomfort (SUDs) scale.
4. Construct a hierarchy of avoided situations with a SUDs rating for each.
5. Work with the client to develop homework assignments based on this hierarchy.
6. Instruct client in *in vivo* exposure procedure:
   a. Client begins with situations that evoke moderate anxiety levels (e.g., SUDs = 50).
   b. Client puts herself into anxiety-provoking (but realistically safe) situation.
   c. Client records time and initial SUDs rating on the *In Vivo* Exposure Homework Recording Form.
   d. Client must remain in situation for 30–45 minutes or until anxiety decreases by at least 50%.
   e. Client records endpoint SUDs rating for the situation.

As with all other techniques described in this book, you should begin by presenting a rationale to the client. In addition, giving examples of the habituation process is a key to motivating the client to practice *in vivo* exposure. The SUDs scale is then introduced in preparation for constructing a list of situations the client finds distressing.

144

Presenting the Rationale for *In Vivo* Exposure

The rationale for the technique can be described to the client as follows:

In this program, we are going to focus on the fears that you are experiencing, and your difficulty in coping, both of which are directly related to your assault. We've just talked about the feelings, thoughts, and memories that are connected with the assault. We've also talked about some of the ways in which you are coping with that distress, such as avoiding situations and memories that remind you of the assault.

Although most of the symptoms that you and I have talked about gradually decline with time after the trauma, some of these symptoms endure and continue to cause marked distress for many victims like yourself. It is possible to speed up your recovery process by understanding what causes your reactions.

A major factor that prevents recovery is avoidance of situations, memories, thoughts, and feelings. It is quite normal for people to want to escape or avoid memories, situations, thoughts, and feelings that are painful and distressing. However, though the strategy of avoiding painful experiences works in the short run, it actually prolongs the posttrauma reactions and prevents you from getting over your trauma related difficulties. [You may want to elicit examples of the client's avoidance, based on the previous discussion of common reactions.]

When you *confront* the painful experiences rather than avoiding them, you will have the opportunity to process the traumatic experience, and the pain will gradually lessen. For example, if you avoid assault-related situations that are objectively safe, you do not give yourself the opportunity to get used to being in these situations. So, you will continue to believe that anxiety stays forever unless you avoid or escape the situations. Also, unless you confront the situations, you may continue to believe that they are dangerous. However, if you confront these situations, you will find out that they are not actually dangerous and that your anxiety will diminish with repeated, prolonged confrontations. As a result of this process, your symptoms will decline. The same is true for painful memories.

Explaining Habituation

It's important to give a clear explanation of habituation, since this is the desired goal that can motivate clients to continue with the exposure procedures. Describe habituation for the client as follows:

Almost always, as I've just mentioned, repeated exposure to anxiety-producing situations results in an eventual decrease in anxiety. We call this process "habituation." Because of this process, you will find out that even if you are very anxious in certain situations, exposing yourself repeatedly to these situations and staying in them long enough will result in a gradual decrease in your anxiety and distress.

Use the following examples to illustrate this point to the client:

EXAMPLE 1

Let's talk about an example that illustrates how habituation works. A little boy was sitting on the beach with his mother when an unexpected, forceful wave from the ocean washed over them. The child got extremely upset and cried that he wanted to go home. The next day when it was time to go to the beach, the little boy began crying and refused to go. He kept saying, "No . . . no . . . water come to me." In order to help him overcome his fear of the water, his mother took him for walks on the beach over the next few days. She would hold his hand and gradually help him walk closer to the water's edge. By the end of the week, the boy was able to walk into the water alone. With patience, practice, and encouragement, he had habituated to his fear of the water. If he had not been helped to expose himself gradually to being near and in the water, in all likelihood his fear would have remained unchecked, and he would have avoided the water indefinitely. We can get over scary situations if we do it the right way.

EXAMPLE 2

Another example is a taxicab driver who lived in New York and who developed a fear of driving across bridges. This fear created serious problems with his work, since he was unable to drive customers across bridges. Each time he approached a bridge, he pretended that something was mechanically wrong with the taxi and called another cab to take his customers to their destination. The taxicab driver, with the support of a therapist, practiced driving over bridges daily. Within a week's time, he was able to go across the bridge with the therapist following him in another car. And in 2 weeks, with repeated practice, he was able to drive over small bridges by himself.

Now, continue to explain the technique of *in vivo* exposure to the client:

These are a few examples to help you understand how systematic confrontation with a feared situation can reduce your level of discomfort. Because you have experienced a traumatic event, you may need more time to confront fears related to your assault. But with time, practice, and courage, you will be able to confront the things that now make you afraid. For this reason, we will ask you to work throughout your treatment on confronting many relatively safe situations that you are now avoiding.

Today, in order to help you stop avoiding situations and people that were once enjoyable or important to you, we are going to work together to make a list of situations that you have been avoiding since the assault. I call this list "the hierarchy." I also want to find out from you how much distress or discomfort these situations would cause you if you weren't avoiding them. Therefore, I will teach you a method to indicate your level of distress. Of course, we will not ask you to confront unsafe situations.

The goal is not to help you view dangerous situations as safe, but rather to help you stop avoiding situations that are realistically quite safe.

Introduction to SUDs

Use the following explanation of the SUDs scale before beginning to construct a hierarchy of feared and avoided situations. Evaluate the safety of each situation before you include it on the list, to ensure that unsafe situations are not included (e.g., walking in an unsafe neighborhood at night, approaching an unfamiliar man on a street corner and talking with him).

In order to find out how much discomfort certain situations cause you, we need to use a scale that you and I are familiar with. We call this the SUDs scale (SUD stands for "subjective units of discomfort"). It's a 0-to-100 scale. A SUDs rating of 100 indicates that you are extremely upset, the most you have ever been in your life; a SUDs rating of 0 indicates no discomfort at all, or complete relaxation. Usually when people say they have a SUDs rating of 100, they may be experiencing physical reactions, such as sweaty palms, palpitations, difficulty breathing, feelings of dizziness, and anxiety. How much discomfort are you feeling now as we are talking? What do you think your SUDs level was during the assault?

Teach the client how to make adjustments in SUDs, if necessary. For example, you might say something like this if it seems appropriate: "You don't appear to look as anxious now as I would expect someone to look with a SUDs rating of 70. Remember the entire scale is measuring distress, so even a 10 tells me you're not completely relaxed." Once the client seems to have a good grasp of the SUDs concept, say:

We are going to be using SUDs ratings to monitor your progress during *in vivo* exposure. It is almost like an anxiety thermometer, and I'll be "taking your distress temperature" every few minutes. We will use this scale during exposure to monitor change in your anxiety.

Constructing a Hierarchy of Avoided Situations

Having presented the client with the rationale for the *in vivo* exposure procedure, given examples of habituation, and introduced the SUDs scale, you can now proceed to elicit specific examples of the situations, people, and places that she avoids because of her assault. Use the *In Vivo* Hierarchy Form to help develop a list of situations that the client is avoiding, and to help her rate the intensity of anxiety she experiences when she imagines she is confronting these situations. Follow the example of Melanie's forms (see Figures 9.1 and 9.2 later in the chapter).

Typically Avoided Situations for Assault Survivors

If the client is having trouble coming up with situations that she is avoiding, you may suggest a few from the following list of situations that are typically avoided by assault survivors:

1. Seeing an unfamiliar man, especially of the same race as the assailant.
2. Someone standing close to her.
3. Being touched by someone (especially someone unfamiliar).
4. Someone coming up behind her.
5. Walking down a street.
6. Being alone in her home (day or night).
7. Getting into her car at night.
8. Being in a crowded mall or store.
9. Talking to men or strangers.
10. Being in a car stopped at a stoplight.
11. Being in a parking lot.
12. Going out at night with friends.
13. Reading about an assault in the newspaper or hearing about an assault on television.
14. Talking with someone about the assault.
15. Seeing the names and pictures of assailants.
16. Going to the building or street where she was assaulted.
17. Riding public transportation.
18. Hugging and kissing significant others.
19. Having sexual or physical contact.
20. Wearing clothes similar to those worn during the assault.

Remind the client that she need not include every situation that frightens her or that she avoids on the hierarchy. This is supposed to be a representative list to teach her the idea behind *in vivo* exposure therapy—namely, that when she repeatedly confronts feared situations that are realistically safe, her anxiety will decrease. You will want to make sure that there are items representing SUDs levels of 50, 60, 70, 80, 90, and 100 (or thereabouts), as these will be a major focus of treatment.

Case Example of Hierarchy Construction

Melanie was raped on her college campus while walking home from the library one evening, approximately 2 years prior to presenting for treatment. After the rape, in addition to having other PTSD symptoms, she was very avoidant. She avoided leaving her dorm room after dark, even when accompanied; this restricted her activities extremely. She slept with the light on, much to the annoyance of her roommate. She would not listen to or read anything that referred to a woman's being assaulted, even refusing to complete some class assignments. She also no longer wore yellow sweaters or Reebok athletic shoes, since she was wearing them at the time of the assault. In therapy, the rationale for *in vivo* exposure was explained and discussed, and she agreed with its necessity. The transcript that follows describes the construction of Melanie's personal hierarchy.

THERAPIST: We want to make a list of some of the situations that you avoid since the assault, or that you feel very uncomfortable if you find yourself in. The list doesn't have to be exhaustive, just representative. I'll ask you to give each situation a rating on the 0–100 SUDs scale of how uncomfortable or scared you think you'd be in that situation, where 0 indicates no anxiety and 100 indicates extreme discomfort—probably how you felt during the assault. It will be our working list, so don't get worried that these ratings are written in stone. Sometimes it's easier to start from the top. What's a realistically OK situation to be in that you avoid? What's the worst for you now?

MELANIE: Uh, that could be several things. I won't go to the library if I can help it. I definitely won't go to the library at night. Actually, I don't like to go anywhere at night. I like to stay in my dorm room with lots of lights on and lots of people around the place. I get pretty scared if there's no one around the dorm.

THERAPIST: OK, let me stop you there for now. Those are all very important situations to include on our hierarchy. Out of those, which is the scariest—the one you avoid the most?

MELANIE: I guess that would be going to the library. If I can, I do my work on-line or get someone else to check out what I need. I've only been back there one time since the assault, and I freaked out and had to leave without getting my work done. I could never go there at night.

THERAPIST: So it sounds like going to the library at night would be at the top of the hierarchy. On that 0–100 SUDs scale, how much would you rate going to the library at night?

MELANIE: I don't think I could do it. Campus security even tells people now not to walk alone to the library or on campus at night.

THERAPIST: That's a good point. If it's not a good thing to do, I certainly won't recommend it or put it on the hierarchy. But I find it hard to believe that no one goes to the library at night any more.

MELANIE: Oh, people still go. They just say not to walk alone.

THERAPIST: OK, good. So how much would you rate going to the library at night with someone you trust?

MELANIE: I'm scared I would freak out again. I'd have to say 100.

THERAPIST: That's OK, we just need to make the list now. So let's write that down at the top. You also mentioned that you don't leave your dorm at night. Is that right? How much on this 0–100 scale would you rate leaving your dorm at night, say, with someone you trust?

MELANIE: That would be pretty scary, too. I've tried that a couple of times, not recently, and I was too scared, so I just stopped doing it. You asked how much? I guess that's pretty close to going to the library at night. Let's say 95.

THERAPIST: OK, we'll put that down. You also mentioned just going to the library—that you avoid that. How much do you think it would bother you to go to the library during the day with someone else?

MELANIE: That's pretty scary, too. I guess I'd say 95.

THERAPIST: Is it more or less scary than going out at night with people?

MELANIE: I guess it's not quite that scary, but it's close. What did I rate going out at night as? 95? OK, let's say 90 for the library, then.

THERAPIST: OK, we're moving right along. Let's write that down. You also mentioned not liking to be at the dorm without lots of lights on and people around. Should we put those on our hierarchy, too? How about just having a reading light on? And what about sleeping? Do you sleep with the lights on or off?

MELANIE: On. My roommate is really getting sick of it, too. I even bought her one of those eye mask things to wear at night to try to shut the light out, but she says it's uncomfortable.

THERAPIST: So it sounds like this is a good thing to work on—getting used to fewer lights on and sleeping without any lights on. How much would that bother you, to sleep without any lights on?

MELANIE: Oh, my gosh! In the dark? I have a confession: I keep a flashlight in my night table drawer just in case the lights go out. What about that? Do I have to give that up?

THERAPIST: Does it cause any problems for you?

MELANIE: No. Other people I know keep flashlights around, too.

THERAPIST: Then why don't you keep yours, too? How about sleeping in the dark?

MELANIE: Well, I used to before all this, and it never bothered me. I used to sleep better, too. I guess I can try it. Let's say 80. And having fewer lights on when we're up probably wouldn't be as bad. Say around 60.

THERAPIST: You're doing great with this. Let's write those down. [Figure 9.1 is the *In Vivo* Hierarchy Form filled in with the situations discussed up to this point.]

In Vivo Hierarchy Form

Name Melanie_____ Date 11/10/96_____

Item	SUDs
1.	
2.	
3.	
4.	
5.	
6.	
7.	
8.	
9.	
10.	
11. Only necessary lights on	60
12.	
13. Sleeping in the dark	80
14. Going to the library, day, accompanied	90
15. Going out at night with people	95
16. Going to the library at night with someone	100

FIGURE 9.1. *In Vivo* Hierarchy Form, filled in with Melanie's first few avoided situations.

THERAPIST: OK, what else do you avoid?

MELANIE: Um, I don't know.

THERAPIST: Let's think. Are there things that didn't use to bother you before the assault that bother you now?

MELANIE: I had trouble doing an assignment the other day because the reading had one scene where a girl was assaulted, and I didn't finish reading it and I didn't write the report. I wanted to ask the teacher for help—to tell him why I couldn't do it and ask for another assignment—but I couldn't do that, either.

THERAPIST: Sounds like those would be good things for us to work on. How much would you rate reading about someone being assaulted? In books, newspapers, seeing it on TV? Are all those the same?

MELANIE: Yeah, they would all be about the same. I didn't even really try to finish that reading. As soon as I read she was gonna get hurt, I just stopped. I guess if I had finished it, it probably would have been about a 50. I leave when the news comes on TV, too, just in case they'll report a rape. I guess that would be around the same.

THERAPIST: You're doing a great job here. Let's put those down. OK, what else?

MELANIE: I can't think of anything.

THERAPIST: I think I remember when you first came in, and we were asking you about avoidance, that you said there were certain clothes you didn't wear any more. Is that true?

MELANIE: Yeah, I guess. The police still have the clothes I was wearing that night. I guess they have them. I don't want them back. Maybe they gave them to my parents, I don't know. But I had on my favorite yellow sweater and Reeboks. My mom, when we were shopping, bought me a pretty yellow sweater, but I haven't worn it. I don't want to wear a yellow sweater. I had an old pair of Reeboks, too, that I don't wear any more. Now I wear Nikes. Is that what you mean?

THERAPIST: Exactly. Can you see that there's nothing about a yellow sweater or Reeboks that can hurt you? It's just because in your mind they are associated with the assault that you don't want to wear them.

MELANIE: Yeah, I see.

THERAPIST: Good. Let's put them on our list. How much do you think it would bother you to wear a yellow sweater and Reeboks? Are they the same?

MELANIE: Yeah, they'd be the same. Let's see . . . wearing a yellow sweater and Reeboks. I just haven't; it probably wouldn't be too bad. Let's say around 50.

THERAPIST: OK, do you think that would be easier or more difficult than reading or watching TV about someone getting assaulted?

MELANIE: A little harder, but not much.

THERAPIST: So wearing a yellow sweater and Reeboks would be a little more difficult than reading or watching TV about someone who was assaulted?

MELANIE: Yes.

THERAPIST: OK. You also mentioned that you wanted to tell your professor what happened to you, why you couldn't do your assignment, but you couldn't. Is that right?

MELANIE: Yeah, I couldn't.

THERAPIST: In general, do you have a hard time talking about what happened to you? Can you tell people you think should know?

MELANIE: Well, most people around here already know. It was in the paper, and I was in the hospital for a while, and you know how people talk. But nobody says anything to me about it, and I never talk about it. It would be hard to talk about it.

THERAPIST: Are there people you think it would be helpful for you to talk about it with?

MELANIE: Sometimes. If I told that teacher, I probably wouldn't have failed that assignment. I've kinda pushed people away; maybe I'm scared they would want to talk about it. I've done that with my sister. We used to talk about everything, but not any more. Same with my best friend back home, ever since this happened.

THERAPIST: Sounds like we should add that to our hierarchy, too. How much do you think it would bother you to talk with your sister or best friend about what happened to you?

MELANIE: Um, that would be pretty hard. Say about 80, I think.

THERAPIST: OK. Would that be easier or more difficult than sleeping in the dark?

MELANIE: Oh, sleeping in the dark would be scarier.

THERAPIST: Would it be easier or more difficult than turning some lights off, only keeping the necessary lights on?

MELANIE: That would be easier. The lights.

THERAPIST: OK. Let's put that in the middle, then—talking to your sister and best friend about what happened to you. Would they be the same?

MELANIE: Yes, they'd be about the same.

THERAPIST: What about telling someone like your teacher?

MELANIE: Well, I'd be so embarrassed to tell him to his face. I was thinking about writing him a note and telling him. Would that work?

THERAPIST: Sure. I think it's important to be able to talk to people to their faces if you want to, but you're going to do that with your sister and best friend, so I think it's OK to write it to your teacher. How much would that bother you?

MELANIE: I don't think that would be too bad. Say about a 40.

THERAPIST: OK. Let's write all of these down. [Figure 9.2 is the *In Vivo* Hierarchy Form filled in with all of these situations.] You've done a great job making this hierarchy. I think we have some real important things down here, and they're all things you can do and all things that I think will free you up a little. I think we have enough to start with now. If other things come up, we can add them to the list. We're going to take it one step at a time.

Developing *In Vivo* Homework Assignments

Review the *in vivo* hierarchy list with the client, and decide together which situations she will confront during homework. Start with situations that have been given SUDs rating of between 40 and 60. By the end of treatment, the client should be practicing daily all the situations listed on the hierarchy.

See the next section for guidance in instructing the client about *in vivo* exposure. Give the client the Model for Gradual *In Vivo* Exposure handout (Figure 9.3). In many cases, the client will feel more comfortable in certain situations if she is accompanied. This is fine. We sometimes refer to this person as the client's "coach." This doesn't mean that the coach should push, "guilt-trip," or cajole the client. He or she should be there as a physical presence to help the client feel safer, but can be supportive too. The coach should *not* be

·*In Vivo* Hierarchy Form

Name Melanie   Date 11/10/96

Item		SUDs
1.		
2.		
3.		
4.		
5.		
6.		
7.		
8.	Writing teacher note about assault	40
9.	Reading/watching TV about a rape	50
10.	Wearing yellow sweater/Reeboks	55
11.	Only necessary lights on	60
12.	Telling sister/best friend about assault	70
13.	Sleeping in the dark	80
14.	Going to the library, day, accompanied	90
15.	Going out at night with people	95
16.	Going to the library at night with someone	100

FIGURE 9.2. *In Vivo* Hierarchy Form, filled in with Melanie's avoided situations (as of end of discussion).

someone who is inconvenienced by the client's avoidance, and may therefore have his or her own agenda to get the client over this as quickly as possible. You and the client should discuss the choice of a coach. The client should try to choose a patient, kind, nonjudgmental person who will be there to assist the client in whatever way she wants to be assisted.

In developing homework assignments, you should also discuss the safety of situations with the client. Help her decide which situations are safe for *in vivo* exposure and which should be avoided. Use the following two examples to illustrate this process.

CASE EXAMPLE 1

Betty lived in a dangerous inner-city neighborhood. Most of the people she knew had been the victims of crimes. She had lost many dear friends to crime in her neighborhood. Gangs and drug addicts ruled her streets. When she left her apartment during the evening, she needed to be accompanied by someone. Because of the potential danger involved, the therapist, together with Betty, developed a list of supportive individuals who could accompany her on her exposure *in vivo* homework.

CASE EXAMPLE 2

Veronica was raped in a public parking garage close to her place of employment. Consequently, she avoided going to work because she was afraid of using the only parking garage available to her. In order to help her return to work and use this parking garage, the *in vivo* exposure assignment included visits to the garage. In order to decrease the probability that Veronica would be revictimized (because the garage was located in a high-crime area), it was suggested that she arrange to be escorted by the security guards who worked in the garage.

Instructing the Client about the *In Vivo* Exposure Procedure

In vivo exposure begins with situations that evoke moderate levels of anxiety (e.g., SUDs = 50), and gradually progresses to situations that provoke maximum fear (SUDs = 100). During an *in vivo* exposure exercise, the client is instructed to remain in the situation for 30–45 minutes or until her anxiety decreases considerably. Emphasize the importance of remaining in the situation until her SUDs decreases by at least 50%. You do not want her to experience a sense of relief upon leaving the situation, because this will reinforce the habit to avoid feared but safe circumstances. You want her to leave feeling relatively comfortable with that situation. *Most importantly, you want*

Model for Gradual *In Vivo* Exposure

Instructions:
Use this example to help you design your *in vivo* exposure assignments. Remember that it is important for you to remain in the situation for 30 minutes or until there is a 50% decrease in your SUDs level. Record your SUDs level before and after the exposure, using the homework sheet.

Example: Going to a shopping mall
1. Your coach accompanies you to a shopping mall, and you walk around the mall together.
2. Your coach accompanies you to the mall and stays in a a specific area of the mall while you walk around alone.
3. Your coach accompanies you to the mall and stays in a specific area while you walk into some stores alone.
4. Your coach drives you to the mall and stays in the parking lot while you walk around the mall alone.
5. Your coach drives you to the mall and leaves the parking lot for 30 minutes while you walk around the mall alone.
6. You go to the mall alone, and your coach waits by a telephone in his or her home.
7. You go to the mall alone and don't tell your coach.

FIGURE 9.3. Model for Gradual *In Vivo* Exposure handout.

the client to experience habituation. Characteristics of the situations, such as time of day and the people that are present, can be adjusted to achieve the desired level of anxiety during exposure. For one client, Martha, going to the mall with her mother evoked a SUDs rating of 60, whereas going alone evoked a SUDs rating of 85. A second client—Belinda, a female physician who was raped by a male—reported a SUDs level of 100 while conducting physical exams of her male patients, but that her SUDs rating decreased to 60 when a nurse was present during the exams.

Once the situations for practice have been determined (see above), explain the procedure to the client as follows:

When you are practicing in the mall, for example, you may initially experience anxiety symptoms, such as your heart beating rapidly, your palms sweating, and feeling faint; you may want to leave the situation immediately. But in order to get over the fear, it is important that you remain in the situation until your anxiety decreases. Once your anxiety has decreased at least 50%, then you can stop the exposure and resume other activities.

However, if you leave the situation when you are very anxious, you are again convincing yourself that the situation is very dangerous and that something terrible is going to happen to you. And the next time you go into that situation, your level of anxiety will be high again. However, if you stay in the situation, your anxiety will decrease, and eventually you will be able to enter it without fear. The more frequently you practice each situation on your list, the less anxiety you will be experiencing. As a result, you will feel less of an urge to avoid situations and people that are now distressing for you.

Finally, show the client how to record her SUDs during exposure homework on the *In Vivo* Exposure Homework Recording Form (Figure 9.4).

Using *In Vivo* Exposure in Sessions

Sometimes a client's *in vivo* exposure hierarchy includes items that can be accomplished during a therapy session. Examples include such items as greeting men or making eye contact with them (if there are any men in the clinic or vicinity), lying on one's back with eyes closed, sitting in a waiting room with unfamiliar people, sitting at a table in a cafeteria by oneself, and so on. These situations may be first attempted as a part of the therapy session with your support, if it seems useful. The client will then continue to practice that particular exposure for homework.

For other clients, the *in vivo* hierarchy may not include any items that are easily conducted in session. For these clients, the discussion of *in vivo* exposure in sessions will focus on the completion of homework and the planning of upcoming assignments.

***In Vivo* Exposure Homework Recording Form**

Date _____

Name _____

Situation practiced_____

Instructions: Before performing the *in vivo* exposure, please answer the following questions in the spaces provided.

1. What is the worst that could happen in this situation?

_____
_____

2. What is the likelihood that this could happen?

_____
_____

3. Evaluate the evidence for or against the likelihood of this happening.

_____
_____
_____

Ratings before and after In Vivo *Exposure*

	Time	SUDs
Before	____	____
After	____	____

Comments_____
_____
_____

FIGURE 9.4. *In Vivo* Exposure Homework Recording Form.

10

Imaginal Exposure: Reliving the Trauma

Some clients express hesitation when they first learn that treatment will involve engaging fully in reliving the assault and in complying with assignments to confront feared situations or images. Such hesitation can be overcome by explaining to the client that the confrontation of the feared thoughts or images will be done gradually. Accordingly, during the first two sessions of imaginal exposure, the client should be allowed to determine the level of detail with which she recounts the narrative of her assault. In the third and subsequent imaginal exposure sessions, you should encourage her to describe the event in more detail by probing for the emotional and physiological reactions that accompanied the assault. It is important for the client to feel in control of the process of remembering the assault and the feelings associated with it; therefore, give her permission to approach the memories slowly.

In addition, you should ensure that the client will not leave the reliving sessions with high anxiety. Treatment sessions should be planned so that there will be sufficient time at the end to calm the client and to give her the opportunity to discuss her reliving experience and new insights she has achieved from it. Thus, it is very important to encourage the client to talk about her reactions to reliving the assault, and to discuss new details and associations that have emerged. Reintroduce breathing retraining after the imaginal exposure if necessary. It is also important for you to be available to talk to the client on the telephone between sessions, in the event that either imaginal or *in vivo* exposure exercises cause her extreme distress. Let her know that she may initially feel as if she is getting worse; she may find herself thinking about the assault more and experiencing more symptoms. This is normal, but she should be able to contact you for reassurance.

Overview of Steps for Teaching Imaginal Exposure

1. Present the rationale for imaginal exposure to the client.
2. Be alert to the client's anxiety; give her reassurance.
3. Explain that the session will be audiotaped so that the client can listen to it as homework.
4. Ask the client to close her eyes.
5. Ask client to recall the trauma vividly, speaking in the present tense.
6. In the first and second exposure sessions, allow the client to approach memories gradually. In the third session, begin asking directive questions.
7. Every 10 minutes, ask the client for a SUDs rating and record on Therapist Imaginal Exposure Recording Form.
8. Continue for 30 to 60 minutes.
9. Allow time in the session, after exposure, for the client to calm herself. Use the breathing retraining method if necessary. Encourage the client to talk about her reactions to reliving the assault.
10. Be available to talk to the client by telephone between sessions.

Presenting the Rationale for Imaginal Exposure

Present the client with the following rationale for imaginal exposure:

Today we are going to spend most of the session having you relive the memory of your assault in your imagination. It is not easy to understand and make sense of traumatic experiences. When you think about the rape or are reminded of it, you may experience extreme anxiety and other negative feelings, such as shame or anger. The assault was a very frightening and distressing experience, so you tend to push away or avoid the painful memories. You may tell yourself, "Don't think about it; time heals all wounds," or "I just have to forget about it." Other people often advise you to use these same tactics. Also, your friends, family, and partner may feel uncomfortable hearing about the assault, and this may influence you not to talk about it. But as you have already discovered, no matter how hard you try to push away thoughts about the assault, the experience comes back to haunt you through nightmares, flashbacks, phobias, and distressing thoughts and feelings. These symptoms signal us that your assault is still "unfinished business." In this part of treatment, our goal is to help you process the memories connected with the assault by having you remember them for an extended period of time. Staying with these memories, rather than running away from them, will help decrease the anxiety and fear that are associated with them. It is quite natural to want to avoid painful experiences, such as memories, feelings, and situations that remind you of the assault. However, as we have already discussed, the more you avoid dealing with the memories, the more they disturb your life. Our aim is to help you gain control over the memories instead of having the memories control you.

You may find the following analogies helpful in demonstrating this point to the client:

ANALOGY 1

Suppose you have eaten a very large and heavy meal that you are unable to digest. This is an uncomfortable feeling. But after you have digested the food, you feel a great sense of relief. Flashbacks, nightmares, and troublesome thoughts continue to occur because the traumatic event has not been adequately digested. Today you are going to start digesting or processing your heavy memories so that they will stop interfering with your daily life.

ANALOGY 2

Imagine that your memory is like a very elaborate file cabinet. Past experiences are each filed into a proper drawer. In this way you can organize your experiences and make sense of them. For example, you have a drawer for restaurant experiences. Every time you go to eat in a restaurant, you file the memory in this drawer in your mind. This is the way in which you remember how to behave in a restaurant, what to expect, and how to evaluate the quality of the food and the services. But in what drawer should you put your assault experience? How should you make sense of it? Part of recovering from a traumatic experience is being able to organize these distressing feelings and memories and find a drawer for them, so you can move on with the business of your life.

ANALOGY 3

Have you ever lost someone that you loved as a result of death or breakup? Could you tell me what that was like for you? [Encourage the client to share her experience with you.] Immediately after the loss you may have felt numb, then extremely sad and pained; you may have also been angry. The way to get over the pain was to experience it, to grieve. After some time, the loss of that person will still be sad, but it probably won't cause as intense pain as it used to, and you may be able to think about him or her without crying. We think that this process of grieving is similar to what a person experiences following a trauma. All of these feelings are part of a natural process that an individual may experience after a traumatic event. In fact, it is important to experience all emotions that are connected to a trauma, in order to process them and get to a point in which the memories are not so devastating.

Now continue presenting the rationale as follows:

What we are going to do today is to begin helping you process the memories associated with your assault. The goal of imaginal exposure as well as *in vivo* exposure is to enable you to have thoughts about the rape, talk about it, or see triggers associated with it without experiencing intense anxiety that disrupts your life. This part of the program includes having you confront situations and memories that generate both anxiety and avoidance. Gradually, the memories will become less painful. You will get used to them. Remember, we call this "habituation."

Repeated reliving of the trauma will also help you in other ways. It will teach you that remembering is not the same as reexperiencing the trauma. In other words, it will help you discriminate between remembering the trauma and being traumatized again. There is no danger in remembering, and therefore there is no good reason to become overwhelmed with anxiety every time you think about the rape. Also, repeated reliving will teach you that you are not going to lose control or go crazy if you engage with the traumatic memory. On the contrary, through repeated reliving of the rape, you are going to gain control over your memories instead of being controlled by them.

And finally, repeatedly engaging with the traumatic memory will allow you to differentiate between the traumatic event and other events that are similar but not dangerous. For example, now you are afraid of all bald men because you were raped by a bald man. Through repeated reliving of the rape, you will realize that baldness itself is not dangerous. Before we begin, do you have any questions about anything that I have said?

You may find it helpful to summarize the rationale for this treatment with the following points:

1. *Emotional processing.* Repeated reliving helps organize the memory and process the trauma. You will learn that thinking about the assault is not dangerous, and that being anxious or upset is also not dangerous.

2. *Habituation.* Repeated reliving of the experience for long periods of time will lower anxiety, and disconfirm the belief that anxiety will last "forever." The more often and longer that you do it, the better it will work.

3. *Discrimination between and remembering and being retraumatized.* Repeated reliving will help you realize that remembering the trauma is not akin to being raped again.

4. *Increased mastery.* Exposure enhances your sense of self-control and personal competence. You feel progressively better about yourself as you stop avoiding and begin mastering your fears.

5. *Differentiation.* Exposure will decrease the generalization of fear from the specific assault to similar but safe situations.

The Imaginal Exposure Procedure

Explaining the Procedure to the Client

It is typical for clients to have some trepidation about the imaginal exposure procedure. Reassure your client and present the following explanation:

I'm going to ask you to recall the memories of the assault. It is best for you to close your eyes, so you won't be distracted and so you can envision these events in your mind's eye. I will ask you to recall these painful memories as vividly as possible. We call this "reliving." I don't want you to tell your story about the assault in the past tense. What I would like you to do is describe the assault in the present tense, as if it were happening now, right here. I'd like you to close your eyes and tell me what happened during the assault in as much detail as you remember. We will work on this together. If you start to feel too uncomfortable and want to run away or avoid it by leaving the image, I will help you to stay with it. We will audiotape the narrative so you can take the tape home and listen to it for homework. From time to time, while you are reliving the assault, I will ask you for your anxiety level on the 0-to-100 SUDs scale, where 0 indicates no anxiety or discomfort and 100 indicates panic-level anxiety. The rating should indicate how anxious you are at the time I ask, sitting here in my office—not how you felt during the assault. Please answer quickly and don't leave the image. Do you have any questions before we start?

Case Example: Helping a Client Get Started with Imaginal Exposure

The following brief case example is provided to demonstrate how to help a client handle her discomfort about starting the imaginal exposure scene.

> THERAPIST: Do you have any questions before we begin?
> CLIENT: No.
> THERAPIST: You are looking a little apprehensive. How are you feeling?
> CLIENT: I am feeling very scared. I haven't told this story to anyone except the police.
> THERAPIST: I imagine the thought of doing this is very frightening. In fact, we even have a term for this. It is called "anticipatory fear" or "anticipatory anxiety." Remember how I have talked about processing and habituation. Eventually, imagining the assault and talking about it will become easier for you. However, the way to get to that point is through repeated practice. In the beginning, reliving the assault may be very anxiety-producing; in fact, you may notice increased flashbacks, troublesome thoughts, and difficulty sleeping in between sessions. This is a signal that you are beginning to process or digest the assault. I want you to know that I will be here to help you 100%. It is important for you to realize that this type of treatment has helped many survivors of rape and other types of assault, and that it will become easier with time.

Case Example: An Early Imaginal Exposure Narrative

Emily was raped in her apartment on a Wednesday night. She had run out to the grocery store after work. She had returned home, put her groceries away, and encountered an intruder. Here is a transcript of her narrative from an early imaginal exposure session:

I'm in my kitchen . . . and I hear a noise . . . and I turn around, expecting to see the cat that I think just jumped up on the counter, and instead I see this man . . . and I can't believe it . . . and he's looking at me . . . and he's coming towards me . . . with his hands out like . . . telling me not to scream and he won't hurt me . . . and I'm begging with him not to hurt me . . . and he just keeps saying, "Don't scream and I won't hurt you." . . . Back and forth we keep this up, and he tells me to go to the bedroom and sit on the bed.

I'm sitting on the edge of the bed, thinking, "Who is this man?" and thinking, "It's impossible he is in my house." . . . I was just gone for several minutes . . . that's about all I feel . . . I'm scared . . . I'm just feeling scared . . . and I'm just shaking . . . and I'm holding on to my can of soda as tight as I can . . . and he makes me lay back. I lay back on my bed . . . and I'm staring at the ceiling, and he takes the can out of my hand and he puts it down . . . and I'm hearing him do something, and I turn my head to the right and I see his penis out of his pants . . . and I'm shocked . . . I never expected to see that . . . and he's telling me to touch it . . . it seems like a long time passes and I cannot move my hand.

And now . . . and now he's moving my hand . . . and he throws off my hand . . . because he is frustrated. And he comes around to the other side of the bed and he's kneeling down . . . and it's like this is just happening to me but I'm not thinking . . . I'm not wondering what he's doing . . . it's just happening . . . one right after another . . . until I feel his mouth on my vaginal area and I'm beginning to just . . . I'm just talking to myself and I'm telling myself, "It will be OK . . . just let me get through this alive . . . this is not happening."

And then he's standing up but kind of toward me . . . like leaning on me . . . and my thoughts are "What is he doing now?" I'm sensing that he's having trouble doing whatever he's doing . . . I'm not real sure . . . until I can feel that he just begins to rape me . . . and he's coming towards me and he's kissing me on my lips . . . and he's just sloppy . . . and he smells like alcohol and sweat . . . and I just . . . I'm almost playing dead . . . and then he lowers down and pulls my bra over and he's just kind of slobbering on me . . . and my eyes are shut . . . and my ears are ringing.

And then he leans up and he says, "Tell me you love me," and he's kind of saying it in a real harsh voice . . . and I'm telling myself, "Don't do it," and he's saying it again . . . and he's getting mad . . . he's repeating again and again, "Tell me you love me," and I quick respond, "Yes." I'm more angry at him asking me to tell him I love him than I am about him raping me . . . 'cause before I could pretend that this just wasn't happening, but now I am mad . . . I'm feeling mad . . . I'm feeling like I'm being forced to say yes.

And I continue to stare at him . . . and he's so scary I start to cry, and I'm asking him why he's doing this to me . . . he just gets up . . . stops raping me . . . I'm sitting up . . . and he says, "Have you got any money? and I say, "Yes." And then I turn over looking for my purse and I find five dollars . . . and I give it to him . . . and he's telling me to stay in the bedroom and lock the door . . . so I just respond . . . and while I'm sitting in my bedroom I'm hearing him on the other side of the door . . . and I shake more . . . all over . . . I cannot control it . . . I'm so scared that he's coming again . . . and then I don't hear him any more, so I sit there and just stare at the wall.

And after about 10 minutes I get up and run through the living room and leap down the steps and run across to my neighbor's and ring the doorbell repeatedly until my neighbor answers the door . . . and she has this look of shock on her face . . . and I quickly say, "I've just been raped," and she lets me inside . . . I'm in shock . . . I can't think what just happened . . . and I'm afraid that he's still close by and can get to me . . . I'm scared . . . it's as if I have no control in my life 'cause I won't stop shaking . . . no matter what I do . . . my whole body . . . it won't stop shaking . . . and then I just call the police and then it's just . . . so disorganized . . . just . . .

Police arrive . . . I'm not looking around . . . I'm just staring at my legs . . . my feet . . . and part of me is very relieved. The police keep saying I don't have to go to the hospital . . . I don't have to cooperate . . . I don't have to tell them anything . . . I just keep telling them, "Whatever it takes to get him caught . . . I'll do whatever it takes to get him caught." I just can't say that enough to them . . . I'm crying almost the whole time I'm at my neighbor's . . . I finally calm down when the ambulance gets there . . . I'm feeling calm when the ambulance gets there . . . and I am stepping into the ambulance all by myself. I'm not sure what is happening . . . and there is police just going all over the place . . . I'm cold . . . I'm shaking, cold . . . numb . . . I'm in shock. I don't cry any more; I just stare out the back window of the ambulance the entire drive . . . and I can hear the people in the ambulance telling me to relax . . . just feel . . . numb.

Emily described feeling emotionally numb at times during and after her assault; it is interesting that this is a reaction she described during her imaginal exposure as well. In later sessions, her therapist worked on helping Emily to feel all of the emotions associated with her assault while reliving it, to aid in her emotional processing of this trauma.

SUDs Recording, Repetitions, and Discussion

Use the Therapist Imaginal Exposure Recording Form (Figure 10.1) to record the client's SUDs ratings every 10 minutes. In the first imaginal exposure session, allow 60 minutes for the exposure. (Exposures in later sessions are usually somewhat shorter; see below.) If it takes 15 minutes for the client to recount the assault, then ask her to start from the beginning and go through it again, repeating it four times. If it takes 20 minutes, she will be able to repeat it three times, and so on. After about 60 minutes of imaginal exposure, terminate the first exercise by asking the client to open her eyes and take several deep breaths. Talk about the experience of reliving the

---

Therapist Imaginal Exposure Recording Form

Client #   619   Date   9/2/97

Exposure #   3   Session #   5

Description of exposure in imagination   returned home and intruder in home, rapes her on

her bed, goes to neighbor's

Start time 1:15   SUDS

10 minutes   70

20 minutes   100

30 minutes   80

40 minutes   70

50 minutes   60

60 minutes   50

Comments

reported feeling numb at times, helps her to describe her thoughts and fears

---

FIGURE 10.1. Therapist Imaginal Exposure Recording Form.

assault with her. Did she remember things she had not previously recalled? Was it easier or more difficult than she thought it would be? Was there something you could have done to help her? What does she feel? What does she think?

Additional Guidelines and Suggestions

Therapeutic Comments during Exposure

The following comments are helpful during imaginal exposure (and during review of the *in vivo* exposure homework as well; see Chapter 9) to encourage the client:

    1. "You are doing fine. Stay with the image."
    2. "You've done very well. It took some courage to stick it out even though you were quite afraid."
    3. "Stay with your feelings."
    4. "I know this is difficult. You are doing a good job."

5. "Stay with the image. You are safe here."
6. "Feel safe and let go of the feelings."

If the client's anxiety *does* decrease within the session of exposure, these comments may be made:

1. "You see, your anxiety decreases if you just continue to stay in the fearful situation."
2. "I want you to notice that you are much less anxious than you were in the beginning of the session."
3. "I can see that you are more relaxed today than last time when you confronted the distressing circumstances. As you can see, the more you confront this situation, the less it is associated with anxiety. Does it seem as bad to think about it as it used to seem?"
4. "You see, you exposed yourself to your fears, and nothing terrible has happened. Does this situation seem as dangerous or as unpleasant as it used to seem?"

If the client's anxiety *has not* decreased within the session of exposure, these comments may be helpful:

1. "Your anxiety persisted. This often happens, especially in the first sessions. I want you to continue at home exposing yourself to memories of the trauma, using the tape, for an hour each day."
2. "You were feeling very anxious today during the imaginal exposure. You did a great job facing the memory. You were not sure that you would be able to do this. You can give yourself a big pat on the back."

Later Exposure Sessions: How to Habituate the Most Fearful Assault Memories

During the third and subsequent imaginal exposure sessions, you will be asking specific questions about the client's thoughts, feelings, and physical reactions while she is reliving the assault. Identify the parts of the scenario that are the most anxiety-producing for the client. We refer to these memories as "hot spots." They need repeated exposure in order for habituation to occur. During the last few sessions, you should expect SUDs ratings during imaginal exposure to range from 20 to 30, and finally from 15 to 20. At this point, "hot spots" should be peaks of anxiety with SUDs ratings over 20. These portions of the memory are then reviewed in a repetitive fashion (as many as six or seven times) during a single session.

In these later sessions, conduct imaginal exposure for 30–45 minutes and record SUDs every 10 minutes. Encourage the client to slow down during the recollections eliciting intense distress (i.e., the "hot spots"). Below is a list of questions that you can ask the client in order to facilitate confrontation with fear-evoking cues during imaginal exposure:

- "What are you feeling?"
- "What are you thinking?"
- "Are you experiencing any physical reactions? Describe them."
- "What is your body feeling?"
- "What are you seeing/smelling/doing now?"
- "Where do you feel that in your body?"

Problems That May Arise during Imaginal Exposure

Sometimes a client may have difficulty expressing her feelings. She may be afraid to start to cry because she imagines she will never stop. A few clients may feel inhibited in your office, worrying that others outside the office might be able to hear them, especially if they become emotional. Others have just become so used to cutting themselves off from their feelings that it's difficult for them to let go. Provide reassurance, and proceed with the review of the memory of the assault.

Also, in order to maintain control, a client may engage in avoidance behavior during imagery. For example, she may become quiet and may turn her head to the right or left while avoiding extremely upsetting memories (e.g., memories of the assailant's face, being threatened with a weapon, being forced to perform oral sex, or the time of penile penetration). You should ask at this point, "What's happening now?", and encourage the client to confront the difficult image. Another effective method is to ask the client to use the "slow-motion technique." This involves focusing on the image and asking the client to express her thoughts, feelings, and physical reactions as if things are happening in slow motion.

Finally, if a client is having difficulty expressing her feelings, you can say in an encouraging tone, "Allow all of your feelings to be expressed. There is no reason to censor feelings of anger, sadness, guilt, shame or fear." Or you can say the following:

The last two times that you reviewed the memory of your assault, I noticed that you seemed to have difficulty letting go of your feelings. I want to remind you that you are safe here, and that it is important for you to release your feelings that are associated with the memories. Is there anything that I can do that will be helpful to you in this process? Do you have any ideas about why it is difficult for you to fully express your feelings in here?

As we have mentioned earlier, you need to express confidence that you will be able to handle, and help the client handle, whatever comes up. Sometimes a client is frightened of what she may remember during imaginal exposure. You will need to reassure her about this. Sometimes it helps to remind her that whatever she remembers, it does not change what happened: She survived, and therefore she obviously did the right thing for survival. We have not yet encountered a client who remembered details during imaginal exposure that she could not cope with. One of our patients described each session of imaginal exposure therapy as "peeling a layer off of an onion, and after a few sessions, you get to the stinky part in the middle, and then it doesn't stink any more."

Ending Exposure and Assigning Homework

After each reliving, discuss what happened with the client, as noted previously. Was it as bad as she thought it would be? How is she feeling now? Encourage her to sit in your waiting room for a few minutes at the end of a session if she wants to unwind before leaving. Praise her courage, and discuss her responses. Finally, assign homework, including reliving at home with the use of the audiotape recorded in the session. Discuss plans for imaginal exposure at home. Is there a private place where your client can listen to the tape, and where no one else can hear or will disturb her? Portable tape players with earphones are useful for privacy. We don't encourage letting significant others listen to the tapes, for various reasons. First, we don't want our clients monitoring what they say because they are thinking about an audience; second, it may be very upsetting for other people to hear with no therapist present to help them. In unusual circumstances, though, it is allowed. Also, ask your client to record her anxiety level and any comments each time she practices; the Exposure Homework Recording Form (Figure 10.2) is used for this.

Case Illustrations

Below are two additional cases illustrating imaginal exposure. The first contains several brief excerpts from an actual exposure session, with commentary. The second features another complete imaginal exposure narrative, with the therapist's prompts and probes.

Case Example: Session Excerpts with Commentary

Susan was a 31-year-old married white woman in graduate school. She was upstairs in her townhouse studying for a test when her husband left to make a

---

Exposure Homework Recording Form

Client Susan   Date 9/6/95

Description of exposure in imagination Starting from the minute I realize he will rape me
and ending at the time I heard a knock on the door

Date   9/7/95

Before imaginal exposure: SUDs   45

After imaginal exposure: SUDs   65

Comments It was difficult in the beginning and then it became easier

Date   9/8/95

Before imaginal exposure: SUDs   25

After imaginal exposure: SUDs   60

Comments It was not as difficult as yesterday

Date   9/12/95

Before imaginal exposure: SUDs   10

After imaginal exposure: SUDs   50

Comments It is becoming more difficult to be as upset as I used to be

Date

Before imaginal exposure: SUDs

After imaginal exposure: SUDs

Comments

Date

Before imaginal exposure: SUDs

After imaginal exposure: SUDs

Comments

FIGURE 10.2. Exposure Homework Recording Form.

quick trip to the store. A black man in his 20s then entered her house, robbed her, and raped her at what she thought was knifepoint. She was hit and threatened when she screamed. After the rape was completed and the rapist was adjusting his clothing, Susan made a dash for the door and was caught in a struggle, but managed to escape.

Susan presented for treatment approximately 1 year following this incident, complaining of nightmares, fears of being alone, avoidance of sex with her husband, hypervigilance, jumpiness, and decreased concentration (with consequent difficulties in school). She reported avoiding taking the dog for walks after dark, avoiding being downstairs in her house when alone, constantly checking locks, and avoiding discussing the assault. Treatment consisted of prolonged exposure—imaginal exposure as described in this chapter, and *in vivo* exposure as homework.

Susan responded well to treatment. She complied with treatment instructions in carrying out all exposures, despite high anxiety. Her anxiety decreased both within sessions and between sessions, as indicated by her SUDs ratings and observable discomfort. She maintained treatment gains at follow-up assessments 3, 6, and 12 months after treatment, and became highly functional as reflected in her professional and family achievements.

Excerpts from Susan's imaginal exposure narratives follow.

I see this person in the doorway of the stairwell and he seems to be rushing at me . . . and my heart's pounding . . . I'm really surprised . . . and I know I'm really in trouble . . . He has this thing at my head and he says if I scream, which I don't 'cause I got fingers practically down my throat . . . that he'll shoot me.

In this excerpt, Susan described the scene in the present tense. She included physiological reactions ("my heart's pounding"), appraisals ("I know I'm really in trouble"), actual threat ("he'll shoot me"), and detailed stimuli and action. The inclusion of all these stimuli and response elements in a client's imagery scenarios has been found to enhance the activation of the fear structure. When only stimuli are described (and not responses), fewer fear responses have been observed. As noted in Chapter 5 of this book, enhanced activation of fear has been found to be positively related to treatment gains.

He says, "Where did your husband go?", and I say, "Just out to do something very quickly. He'll be right back." And he says, "I've got my buddy waiting for him." And that really scares me, because it seems like now this is some type of horror story or something . . . that we're both going to be hurt.

Here, the assailant made a threat that extended into the future and involved her husband. Now Susan's trauma was broadened; she was in the position of considering the future consequences of her actions, as well as the safety of her husband.

He says, "Get on the bed," which again surprises me . . . I didn't expect that . . . it's the first time I suspect rape. So I get on the bed . . . I don't see any choice, any way to escape . . . I think there is somebody downstairs.

Many rape victims report that they were surprised when they realized they were going to be raped and not just robbed. Unpredictability ("I didn't expect that") and uncontrollability ("I don't see any choice, any way to escape") have been hypothesized to underlie the development of PTSD (Foa et al., 1989, 1992). When detected, the expression of unpredictability and uncontrollability should be included as part of the scenario. The fight for control is expressed in the following excerpt:

He whacks me across the face . . . and he says, "Don't scream any more." I think this man is really dangerous . . . he really can hurt me and I have to be careful . . . so I have to figure out how much anything I try to do is going to provoke him and not let it get that far.

Susan's attempts to call for help through screaming were punished, which prompted her to try different strategies. Many victims become passive during the assault, which may help them to survive by not provoking their assailant, especially when a weapon is present. No one is prepared to confront a rapist, and therefore the response of the victim during the rape relies totally on momentary improvisation. Therefore, the therapist must not convey any judgment regarding the victim's actions.

He's pushing too low and I feel burning, sharp, cutting, and then it goes in . . . and I don't really feel it after that, just like movement . . . he says, "When I'm done with you . . . my buddy's coming up." That's just another terrifying moment . . . I want to get out, I can't have that . . . another person . . . going to hit me . . . I'm saying, "No, no, please don't hurt me, no, no," and I hate it; I hate whining. I hear myself saying it and I wish I would stop . . . it's like I can't make myself stop.

Here, Susan was describing some dissociative reactions, which are very common at the time of an assault. Susan's dissociative responses were minimal ("I don't really feel it after that," "I hear myself saying it"), but more blatant dissociation is also common among rape victims. This may include a sense of leaving one's body and watching the assault as an outsider. An extreme dissociative reaction involves psychogenic amnesia (inability to recall important aspects of the situation). In these cases, imaginal exposure has been found to be helpful in aiding recall of details that were previously inaccessible. For example, during the third session of imaginal exposure, one patient recalled for the first time that her assailant cocked the pistol he was holding to her head and threatened to pull the trigger if she did not perform fellatio. Thereafter, she was able to describe her assault in detail, and within six sessions her fear dissipated.

He comes off of me, says, "Kiss it," which I don't wanna do . . . my mouth's bleeding and it hurts . . . it just looks evil and I think it's dirty . . . and I don't want to do it, but he pushes me down and I'm afraid I'm going to be hurt . . . so I just do it.

Susan was again describing a perceived lack of control and a fear of further injury. In this particular session, she did not describe the fellatio in detail. In subsequent sessions, however, she included a detailed description of the assault, including her responses. It is important to prompt all memories, including olfactory, visual, auditory, and tactile.

I'm shaking now, it's cold . . . and I'm embarrassed. It's very peculiar . . . it's like I'm again suspended, and I'm nude in my bedroom with someone I don't know . . . it's like this same feeling when you dream that you're at work, but you're not dressed correctly, like you wore your pajamas to work or something . . . sort of a little panic and embarrassed and you don't want anyone to see you.

This is a rich description of the feelings that can arise during an assault. The embarrassment and shame Susan described are common in rape victims and probably inhibit disclosure; in turn, this may hinder emotional processing.

Case Example: Imaginal Exposure Narrative with Prompts/Probes

Althea was raped by an acquaintance who offered to give her a ride home after a party. She felt a great deal of shame and didn't tell anyone what had happened to her until she requested therapy, almost 6 years following her assault. A full transcript of one of her imaginal exposure narratives, with the therapist's prompts and probes, follows.

ALTHEA: I'm at a party with Laura . . . we're having a nice time . . . the party is really crowded . . . it's getting late so we are looking for a ride to go home . . . she asks Jimmy to give us a ride home. Jimmy is her brother's friend . . . he's taking us home. He takes her home first . . . he tells me he's gonna take me home last because he lives nearer to me . . . he's driving and he passes my street . . . he says he's just going to get gas, but he doesn't stop at a gas station . . . he says he's just driving. Now he's putting his hand on my knee . . . he's rubbing my knee . . . I'm moving his hand away . . . he's driving further . . . he's driving to a wooded area. He tries to kiss me and I push him away . . . I tell him no . . . he tries again and I tell him no . . . so he's pushing me down towards the seat. I'm struggling with him and I get out of the car . . . I start walking . . . it's very dark and wooded . . . so he drives behind me . . . he gets out of his car . . . and he tells me, "OK, I'm gonna take you home." Then all of

a sudden he comes near me and throws me down on the ground . . . I'm struggling . . . and I'm fighting and I'm hitting him in the top of his head. But he
doesn't stop . . . he's tearing my blouse . . . he tells me if I tell anyone they won't
believe me . . . he tears my skirt . . . and he's on top of me . . . and I'm fighting
him and I'm fighting him and he's hitting me in my face . . . and he's fighting
me and fighting me. And as time goes on I'm getting tired of fighting him . . .
so I give up the fight . . . I can feel him kissing me . . . touching me . . . and was
pulling at my underwear.

THERAPIST: He's *pulling* at my underwear.

ALTHEA: He's pulling at my underwear . . . he tears them off . . . he unzips
his pants . . . he pulls his underwear down. I'm screaming, yelling . . . I'm telling him to stop but he won't stop . . . I'm scared if I yell any more that he'll
seriously hurt me. We stayed there for a couple of hours . . . and then he finally
takes me home . . . I can't continue any more.

THERAPIST: Just try. You're doing great.

ALTHEA: He pushes . . . he grabs me . . . he is trying to kiss me again . . .
he pushes me down on the ground. I'm fighting him . . . my heart is beating
real fast . . . I'm really nervous. I'm hitting him in his head and in his face . . .
but he doesn't stop. He tears my shirt . . . and he starts to kiss me . . . then he
tears my skirt . . . and he's starting to get on top of me . . . he tears my panties
. . . (*She hesitates.*)

THERAPIST: You are doing real good. Just try to stay with it. It's very important to stay with it and not escape when you're feeling real anxious. Try to
stay with it.

ALTHEA: I feel him pulling at my legs . . . he's trying to part them . . . I'm
very nervous and I'm very scared. He tells me not to scream any more . . . he
tells me no one can hear me . . . he's beginning to unzip his pants and pull his
pants down. I can feel him . . . I can feel him forcing his way on top of me . . .
I can feel him pushing to get his penis inside of my legs. I'm crying . . . I'm
asking him to stop . . . but he doesn't stop . . . I'm telling him that I'll tell someone . . . he says no one will believe me. So at that point I just give up the fight
. . . because I'm getting scared that he's gonna really hurt me. We stay there
for a couple hours . . . he's having sex with me more than once . . . he's having
sex with me for at least three times . . . I'm crying . . . my back is dirty . . . I
have sand all over me. It's almost morning and he decides that he's gonna take
me in . . . take me home . . . he tells me no one will believe me . . . he tells me,
"And if you do tell, they'll say you asked for it."

THERAPIST: What is your level right now?

ALTHEA: 80.

THERAPIST: OK, you are doing real well. You're doing fine. I know it's
tough. Take it easy. You are doing real well.

ALTHEA: He drives beside . . . the street where I live and lets me out of
the car . . . he goes home. I take my keys . . . it's almost daybreak but not yet

. . . I take my keys . . . I go into the house. Everybody is sleeping and I go into the bathroom . . . 30 minutes later I hear my mom walking around . . . she wants to know where I have been. I tell her that I stayed with my girlfriend Laura . . . she asks me, "Why are you looking all wild?" She says that I'm looking wild . . . she tells me . . . she asks me, "How did you get sand in your hair?" I tell her . . . I told her I fell . . . she really . . . I don't think she really believes me. We argue for a while . . . then finally she goes back to bed and I take a shower . . . I shower for about an hour and a half. And then I go to my room . . . I stay in my room all day . . . during the day I don't take any phone calls from anyone. My girlfriend Laura comes by to see me . . . she asks me, "What time did you get home?", because she called and no one answered the phone when she thought I was home. I tell her that we went to another . . . to a club . . . and she believes what I tell her. As the day goes on, I feel afraid . . . I feel scared . . . I'm wondering if he's gonna tell anyone . . . I feel dirty . . . I feel ashamed.

THERAPIST: What's your level at this point?

ALTHEA: About 90.

THERAPIST: Let's start from the beginning again, OK?

Vicarious Traumatization of the Therapist

"Vicarious traumatization," sometimes referred to as "secondary traumatization," occurs when someone hearing about a trauma or helping in the aftermath of a trauma becomes emotionally affected. We often hear about the toll this takes on emergency workers, such as firefighters, police officers, or Red Cross workers. Even though these people were not the victims, trauma has nonetheless touched their lives and left its emotional scar. Working with trauma survivors in therapy is very taxing for those of us who do this work. In the midst of imaginal exposure therapy, we hear all the gory details of life's worst moments, and some of them are hard to shake.

Somehow, as trauma therapists, we need to find the right balance between empathic responses to our clients' pain and professional distance that allows us to respond in a manner that is therapeutic for the clients. We have all teared up or felt a lump in our throats when we hear some of our patients' accounts. But we have also had the experience of hearing atrocities and of responding intellectually and (we hope) therapeutically, while feeling emotionally unaffected. Somewhere in the middle probably lies the optimal balance. Our work is very similar to that of hospital staff members caring for medical trauma survivors or cancer patients. It is hard for most compassionate people to see and hear these things without feeling very upset, sometimes being devastated, and thinking, "There but for the grace of God go I." But we need to remember that we are the trained professionals; although we weren't responsible for what happened to our patients, we have accepted the responsibility of trying to help them recover.

Even in the worst atrocities, there are opportunities for the resilience of the human spirit to shine through. These experiences may be perceived as "gifts" that are only available to those of us who are working "in the trenches." Seeing an assault victim who accepts what has happened to her with dignity and self-respect, and who sometimes even finds a positive message in it, is an example of such an uplifting experience. Working with a terminally ill cancer patient who is leaving behind a legacy of love and integrity and is dying with such dignity as to make us marvel that such people exist is another example of such a gift. We truly gain an understanding of what people are capable of, both good and bad, and we are doing something that not everyone can do.

Remember, you deserve praise, too! You can never be completely sure what is going to come up when you are beginning imaginal exposure therapy with a new client, so you may often feel some trepidation (well hidden, of course!). Each time, however, it should get easier for you, and thus for your client. It is very helpful if there is someone *you* can talk to and debrief with— for example, another therapist doing similar work. Of course, you need to make sure that any person you choose to "unload on" can handle it, or you may end up vicariously traumatizing a friend or loved one. It is also a good idea to have a mix of patients or professional activities to help keep your work in perspective. If you start to feel burned out, or to feel that your ability to respond therapeutically is compromised, you may need to take a break. This break may be from seeing all patients, or just traumatized patients. Your clients need an emotionally healthy therapist, and you do both yourself and your clients an injustice if you try to go beyond your limits. Take care of yourself!

11

Cognitive Techniques I: Cognitive Restructuring

Theoretical Bases for Cognitive Restructuring

Emotions, Thoughts, and Beliefs

Cognitive restructuring is based on the cognitive theory of emotional disorders, developed by Beck and his colleagues (see Chapter 5). This theory supposes that emotions are produced by the interpretation of events rather than by the events themselves. Thus, the same event can be interpreted in different ways and consequently can evoke different emotions. The example given in Chapter 5 illustrates this: A woman who is in bed and hears a noise at the window will become afraid if she thinks it is a burglar trying to invade her home. However, if she thinks it is just the wind, she will not become anxious, but rather slightly annoyed to be awakened.

Each emotion is also said to be associated with a particular type of thought or belief. In anxiety, the characteristic thoughts (interpretations) are concerned with perceived danger or threat. In anger, the thoughts are concerned with perceiving other people as having behaved in a way that is wrong and unfair. In guilt, the thoughts are concerned with perceiving oneself as having behaved (or thought) in a way that is wrong and unfair. Finally, in depression or sadness, the thoughts are concerned with a perceived loss of something that is crucially important.

Some examples of automatic thoughts in assault victims include the following:

Emotion	Automatic Thought
Anxiety	"That man is going to attack me."
	"This street is dangerous."
	"I'm losing my mind."

Guilt/shame	"It was my fault." "I am a bad mother/wife/friend." "I could have stopped it."
Anger/rage	"It's not fair." "Why me?" "I should get more help." "Nobody gives a damn."
Sadness/hopelessness	"My life's over." "I'll never be the same again." "I will never be close to people again."

In everyday life people experience a wide range of events involving danger, loss, or violation of rules of fairness, and these events lead to normal emotional responses. However, when the emotional responses are more intense and/or more prolonged than usual, it is assumed that people's thinking is to some extent distorted or dysfunctional. Therapy then focuses on helping people to become aware of their excessively negative thoughts and to modify them. In this way, excessive emotional reactions and associated problematic behaviors can be overcome.

Distinguishing Negative Automatic Thoughts from Dysfunctional Beliefs

Two different levels of disturbed thinking can be distinguished.

"Negative automatic thoughts" are those thoughts or images that go through a person's mind during a situation that provokes an emotional response. For example, a trauma victim who feels that she is a poor coper when facing a stressful situation might have the automatic thoughts "I can't take it any more," "I am falling apart."

"Dysfunctional beliefs" are general assumptions people hold about the world and about themselves that cause them to interpret specific events in an excessively negative and dysfunctional manner. For example, a belief that the world is an extremely dangerous place makes a person particularly likely to interpret situations or people as harmful. Unlike negative automatic thoughts, which the person can usually recognize, dysfunctional beliefs do not always enter the person's consciousness in the distressing situation. Instead, they may need to be elicited by detailed questioning. With respect to rape victims, a good example of the distinction between automatic thoughts and dysfunctional beliefs can be found in the feelings of guilt and self-blame that often follow a rape. When thinking about the rape and feeling guilty, a victim may have the automatic thought "It was my fault." After careful questioning, she may recognize that before the rape she had the belief "I am the kind of person who can always take care of myself," or "I am the kind of person who always gets in trouble." Thus, automatic thoughts can often be a manifestation of a broader assumption or belief.

When doing cognitive restructuring, the therapist focuses on both the negative thoughts and the dysfunctional beliefs of the client. It is usually more effective to work on the client's more general beliefs, since they will affect a broader range of situations than specific negative automatic thoughts. However, you will need to work with at least some of the specific thoughts, both to show the client how to modify these and to determine what the underlying beliefs are. The dysfunctional beliefs that are common in PTSD (and a few of the negative thoughts that reflect them) are summarized below.

Common Dysfunctional Beliefs (and Associated Negative Thoughts) in PTSD

PRETRAUMA BELIEFS ABOUT ONESELF

As discussed in Chapter 5, recovery from trauma is severely hindered if a person's pretrauma beliefs lead her to interpret the trauma as a sign that she is inadequate or incompetent. This can happen in two ways. First, if the person already had a negative view of herself before the trauma, the trauma may be taken as final proof that this view is correct. Second, if the person has viewed herself as particularly invulnerable and strong before the trauma, this view may be contradicted by the trauma and by her reaction to it.

PRETRAUMA BELIEFS ABOUT THE SAFETY OF THE WORLD

PTSD is likely to occur (1) if before the trauma the person had the view that the world is a dangerous place and the trauma has validated this view; or (2) if the person had the view that the world was entirely safe and the trauma has shattered this belief. In both cases, the person is likely to overgeneralize from the trauma in a way that leads her to believe that she is always in danger and that there is no safe place in the world. This leads to chronic hyperarousal, extreme fear, and avoidance. Typical specific beliefs reflecting the general belief of danger would be that all men are potential rapists, that dating is dangerous, that sleeping with the light off is dangerous, that living alone is asking for trouble, and that wearing skirts and dresses encourages men to rape.

BELIEFS ABOUT REACTIONS DURING THE TRAUMA

Some victims interpret their emotional responses and behaviors during the trauma in a way that generates a negative view of themselves, and this view interferes with recovery. For example, a rape victim may interpret the freezing response and the confusion that occurred during the rape (and that are common fear responses) as signs of incompetence or poor coping ability, and this will produce negative thoughts or beliefs (e.g., "Other people would have struggled and prevented it," "I can't trust my body," "I can't trust myself," "In stressful situations I fall apart"). Dissociation during a rape can be processed in a similar way and can also be taken as a sign of vulnerability to insanity.

BELIEFS ABOUT INITIAL PTSD SYMPTOMS

Some trauma victims interpret the normal initial symptoms of PTSD in a way that is likely to make the symptoms persist. For example, if a rape victim thinks that intrusive recollections of the rape or flashbacks mean that she is losing control or going crazy, she is likely to try hard to push the intrusions out of her mind. Paradoxically, this attempt at thought suppression is likely to increase the frequency of the intrusions, and hence to strengthen her belief that she is going crazy. This will further increase her fear of the intrusions and strengthen her suppression attempts, creating a vicious circle that maintains the symptoms. Another example concerns numbing and detachment from others. This can be interpreted as a sign that the person will never experience normal feelings again and may contribute to self-critial thoughts and beliefs (e.g., "How can I not love my children/husband?", "I must be a horrible person," "I have died emotionally," "I'll never recover," "I'm no longer the same person").

BELIEFS ABOUT THE REACTIONS OF OTHERS

Unfortunately, some people do not always respond to a rape victim in a supportive way. Some people care a great deal but don't want to discuss the rape because it pains them or they believe it will increase the victim's pain. The victim may misinterpret this as a sign that other people do not care about her or actually blame her for the rape; again, negative thoughts and beliefs may result (e.g., "I'm all alone," "Everyone thinks it was my fault," "They think I'm overreacting," "I should be able to just put it behind me," "Other people don't want to know"). Such beliefs and thoughts prevent the victim from sharing what happened. Sometimes people really *are* critical of a victim and her persistent symptoms, and the victim may agree with this unfair criticism.

Aims and Methods of Cognitive Restructuring

In summary, as a result of a traumatic experience, an individual's views of the world and of herself as a person can change drastically. Assault victims with

PTSD perceive the entire world as dangerous and themselves as incapable of coping with stress. They also often believe that the assault is their fault and that they deserved to have been assaulted. Cognitive restructuring can help such a client to correct her mistaken beliefs that the world is entirely dangerous and that she is entirely incompetent. The goal of cognitive restructuring is to reduce anxiety or other emotional distress by teaching clients to identify, evaluate, and modify their negative thoughts and dysfunctional beliefs. Cognitive restructuring aims to teach the client to develop more realistic (new) beliefs about her ability to cope, and about the safety of the world in general and trauma reminder situations in particular.

This technique is described to the client as a collaborative effort of a scientific or detective team (her and you!). Negative thoughts and beliefs are treated as hypotheses. You and the client will work together as a team to collect evidence to determine whether the client's hypotheses (conclusions) about herself and about others are accurate and useful to her.

The Socratic method of questioning is used to help clients evaluate and modify their negative thoughts and beliefs. Homework assignments consist of Daily Diaries, in which the client first identifies "trigger" situations, the emotions felt in those situations, and the negative thoughts and beliefs behind these emotions; she then challenges the beliefs and generates rational responses to them.

Overview of Steps for Teaching Cognitive Restructuring

1. Present the rationale for the technique to the client.
2. Identify a situation that caused the client emotional distress (e.g., "I was in the mall when I saw this man looking at me").
3. Help the client identify her emotions (anxiety, anger, guilt/shame, sadness).
4. Help the client identify the thought that caused the emotion (e.g., "He is looking at me in a funny way").
5. Help the client identify beliefs that underlie the thought by continuing to ask questions (e.g., "So what does this mean, that he looks at you in a funny way?" "He is going to hurt me").
6. Help the client challenge the beliefs by collecting evidence to support or refute them.
    a. If insufficient evidence exists to support the belief continue the discourse by asking questions that aim to help her modify the belief.
    b. If sufficient evidence exists to support the belief help the client restate the belief rationally and adaptively or seek a safety response.
7. Facilitate the process of identifying and challenging negative thoughts, and prepare the client to examine dysfunctional beliefs, by teaching the client about common cognitive distortions.
8. Help the client to identify and challenge the dysfunctional beliefs underlying her negative thoughts (e.g., "Why is this man going to hurt

you?" "Because all men are dangerous, and you can't trust them"),
again through repeated questioning (see Steps 5–6).

Presenting the Rationale For Cognitive Restructuring

The Relationship among Facts, Beliefs, and Emotions

Begin providing the client with a rationale for cognitive restructuring as follows:

Let's discuss what happens to people's thoughts after they experience an assault. After
an assault, which is a traumatic event, your thoughts and beliefs about yourself and
the world can go through a drastic change. Often victims believe that the world is
entirely dangerous and that they are unworthy people who cannot cope. The goal of
this part of treatment is to help you evaluate your thoughts and beliefs about the world's
safety and about yourself, and to identify the unhelpful thoughts and beliefs that make
you feel distressed and prolong your PTSD symptoms.

Let's discuss an example. Before the assault, you may have felt that the world
was a safe place and that you were able to handle challenging situations. Many women
tell us that after an assault they feel anxious about, and afraid of, being alone at home,
going to work, going shopping, or being with a man. Have you had similar experiences? When you experienced these feelings, have you noticed what you were saying
to yourself? [Encourage the client to respond.]

After you have been assaulted, you may feel that the world is a dangerous place.
Let's imagine that there is a continuum of belief about the world's safety, with a belief
that the world is entirely safe on one end of the continuum and a belief that the world
is entirely dangerous on the other end. It is most reasonable to be somewhere in the
middle on this continuum, where you will have an appreciation of the need to ensure
safety but will not be unrealistic in judging the safety of such situations as going to
work, leaving your house, walking down the street, or spending time with people. In
reality, there are situations where you need to implement safety guidelines. There are
certain places or situations where you should not be alone or be trusting. For example,
a woman should not be walking alone late at night in a high-crime area. However,
this does not mean that the entire world is an unsafe place and that you cannot conduct your life with some sense of freedom and safety. After a traumatic event such as
rape or other assault, many women see the world as completely dangerous and begin
avoiding many safe situations and people. The belief that the world is a dangerous
place naturally leads to PTSD symptoms, such as general anxiety, hypervigilance, and
unnecessary avoidance of situations. Do you have the sense that a lot of situations are
not safe?

In addition to thinking that the world is a dangerous place, many assault survivors feel that they are "not in control" and think that they are incompetent and cannot cope with stress. For example, after an assault a woman who was able to handle

the daily demands of her children now finds that she is extremely irritable and unable to handle daily problems. This type of experience leads her to believe that she is unable to cope with normal demands, that she is not a good mother, or that she is losing control. These beliefs bring on an overall feeling of lack of control and incompetence. Also, there can be an increase in the feeling that the person is in constant danger. Do you experience similar thoughts about yourself? [Encourage the client to respond.]

Another common belief after a trauma is that the common reactions to trauma we have discussed before—such as intrusive recollections, flashbacks, and nightmares—are signs of going crazy, and this idea leads survivors to try to suppress recollections and thoughts about the trauma. Paradoxically, however, the more they try to push these thoughts away, the stronger the thoughts become, and the less control survivors have over them. In this way, attempts to suppress thoughts about the trauma actually increase the PTSD symptoms. Do you find yourself working hard *not* to think about your rape? [Encourage the client to respond.]

Inquire about the client's perceptions of the world (other people) and of herself before and after the assault. In particular, you should explore with the client how she coped with severe stress before the assault. Ask her which specific coping devices she used, and what beliefs she had during difficult and stressful times. Prior to the assault, did she have doubts about her abilities to manage such situations, or was she confident in her abilities to handle them? Did she perceive negative experiences with others as unusual, or did she believe that the world was unkind to her in general? Determine her beliefs.

Identifying and Challenging Negative Thoughts and Beliefs

Continue with the rationale for cognitive restructuring as follows:

The aim of cognitive restructuring is to identify, challenge, and modify the unhelpful thoughts and beliefs that cause you intense anxiety, guilt, anger, or sadness. Automatic thoughts occur automatically (hence the name) and are not deliberate thoughts. They are brief and discrete statements that people say to themselves. Automatic thoughts occur at or just below the threshold of our awareness. We are frequently unaware of the fact that we are having these thoughts; sometimes we are aware only of uncomfortable feelings that seem to come out of nowhere. Automatic thoughts reflect underlying beliefs, which are usually not conscious thoughts but influence us greatly.

The skill that you are going to learn in this part of the treatment program is to identify the negative thoughts and beliefs that are creating distress. This is because they may be interfering with your functioning. Most of the time these negative thoughts and beliefs are based on feelings, not on reality or fact. Negative thoughts can come into our minds so quickly that sometimes we aren't even aware that we are having them. When we realize something has "pushed our buttons" and we have overreacted, we have been responding to an automatic thought.

However, negative thoughts and beliefs are problematic because they lead to excessive or unrealistic negative emotions, such as anxiety, anger, guilt, or sadness. We would like to help you become aware of these distressing and uncomfortable thoughts and beliefs, and then consider whether they are helpful or not. We are going to work together on trying to identify your unhelpful thoughts and beliefs and then discuss them in a more objective way.

One way to become more objective is to pretend that we are scientists [you should determine whether the analogy of scientist, detective, or jury member in a court of law is the best] who develop hypotheses and collect evidence to negate or support these hypotheses. Therefore, as we investigate and look for evidence, we need to be objective and attempt to separate feelings from fact or reality. Let's look at a concrete example.

You and the client can now have a discussion like the following:

THERAPIST: The way a person thinks about or interprets events affects how she feels and behaves. For example, let's say you are home alone one night and you hear a loud noise in another room. If you think to yourself, "There's a burglar in the next room," how do you think you will feel?

CLIENT: Oh, very scared.

THERAPIST: And how might you behave?

CLIENT: I'd try to hide or call the police.

THERAPIST: OK, so in response to a loud, unexpected noise in the other room, you might think there was a burglar in the house and become very scared. You would naturally try to find a way to protect yourself. Now let's say that you heard the same noise and think, "Oh, what has that cat got into now?", or "I must have left the window open and the wind has knocked a plant over." How would you feel then?

CLIENT: Well, I might be startled, but I wouldn't be afraid. I might be upset if something valuable was broken, or annoyed that the cat had broken something.

THERAPIST: And what might you do in this instance?

CLIENT: Well, I would go see what the matter was. I wouldn't call the police.

THERAPIST: Exactly. In this example, the exact same antecedent or trigger can lead to two totally different reactions: either fear and acting to protect yourself, or not feeling much of anything and going into the room. What this example illustrates is that there are usually a number of ways in which you can interpret a situation, and the way you interpret the situation affects your feelings and behavior. If we can teach you how to challenge and modify your negative beliefs and thoughts, we can help you change your behavior and feel less anxious. The goals are to help you become aware of the beliefs and thoughts that contribute to your PTSD symptoms.

This is not an easy task, because basically what you as the therapist are asking the client to do is to change the way she thinks. To do that, first you will have to identify all of the steps in her thinking, then identify where she has been unrealistic. We often use the analogy of learning to drive a car: When we first learn, we must concentrate on each step. After a while, we can be doing other things (e.g., talking to the kids, putting on lipstick!) and driving automatically. Our automatic driving habits are not necessarily all healthy (e.g., speeding, rolling through stop signs, or applying makeup on the Interstate), but at this point we hardly give them any thought. If one aspect of how we drive is changed (e.g., learning to drive a manual transmission), we will have to break the process down into all of its component steps and change the ones necessary to make the major change. Eventually, after much practice, the new way becomes automatic. The same process applies to a client's thinking.

Identifying "Trigger" Situations, Emotions, and Negative Thoughts or Beliefs

Having thus presented the rationale for cognitive restructuring to the client, you can proceed with the first few steps of the actual restructuring process — that is, identifying situations (or thoughts about or recollections of situations) that lead to unpleasant emotions; identifying these emotions themselves; and identifying the negative automatic thoughts or the beliefs that precede and cause the emotions. Use the Daily Diary (Figure 11.1) to demonstrate these steps of the cognitive restructuring procedure. Give one copy of this form to the client and have one copy for yourself, and work together with the client. Together you will fill out the first three sections of the form: the situation or the occasion; the emotions she felt, and their intensity (on a 0–100 scale); and the associated negative thoughts or beliefs, and the strength of the belief (on a 0–100 scale). Then, you and your client write down in the proper column information that supports and negates the belief. Finally, you and your client write down the rational belief and degree to which she believes it (on a scale of 0–100).

It is helpful to begin teaching these steps of cognitive restructuring with a non-assault-related example before you proceed to an assault-related example. Ask for examples of situations in which the client's negative thinking led to distressing feelings and avoidance behaviors. During the pretreatment assessment, and during treatment to this point, the client will have reported various troublesome thoughts, emotions, and situations; use this information at this point, as needed. Emphasize that the client should relate all thoughts that pop into her mind during a given situation.

Daily Diary

1. Situation	3. Unhelpful Thoughts or Beliefs	4. Challenge to Negative Thoughts or Beliefs	5. Rational Response
Describe: a. Actual event leading to unpleasant emotion(s) or b. Thoughts or recollections leading to unpleasant emotion(s)	a. Write automatic thought(s) that preceded emotion(s)/ belief(s) that preceded emotion(s). b. Rate belief in automatic thought(s) (0–100).	Ask yourself questions to challenge each negative thought/belief. For instance, list evidence for and against the thought here.	a. Write rational response to thought(s) or belief(s). b. Rate belief in rational response (0–100).

Shopping in mall and saw man that reminded me of the person who attacked me
 	
2. Emotions
a. Circle emotions that you felt
b. Rate intensity of each emotion
 	
                Intensity
                (0–100)
(Fear/anxiety) <u>85</u>
Sadness   —
(Anger)   <u>10</u>
Guilt   —
Shame   —
	He's going to attack me
	75–90
		Evidence for:
		• *he's dressed like the person who attacked me*
		• *he's about the same age and race as attacker*
		• *he reminds me of attacker*
		Evidence against:
		• *I'm in a mall*
		• *I wasn't attacked in a mall*
		• *There are lots of other people around*
		• *I was attacked in a deserted place*
		• *There will be lots of help here if I needed it*
		• *Just because he looks like the attacker it doesn't mean he's dangerous*
		• *He's with a girl; my attacker was alone*
			Just because someone reminds me of my attacker, it doesn't mean he's going to hurt me; I'm not in danger here
			               85

FIGURE 11.1. Daily Diary.

The following are examples of non-assault-related and assault-related situations that often lead to distressing feelings and negative automatic thoughts:

Non-Assault-Related Examples
- A coworker's not saying hello in the morning
- Going for a job interview
- Getting a parking ticket

Assault-Related Examples
- Going out on a date
- Going to the grocery store at night
- Having an argument with a friend or significant other
- Talking with a man

Three Points about Automatic Thoughts

Make the following three points about automatic thoughts to your client:

First, automatic thoughts occur automatically (hence the name) and are not intentional. Instead, they are brief, discrete statements that people say to themselves. The result of these statements can be distress. Sometimes people are not even aware that they are having these thoughts or the uncomfortable emotions the thoughts produce.

Second, the fact that people have these thoughts does not mean that they are true. For example, a person may have the thought "The world is flat," but this does not mean that it is *really* flat.

Finally, negative thoughts are often difficult to identify because they are habitual and rapid. Your troublesome thoughts of the assault play a major role in the emotions that you are experiencing. The thoughts that are associated with the assault can be embarrassing or can produce guilt feelings. It may be difficult for you to discuss these thoughts. You may feel that the only way to cope with these distressing thoughts is to avoid thinking about them and distracting yourself. But in order for you to be able to challenge and evaluate these thoughts, you have to take a good long look at them. I know this may be difficult, but we will work together on this.

Helpful Ways to Elicit Negative Thoughts or Beliefs from the Clients

If the client is having difficulty identifying negative thoughts, ask her to recall the most recent situation in which she experienced anxiety or otherwise felt worse than she needed to feel. Then ask her to verbalize what the trigger was (situation), how she was feeling (emotions), and what she was thinking (negative thoughts). The following questions may also help to elicit these thoughts:

1. "What thoughts come to your mind and seem to be troublesome for you?"
2. "Was there something specific that happened recently that caused you some distress?"
3. "What was going through your mind in that situation?"
4. "What were you saying to yourself?"
5. "What was on your mind at that time?"
6. "Are you aware of what you are thinking right now?"
7. "Often when people are upset, they are saying something negative to themselves. Were you aware of what you were saying to yourself at that time?"

Finally, a client may be able to recognize and verbalize a negative automatic thought that was within her conscious awareness in a given situation, but may not be able to go beyond this to identify additional thoughts or beliefs that were also present in the situation but were just below the level of her conscious awareness. To use the example given earlier in the "Overview of Steps for Teaching Cognitive Restructuring," a client who noticed a man looking at her in a shopping mall may be able to identify the thought "He is looking at me in a funny way," but may not be able to get past this point. In such a case, additional questioning may be necessary to elicit one or more further thoughts or beliefs of which the client may not have been consciously aware — in this example, "He is going to hurt me."

Challenging and Modifying Negative Thoughts or Beliefs

After the client has identified a number of negative thoughts, you begin to teach her how to challenge these thoughts or beliefs and replace them with more helpful, rational ones. This is accomplished by asking a series of questions about the meaning and the accuracy or validity of these thoughts. Because it is often difficult for the client to come up with rational responses to negative thoughts, you can facilitate this process by asking questions that challenge the accuracy of the dysfunctional thoughts. The client's answers to these questions will help her to arrive at rational responses. We refer to this type of questioning as the "Socratic method."

Point out to the client that this process is not the same as "the power of positive thinking." The purpose is not to trade negative thoughts for positive ones. Rather, the goal of challenging negative thoughts or beliefs is to recognize the errors in one's logic and thinking that cause distress. These errors need to be corrected and exchanged for beliefs that are more objective and reasonable, and that reflect reality more accurately. This process should result in the attenuation of the client's negative emotions.

Following a general discussion of this process, provide an example to demonstrate the procedure. Begin by eliciting a situation and a list of the negative emotions that are likely to arise. Ask the client to generate potential thoughts during the session, and to note these down on a Daily Diary form. Next, use the list of questions given below to challenge her negative thoughts, and help her to arrive at a rational response for each of her negative thoughts. Finally evaluate the degree of the client's belief for each negative thought and each rational response, and evaluate the resulting emotions. Ask the client to note her challenges and rational responses in Sections 4 and 5, respectively, of the Daily Diary.

Questions That Help Challenge Negative Automatic Thoughts

Help the client to examine the accuracy of her negative thoughts by asking her the following questions, and having her choose the most appropriate ones. The bracketed words and phrases are the ones the client will use when she asks herself these questions on later occasions.

1. "What evidence do you [I] have for this thought?"
2. "Is there any alternative way of looking at the situation?"
3. "Is there any alternative explanation?"
4. "How would someone else think about the situation?"
5. "Are your [my] judgments based on how you [I] feel rather than what you [I] are [am] doing or have done?"
6. "Are you [Am I] setting for yourself [myself] an unrealistic and unobtainable standard?"
7. "Are you [Am I] overestimating how much control and responsibility you [I] have in this situation?"
8. "What would be the worst thing that could happen?"
9. "If this is true, what does it mean, or so what?"
10. "How will things look, seem, or work in ____ months?"
11. "What are the real and probable consequences of the situation?"
12. "Are you [Am I] underestimating what you [I] can do to deal with the problem or situation?"
13. "Are you [Am I] confusing a low-probability event with one of high probability?"
14. "What are the advantages of holding on to this belief?"
15. "What are the disadvantages of holding on to this belief?"

The goal of examining negative thoughts in this manner is to help the client think and react more objectively, to respond logically rather than emotionally. Common cognitive errors include assuming danger when none is present, feeling degraded and/or guilty because one has been raped, assuming all men are rapists, thinking people cannot be trusted, and feeling rejected easily. To really change one's thinking is a slow process. Emphasize that work during the therapy sessions is just the beginning for the client; she must practice this disciplined type of thinking at every opportunity. If she does so, the new thinking habits will become automatic, and she should feel much more emotionally stable.

Case Example: Identifying, Challenging, and Modifying Negative Thoughts

We now present a case example that illustrates the full process of identifying, challenging, and modifying negative thoughts and beliefs. Note especially the therapist's use in this example of what we have referred to as the Socratic method of questioning, in order to help the client examine the accuracy of her negative thoughts.

THERAPIST: You mentioned that recently you became frightened while shopping. Why don't we use that situation and see how your thoughts were influencing you? Please tell me more about that shopping trip.

CLIENT: OK. I had a few errands to run, and then I needed to go to the grocery store. I had picked up my shoes and was going towards the drugstore. Then I saw him and panicked.

THERAPIST: Who did you see?

CLIENT: I saw a young guy who looked like the one who raped me. I froze, then I ducked into the closest shop and didn't want to come out. It was all I could do to get home after that.

THERAPIST: Was it the man who attacked you?

CLIENT: No, it wasn't him. But he kind of looked like him, was dressed the same kind of way, was about the same age.

THERAPIST: OK, so in response to seeing a man who resembled the assailant, you felt panicked, froze in fear, hid in a store, then avoided the rest of your plans and went home, right? Seeing the man was the trigger. (*Therapist and client write this down under "Situation," and continue to fill in the Daily Diary.*) What emotions did you experience during the shopping? (*Therapist and client write "Fear."*) How strong was the fear? (*They write "80."*) Now let's look at the thoughts that brought out such a strong fear. What were your thoughts?

CLIENT: I don't think I thought anything. I just got scared.

THERAPIST: Let's see. What was bad about seeing that guy that reminded you of the assailant?

CLIENT: I just figured I'd better get out of there.

THERAPIST: Why?

CLIENT: He might see me.

THERAPIST: Why would it be bad if he saw you?

CLIENT: He might hurt me.

THERAPIST: So what thoughts were you responding to?

CLIENT: "I'm in trouble. I'm in danger. I need help."

THERAPIST: Good. Not good that you thought that, but good now that you figured it out. So you see a guy that looked similar to the assailant, and you respond as if *he* is an assailant, poised to attack you, and you're in danger; you responded accordingly. If you really were in danger, you responded as one would expect: You got scared and froze, and acted to try to protect yourself by ducking into the store and then going home. But let's look at the evidence and see if you really *were* in danger or just *thought* you were in danger. What's your evidence that you really were in danger and should have acted to protect yourself?

CLIENT: He looked kind of like the guy that attacked me. He was the same race, around the same age, and was dressed kind of the same — in jeans and fancy tennis shoes.

THERAPIST: Anything else?

CLIENT: I guess that's it.

THERAPIST: OK, what is the evidence that you were not in danger? Is there anything that was different about that guy from the one who attacked you?

CLIENT: Well, this guy was with a girl, and he was talking and laughing with her. And we were in a busy mall in the middle of the day. The guy who attacked me snuck up behind me when I left work at night, where there wasn't anyone else around, and he was alone.

THERAPIST: Any other evidence that you were *not* in danger?

CLIENT: There were people around and stores open. And I don't think he saw me. I saw him first. And I guess a guy is probably less likely to attack someone when he's with a girl.

THERAPIST: Good. So what do you think a court of law is going to decide? Should you have been responding as if you were in danger?

CLIENT: I guess not. It just scared me.

THERAPIST: Right. Insufficient evidence! Throw it out! It's important to see where that fear came from and to understand it, but it's also important for us to be able to decide objectively if we're in danger, not just to assume we're in danger because we feel scared. In this case, you saw someone that reminded you of the assailant, and you responded as if *he* were an assailant ready to attack you. But when you look at it objectively, you see that we shouldn't assume that this guy you saw in the mall is guilty just because he resembles someone who is. Can you see that now? And how much do you believe that you were in danger?

CLIENT: Less than 5, or even 0. It makes sense now. But what about when I get scared?

THERAPIST: You're going to have to exercise at first to practice thinking like this. When you get scared, instead of letting that be a sign to run, maybe you can let it be a sign to try to evaluate the situation objectively. In this case, maybe when you ducked into the store, you could have thought about it the way we are doing now. What do you think would have happened if you'd been able to do this in your head then?

CLIENT: I probably would have realized I didn't need to get so scared, and would have finished my shopping.

THERAPIST: Right. And over time, you can move this thinking process up, so then as soon as something scares you, you can think about it objectively. And eventually, this can be your new way of thinking, and maybe you won't feel scared as much as you have been. So what is your rational response?

CLIENT: Not all men who are similar to the guy who raped me are dangerous. I need to evaluate each situation separately.

THERAPIST: How much do you believe in it? What's your belief rating?

CLIENT: I'd give it 100.

This is a typical example for several reasons. First, the client was not able to identify any thoughts at first on her own. Second, it was an example of assuming danger in a realistically safe situation. And, third, the client did not appear 100% convinced that she could challenge and modify her negative thoughts when she became frightened. This is why we demonstrate the technique first with a non-assault-related example. The closer an issue gets to "home," as it did in this example, the more difficult it is for the client to evaluate objectively.

Using the Daily Diary as Homework

Instruct the client to use the Daily Diary as homework during the following week:

You have now begun learning how to identify, and challenge, and modify your distressing feelings and thoughts. Over the next few days, until we meet again, I would like you to use the Daily Diary form to record some of the situations, thoughts, and feelings that you experience (positive or negative, but especially negative). Try to use the Daily Diary at least three times a day between now and our next session.

Work through one more example during the session to make sure that the client understands the Daily Diary monitoring technique. Instruct the client to bring the filled-out Daily Diary form to the next session. Each session you are working on cognitive restructuring, review the client's Daily Diary and work with her through the examples she has brought to the session. Highlight target areas of difficulty for additional work (e.g., difficulty identifying negative thoughts, reluctance to use this format to record thoughts and feelings). Use these examples to teach her how to dispute her negative thoughts.

Common Cognitive Distortions

In order to facilitate the process of challenging negative thoughts, and also to prepare the client to examine the broad dysfunctional beliefs that underlie these thoughts (see below), present the client with the Common Cognitive Distortions handout (Figure 11.2) and discuss it with her. "Cognitive distortions," as described by Burns (1980), are patterns of dysfunctional thinking that lead to faulty interpretations of situations and thus to negative emotions. The discussion should be interactive, and should be introduced as follows:

"Cognitive distortions" are errors in logic or thinking that result in negative beliefs and thoughts, which in turn trigger negative emotions. I'm going to review with you a handout listing common cognitive distortions that people make. I'd like you to think about these cognitive distortions and let's see if you can identify which of them you use often.

After you have explained the concept of cognitive distortions and gone over the handout with the client, instruct the client to use the handout for homework as follows:

I would like you to read the Common Cognitive Distortions handout several times, until you become familiar with it. I would also like you to use it to identify times when you find yourself making these distortions. As you are filling out the "Challenges to Negative Thoughts" section of the Daily Diary, make a note about which type of cognitive distortion each of your negative thoughts represents.

Identifying and Challenging Dysfunctional (Unhelpful) Assumptions

Once the client has become adept at identifying the negative thoughts that come automatically to her, cognitive restructuring deals with the underlying, more general dysfunctional beliefs. The two broadest dysfunctional beliefs held by rape survivors with PTSD are that the world is unsafe and that they are unable

Common Cognitive Distortions

1. *All-or-nothing thinking.* You believe that the world is black or white, right or wrong, all or nothing. For example if something you do is not totally perfect, you see yourself as a failure. Another example may be that you see the world as either completely safe or totally dangerous. Are you aware of all-or-nothing thinking?

2. *Overgeneralization.* You see a single negative event as proof that negative events will keep happening to you. Perhaps you arbitrarily conclude that the one negative event means something negative about you—for example, "I am going to be raped again," or "Bad things keep happening to me, so I must be a bad person." Do you tend to overgeneralize? Do you have a personal example?

3. *"Must," "should," or "never" statements.* These are inflexible rules for your behavior that you learned when you were growing up, or are expectations that you must live up to. These distortions can create feelings of discomfort, anxiety, fear, sadness, or anger. Some examples are "I should be able to handle this," or "I never should have fought back," or "I must not lose control of myself." Can you think of any "must," "should," or "never" statements that you say to yourself?

4. *Catastrophizing.* This happens when you focus on the most extreme negative consequences of a given situation. You begin to expect disasters to happen; this leads to heightened fear and anxiety. Most instances of catastrophizing are triggered by "what if" thoughts, such as "What if I were in the bathroom and someone came in?" or "What if I were being followed by the man in the grocery store?" Examples of this are as follows: "If this light doesn't turn green, I am going to go crazy and lose control," or "If this man doesn't stop following me, I am going to be assaulted." Can you think of any catastrophizing statements that you say to yourself?

5. *Emotional reasoning.* This type of distortion arises when what you feel determines what you think. Although it is important to pay attention to how you feel, your feelings can lie to you. In fact, if you are anxious most of the time, you can be pretty sure that your feelings are lying to you. Examples of emotional reasoning include the following: "I am very nervous around men; therefore, they must want to hurt me," or "I feel very anxious in this situation; therefore, I am going to go crazy and lose control," or "I feel panic, so the world must be dangerous." Can you think of an example of this in your own life?

FIGURE 11.2. Common Cognitive Distortions handout.

to cope with stress and with their symptoms. Other typical underlying beliefs in such cases include the following:

1. "I must be a bad person, or this wouldn't have happened to me."
2. "I can't trust anybody."
3. "The world is dangerous."
4. "I am vulnerable."
5. "I am helpless."
6. "I have to be in control at all times."
7. "No one is trustworthy."

Methods of Eliciting Dysfunctional Beliefs

There are several methods of eliciting dysfunctional beliefs from the client. You can do this by examining the Daily Diary and identifying recurrent themes. Alternatively, the "downward-arrow technique" can be used (Burns, 1980). The downward-arrow technique consists of asking the following question about a negative thought in a repetitive fashion: "If this were true, what would it mean to me?" After several repetitions, the client should be able to identify the underlying belief of the negative automatic thought.

As Clark (1989) suggests, you can also direct the client to ask questions like the following, and then respond until she discovers the underlying belief:

1. If this thought were true, what would that mean to me?
2. What does that say about me?
3. What would happen then?
4. What would be so bad about that?

Case Example: Identifying and Challenging Broad Beliefs

A case example is presented here to illustrate the use of the Socratic method of questioning to challenge dysfunctional beliefs. The case example first illustrates how to assist a client who has difficulty identifying both thoughts and beliefs. Once both negative thoughts and beliefs have been identified, you will use the Socratic method of questioning to help the client to evaluate the accuracy of her thoughts and their underlying beliefs.

THERAPIST: You may recall that we discussed earlier how your negative thoughts/beliefs may influence your feelings and behaviors. What did you discover by recording your feelings and thoughts in the past few days?

CLIENT: I feel scared and anxious all the time, and I feel that something terrible is going to happen to me again.

THERAPIST: When you were feeling this way, what types of thoughts were you having?

CLIENT: I just felt scared and anxious. I didn't have any thoughts.

THERAPIST: OK, what I'd like to do is have you go back to this situation and imagine yourself at the mall. Tell me what was happening when you began to feel scared.

CLIENT: I was having difficulty breathing and my palms were sweaty, and I felt this overwhelming sense of fear, like something terrible was going to happen.

THERAPIST: So you were saying to yourself, "Something terrible is going to happen." Would you like to work on that thought, because it makes you feel so uncomfortable?

CLIENT: Well, I guess it would be a good idea, since it does make me feel upset when I think that.

THERAPIST: So you are saying that when you were in the mall, you felt that something terrible was going to happen to you. Can you tell me more about that?

CLIENT: I saw a man who looked like the guy who raped me, and all I could think of was that it was not safe there. I ran out of the mall and went home.

THERAPIST: Do you have that feeling about not being safe in other public places?

CLIENT: Yes. That's why I am not going any place alone any more.

When you reach this stage with your own client, use the Daily Diary and write down the client's emotions and thoughts. Use these to determine the client's underlying dysfunctional beliefs. Then, together with your client, evaluate each belief.

As noted earlier, the first step we take in using the Socratic method is to look for the evidence that supports, or does not support, a negative belief. In the present example, what is the evidence that the client is not safe in public places? Obtain a list of reasons that do or do not support the belief.

THERAPIST: It looks as if the negative belief behind your emotions and thoughts is "I am not safe in public places." What evidence can you think of for this belief?

CLIENT: Well, I was abducted in a public parking lot.

THERAPIST: OK, we'll write that down. What other evidence do we have?

CLIENT: I feel scared in public places.

THERAPIST: Now that's a feeling, a very uncomfortable feeling, but does it support your belief that you are not safe in public places? What type of cognitive distortion is that?

CLIENT: That's emotional reasoning, I guess. Well, I hear about other women who get kidnapped on the news or read about it in the paper.

THERAPIST: That's right. But your last statement also sounded like a distortion in logic. Let's use that statement later. For now, I want to focus on your belief that you are not safe in *all* public places. OK, any more evidence to support this belief?

CLIENT: No.

THERAPIST: Is there any evidence to refute or challenge this belief?

CLIENT: There isn't any.

THERAPIST: OK, how long have you been parking in various public parking lots?

CLIENT: Well, I've been driving since I was 16. About 20 years.

THERAPIST: In those 20 years, how many times have you been abducted in a parking lot?

CLIENT: Well, this was the first time, but once is enough.

THERAPIST: OK, so would you agree that being assaulted in public places is a low-frequency event?

CLIENT: Yes, I guess so, but it doesn't make me feel any safer.

THERAPIST: How about looking at your Common Cognitive Distortions handout to identify the type of automatic thoughts and dysfunctional belief you are having?

CLIENT: I guess they would fall into the category of emotional reasoning.

THERAPIST: Good. That's right. It seems like you are getting a sense of how to question your thoughts and beliefs. Would you like to try to come up with a rational response or new belief, based on the evidence that we have reviewed?

CLIENT: Well, I'll give it a try. I'm probably not going to be very good at that.

THERAPIST: What's the evidence that you are not very good at this?

CLIENT: (*Laughs*) Boy, I really have to watch what I say in here.

THERAPIST: This is a new skill that you are learning, and I think you are doing a good job. Shall we get back to looking for a rational belief?

CLIENT: OK. I may feel anxious in public places now because of my rape, but not all public places are dangerous. Besides, I have my Mace with me now.

THERAPIST: Very good. To what degree do you believe this new belief?

CLIENT: I'd give it a 50.

THERAPIST: OK. What is the other 50 due to?

CLIENT: I'm so scared to go places, because in every public place there is a chance that I could be hurt.

THERAPIST: What does that mean to you?

CLIENT: People can't be trusted. No place is safe.

THERAPIST: Do you remember our discussion about how your views of the world and of your ability to cope change after a traumatic event?

CLIENT: Yes.

THERAPIST: Will you summarize this for us? We have reviewed the evidence to support your belief that you are not safe in public places. Have we come up with more evidence to refute the belief or to support it?

CLIENT: I don't know. Intellectually, I believe that it is not very dangerous to be in the parking lot. But emotionally, I'm still scared and feel anxious just talking about it.

THERAPIST: Let's look at your *in vivo* exposure homework from last week. Last week you said that you went to the grocery store; you drove to and from work without keeping your Mace on your lap; and you went out to lunch with a friend. Did anyone approach you or try to hurt you in any way during these excursions?

CLIENT: No. You're right. I guess that every public place isn't very dangerous. It is just a feeling that I have because of what I have been through. I'm

36 years old, and this is the first time that I have been assaulted. I guess that's a pretty low-frequency event.

THERAPIST: Exactly. This is one reason why you are learning you this skill—so you can come up with objective evidence instead of basing your decisions on how you are feeling. It would be just as inaccurate to say that the world is completely safe as it is to say that the world is completely dangerous. Part of our work here is to help you identify and challenge some of your beliefs about yourself and the world that contribute to your feeling anxious and that interfere with your life.

12

Cognitive Techniques II: Thought Stopping and Guided Self-Dialogue

As we have noted in Chapter 6, there is no empirical evidence that thought stopping and guided self-dialogue actually are effective with PTSD. However, they have been used in stress inoculation training (SIT) for rape victims. Therefore, for the sake of completeness, we describe them in this chapter of the book.

Thought Stopping

The thought-stopping technique (Wolpe, 1958) is used to terminate ruminative or obsessive thinking related to the assault. It is basically a distraction technique. For example, one client who was assaulted (described by Veronen & Kilpatrick, 1983) avoided taking a shower because she couldn't hear anything when the water was running. Her ruminative thinking proceeded along the following lines: "Was that a noise that I heard? Someone could be breaking in and I can't hear him. I know someone will be waiting for me when I step out of the shower." If her husband was home, she would continue by thinking, "Someone is holding Ted at gunpoint. I know that he is going to get me."

On the surface, the thought-stopping technique is incompatible with the theoretical concepts underlying imaginal exposure. As noted earlier in Chapter 5, we presume that attempts to suppress intrusive thoughts about the assault paradoxically increase the power of such thoughts, whereas deliberately and repeatedly engaging in these thoughts results in reduction of the distress associated with them and ultimately reduces their frequency.

The aim of teaching the thought-stopping technique is to give the client a technique she can use whenever a distressing thought appears at a time when imaginal exposure cannot be employed, such as in the middle of a meeting with the boss. It can also be used when she is not engaging in constructive exposure about the assault, but rather is scaring herself needlessly. For example, once she has objectively decided that it is OK to go grocery shopping, it only makes her more anxious to keep thinking that she may be in danger. In this case, she would do much better to think distracting thoughts. Thought stopping is intended for obsessions, ruminations, "crying over spilt milk," or "spinning the wheels"—types of thinking that do nothing except distress people. Often if individuals have a problem, it may be upsetting to think about it, but they must think about it if they want to solve it. Thought stopping is not intended for this type of problem-solving thinking, even though it may be distressing. However, thought stopping may be used if a person has gotten into an unproductive mode of thinking—for example, just looping around the same thought or a "woe is me" mode. In this case, it may be better to stop thinking about the problem at this point, but to come back to it at a later time when the person can think more constructively.

Overview of Steps for Teaching Thought Stopping

1. Demonstrate the thought-stopping technique to the client first.
2. Present a rationale for thought stopping to the client.
3. Begin teaching the technique with a non-assault-related example.
   a. The first time, shout "STOP!" yourself.
   b. The second time, shout "STOP!" yourself, but have the client use some imagery and distraction.
   c. The third time, have the client shout "STOP!" silently to herself.
   d. The fourth time, have the client stop her thinking herself while snapping a rubber band against her wrist.
4. Repeat the sequence in Step 3 with an assault-related example.
5. Assign daily practice of thought stopping for homework.

Demonstrating Thought Stopping

Thought stopping is taught by demonstrating how a loud noise can distract the client from upsetting thoughts and images that she is having. *Do not* present the rationale for thought stopping to the client until you demonstrate how the technique works.

Begin by giving the client the following information:

Today you are going to learn a coping skill to help you manage the troublesome thoughts that you are having on occasions that you cannot utilize exposure, such as when you are at work or with friends, or when you are scaring yourself needlessly. During our conversations, you have mentioned thoughts that have been upsetting you. Of those thoughts and images, which are the ones that are likely to occur in such situations?

Elicit a few distressing thoughts from the client. Then proceed as follows:

Now I would like you to close your eyes and focus on that thought. Let yourself get the thought clear in your mind. When you have that thought in your mind, raise your hand [index finger].

When the client indicates that she has the thought in her mind, shout "STOP!" and clap your hands or bang on the desk. When she opens her eyes and looks startled, ask her what happened. Say this to her:

I hope that you weren't too startled by the noise I just made. However, I needed to make a loud noise to demonstrate the effectiveness of this technique in jolting unwanted thoughts away. When you do this on your own later, I want you to mimic me when you shout "STOP!" in your head. It must be dramatic to really get rid of the thoughts, so remember how I shouted and banged.

Proceed to several trials of practice as described below. Eventually, the client will interrupt her own distressing thoughts by shouting "STOP!" to herself or lightly snapping a rubber band on her wrist. As always, assign daily practice of thought stopping at home for homework.

Presenting a Rationale for Thought Stopping

Present the rationale for thought stopping as follows:

We have discussed some of the thoughts that come into your mind uninvited and generate distressing emotions. We have suggested that trying to push them away, rather than confronting them, prevents you from processing the trauma and prolongs your symptoms. Therefore, we taught you how to use prolonged exposure when distressing thoughts enter your mind. However, there are circumstances where you cannot practice imaginal exposure, for example, when the thoughts enter your mind in the middle of a meeting or when you are scaring yourself needlessly. I will now teach you a technique called thought stopping to help stop these thoughts in these circumstances.

In a moment I will ask you to generate a distressing thought. I'd like you to let yourself get into it as much as possible. Then I will shout "STOP!" very loudly, and we'll take it from there.

Practicing Thought Stopping with the Client

1. Begin teaching the thought-stopping technique with a non-assault-related example. Tell your client that you will ask her to think an obsessive thought and then you will shout, "STOP!" Ask your client to close her eyes and deliberately think distressing or troublesome thoughts unrelated to the assault for 35–40 seconds. Try to encourage her to really get into obsessing about it. If she has a hard time coming up with something, you may want to inquire what she's been obsessing about lately. Has anything been running through her head persistently or keeping her up at night?

2. Shout "STOP!" in a loud and commanding voice, while at the same time you clap your hands or hit the desk. (Take care not to knock over cups of coffee or water!)

3. Ask your client what happened, and she will typically reply, "The thought is gone."

4. Repeat, but suggest that the client use some imagery and distraction. Many people like to picture a big red stop sign when they shout "STOP!" As the stop sign goes down, it pushes the "bad" thoughts away, leaving the distracting thought. Come up with what the client will use as distracting thoughts now, in the session. They can be anything, as long as they actively engage the client's thinking and do not cause distress. One client loved Broadway show tunes and would think of every word of every song in her favorite play as her distraction. Another client, a busy woman who enjoyed her work, would try to think of her appointments for the following day or week without her appointment book; she would often figure out what she would wear as well. A third client, who was well educated in English history, would review in her head all of the kings and queens and their years in power. When all else fails, reviewing a favorite song, movie, or book is a good choice. The client needs to decide what her distraction will be while she is there in your office. If, in the throes of obsessing, she is unable to come up with a distraction, this is like an invitation for the obsessions to return. She can change her distraction at a later time if she needs to, but she must always know immediately what she can turn her thinking to.

5. Again, repeat, but ask the client to stop her thinking herself by silently shouting the word "STOP!" Remind her to use the imagery and the distraction.

6. Repeat once more, with the client stopping her thinking herself as above, but suggest she place a rubber band around her wrist (we keep a good supply on hand to give out!). She should snap the rubber band lightly while silently shouting "STOP!" That often helps jolt the thought away, much as the startling effect of your shouting "STOP!" does. If she likes using it, suggest that she can wear the rubber band always, making sure it isn't too tight.

7. Now repeat the sequence for a rape-related example. Do this first with you shouting "STOP!", followed by the client'a shouting it silently in her head.

Guided Self-Dialogue

In Chapter 11, we have discussed at length how to go about identifying the client's negative thoughts, as well as her underlying dysfunctional beliefs. We have outlined a program that teaches the client how to evaluate the accuracy and usefulness of the identified negative thoughts and beliefs, and how to re-place these with more realistic and useful thoughts/beliefs. It is believed that cognitive restructuring eventually produces enduring shifts in the client's most basic dysfunctional beliefs. Consequently, she will be less inclined to interpret situations in a negative way, and will be less likely to have distressing emotions and irrational behaviors.

Another method of dealing with negative thoughts, called "guided self-dialogue," has been described by Meichenbaum (1974a, 1974b). In this tech-nique the therapist teaches the client to focus on her internal dialogue—that is, on the statements that she is saying to herself, her self-talk. The therapist assists the client to identify self-talk that is irrational, faulty, or negative, and to help her replace it with more task-enhancing and adaptive self-dialogue. State-ments and questions are generated for each of the following four categories:

- Preparing for a stressor
- Confronting and managing the stressor
- Coping with feelings of being overwhelmed
- Self-reinforcing for managing a stressor

The aims of guided self-dialogue are to help the client do the following:

- Determine what she is really afraid will happen.
- Assess the actual probability that something terrible will happen dur-ing the stressful situation.
- Manage overwhelming avoidance behaviors.
- Control self-criticism and self-devaluation.
- Engage in anxiety-provoking behaviors.
- Use coping self-statements.
- Use self-reinforcement for attempting the feared behavior (and for en-gaging in the guided self-dialogue procedure).

The questions and statements are tailored to the individual client and her areas of difficulty; however, some general sayings are provided in the Guided Self-Dialogue Examples handout (Figure 12.1). Encourage the client to add

Guided Self-Dialogue Examples

1. Preparing for a Stressor
- "What is it that I have to do?"
- "What am I scared of?"
- "What is the likelihood that anything bad will happen?"
- "How bad would it be if it really happened?"
- "Don't think about how bad I feel; think about what I can do about it."
- "Don't get caught up in myself. Thinking only about my feelings won't help me cope with the situation."
- "I have the support and encouragement of people who have experience in dealing with these things."
- "I have already come a long way toward handling the problem. I can handle the rest."

Here are my favorite questions and statements for preparing for a stressor: _____

_____

_____

2. Confronting and Managing the Stressor
- "I need to take one step at a time."
- "Don't think about how afraid or anxious I am; think about what I am doing."
- "The feeling that I am having now is a signal for me to use my coping exercises."
- "There is no need to doubt myself. I have the skills I need to get through this."
- "Focus on my plan. Relax and take a calming breath. I am ready to go."

Here are my favorite questions and statements for preparing for a stressor: _____

_____

_____

3. Coping with Feelings of Being Overwhelmed
- "When I feel afraid, I will take a breath and exhale slowly, saying to myself, 'calm.'"
- "Focus on what is happening now. What is it that I have to do?"
- "I can expect my fear to rise, but I can keep it manageable."
- "This fear may slow me down, but it will not stop me."
- "This event will pass, and it will be over soon."
- "I may feel scared and anxious, but I can do it."

Here are my favorite questions and statements for coping with feelings of being overwhelmed: _____

_____

4. Self-Reinforcing for Managing a Stressor
- "It was much easier than I thought."
- "I did it—I got through it. And each time will be easier."
- "When I manage my thoughts in my head, I can manage the feelings in my body."
- "I am making progress."
- "I did a good job."
- "One step at a time."

Here are my favorite questions and statements for preparing for a stressor: _____

_____

_____

FIGURE 12.1. Guided Self-Dialogue Examples handout.

further statements that she finds helpful, and to write these down on the hand-out. As the client becomes proficient with guided self-dialogue, teach her to use the technique to handle real-life problems and difficulties. Encourage her to memorize key self-statements to use in anxiety-provoking situations, and to carry them with her to use in such situations. Work with the client first on a non-assault-related example, and then proceed to an assault-related example.

Overview of Steps for Teaching Guided Self-Dialogue
1. Provide the client with the rationale for guided self-dialogue.
2. Discuss the four dialogue categories with the client.
3. Give the client the Guided Self-Dialogue Examples handout and a pencil. Elicit from the client any questions and statements that she wants to add to the ones in the handout, and eliminate any that she does not find helpful.
4. Apply the technique to a non-assault-related situation, working with the client to develop questions and statements for each of the four categories.
5. Apply the technique to an assault-related situation.

Presenting a Rationale for Guided Self-Dialogue

Give the client the following rationale for learning to use guided self-dialogue:

You have learned the coping skills of thought stopping and cognitive restructuring to help you manage distressing thoughts. Today I'm going to teach you another coping skill that will help you in managing thoughts and beliefs. This technique is called "guided self-dialogue." This skill focuses on your self-talk—that is, what you are tell-ing yourself—and will teach you to prepare and cope with difficult situations more easily. Very often, when something is coming up that stresses us, we can make it worse by what we are telling ourselves.

For example, if someone has a job interview coming up, at some level she may be telling herself, "They're going to laugh me out of there." This type of thought will make her even more nervous as it gets closer, and she may even cancel the interview. However, this type of thinking is not very realistic. In this example, it is unlikely that the person would have applied for the job unless she thought she could do it. And it is unlikely that the employer would have asked for an interview unless she looked like an appropriate candidate. So she may not get the job, but it is unlikely that they will laugh her out of there. By adjusting her self-talk, she will become less anxious about the interview, which also may help her come across more favorably. We will develop a list of questions and statements that will help you control your distress before and during stressful situations.

Discussing the Dialogue Categories and Using the Handout

Begin discussing the four dialogue categories with the client as follows:

There are four steps that you can take to manage your reactions in stressful situations. The first step is called "preparing for a stressor." In this situation, a question that you can ask yourself is "What is the likelihood that anything bad will happen? You should then try to determine, as accurately as possible, the actual probability that what you are scared of will occur. Then ask yourself, "How bad it would be if it really happened?" To answer this question, I often think in terms of a continuum of bad things from 0 to 100. I might give a rating of 0 to something like breaking a fingernail or mildly stubbing a toe; it's not great, but in the scheme of things it is insignificant. I might give a score of 100 to something like serious harm or death to myself or a loved one. I like both to weigh the probability of the bad thing, and to rate how bad it would be if it really happened.

It is also helpful to de-focus on your anxiety at this point. There are statements to try to help you do this. When we get into "woe is me" thinking, focusing on how bad we feel, mostly it just tends to make us feel worse and doesn't help in any way. For example, if you are getting ready for something you're very excited about and you stub your toe, you almost don't notice it. But if you've had a lousy day and are tired and depressed and stub your toe, you could almost sit down and cry about it. The actual pain is no worse in one situation or the other. Only your focus on it is different.

The second step is called "confronting and managing the stressor." Here, self-dialogue is helpful in managing the anxiety that you experience just before or at the beginning of the stressful situation. For example, you are sitting at home worrying about going to work that day. Quite often, your anticipatory anxiety is far worse than the anxiety that you experience once you have really gotten into a situation. These statements will help you manage your anxious thoughts. Very often, people react to anxiety with more anxiety; these statements (and this program in general) will try to let you use your anxiety as a cue to use coping strategies to manage it. For example, when you notice your heart racing, say to yourself that this is a cue to use your breathing technique to slow it down.

The third step is called "coping with feelings of being overwhelmed." We will help you develop statements for reducing this anxiety while you are in the stressful situation. An example of this would be self-dialogue to use when you have actually begun your work for the day and start to feel anxious and uncomfortable. We like for people to remind themselves that if they have *chosen* to be in a situation, that usually means they can handle it. We very rarely *choose* to put ourselves in situations we can't handle. [Note: Clients don't choose to be assaulted, even if they chose to be in the location where they were assaulted. Some clients may require some elaboration on this.] The situation may be challenging, but if we have decided to do something, we usually can.

The fourth step is called "self-reinforcing for managing a stressor." It's important to pat yourself on the back when you have done something that was stressful for you. Just as you would praise a child who had done something that was difficult for her no matter how she actually did, you deserve praise as well. What do you usually say to yourself when you've done well? [Encourage the client to respond.]

First, we'll work together on helping you develop some questions and statements that you can say to yourself during each of these four steps. We'll use a handout to help us with this. Next, we will focus on applying this skill to a non-assault-related situation. Then we will proceed to an assault-related example.

Let's go through the handout now to identify the statements that will be most helpful to you at each step. While we do this, I want you to feel free to add any self-dialogue that you already use to each list, or to develop new sayings. Also, if you dislike any of the statements on the handout, or feel they don't apply to you, scratch them out. Do you have any questions before we begin?

Now give the Guided Self-Dialogue Examples handout to the client and work through the examples. Discuss each statement and edit as necessary.

Applying the Technique to Stressful Situations

To demonstrate how to apply the guided self-dialogue technique to an actual stressful situation, begin by eliciting a non-assault-related example from your client. If she has difficulty coming up with a situation, the following list provides examples of situations you can use to illustrate steps in guided self-dialogue.

Examples of Non-Assault-Related Stressful Events
- Talking to a child's teacher at school
- Having the in-laws over for dinner
- Going for a job interview

After helping the client develop statements to cope with a non-assault-related situation, do the same with an assault-related situation.

Examples of Assault-Related Stressful Events
- Being alone at home
- Going to the mall alone
- Talking with people about the assault
- Going out on a date
- Going to the gynecologist for an annual exam
- Testifying against the assailant at trial

Case Example: Using Self-Guided Dialogue

Mary was experiencing anxiety and fear about returning to her workplace, because she had been assaulted after she left the office one night. She was having trouble concentrating, and repeatedly experienced distressing thoughts and images of the assault. These reactions contributed to her fears about losing control at work and making a fool of herself in front of her coworkers.

The following list provides the guided self-dialogue that Mary developed to assist her in this stressful situation. Mary selected some questions and statements from the handout that she found most helpful, and then added others of her own.

Stressful Situation: Returning to Work

1. Preparing for a Stressor
   - "What is the probability that I will lose control at work?" (Mary's response: "Very low. I've never lost control at work or anywhere else before.")
   - "Don't think about how bad I feel; think about what I can do about it."
   - "I have managed difficult situations in the past. I can get through this one."
2. Confronting and Handling a Stressor
   - "One step at a time; I can handle this."
   - "Relax. Focus on the plan."
   - "This is a cue for me to use my breathing and relaxation exercises."
3. Coping with Feelings of Being Overwhelmed
   - "I can expect my fear to increase, but I can keep it manageable."
   - "This anxiety will pass."
   - "I have worked here for a long time, and people have always been supportive and helpful."
   - "This is a cue for me to use the thought-stopping technique."
4. Self-Reinforcing for Managing a Stressor
   - "It was much easier than I thought to cope with this situation."
   - "I did a good job."
   - "I'm going to treat myself by buying a new pair of earrings."

13

Relaxation Training: Deep Muscle, Cue-Controlled, and Differential Relaxation

The aim of training the client in relaxation skills is to provide her with further means of alleviating her anxiety and fear. First you will teach her deep muscle relaxation (Bernstein & Borkovec, 1973), and then cue-controlled and differential relaxation. Because deep muscle relaxation is both the most basic and the most extensive of these relaxation techniques, and because a knowledge of this form of relaxation is essential to learning the other two techniques, we devote the bulk of this chapter to discussing deep muscle relaxation.

Overview of Steps for Teaching Relaxation Skills
1. Present a rationale for learning deep muscle relaxation.
2. In a properly equipped therapy room, prepare the client for deep muscle relaxation training.
3. Demonstrate the muscle groups to be relaxed and the order in which this is to be done, by engaging in the tension–relaxation procedure for each group along with the client.
4. Have the client do the breathing retraining exercise after the completion of each major muscle group (e.g., all neck muscles).
5. After the completion of tension and relaxation for all muscle groups, have the client engage in pleasant imagery.
6. Present a rationale for cue-controlled relaxation.
7. Have the client practice relaxing on cue.
8. Present a rationale for differential relaxation.
9. Have the client experiment with differential relaxation during various activities.

Deep Muscle Relaxation

During deep muscle relaxation, the client will learn to discriminate between tension and relaxation, and to associate a cue word (e.g., "relax," "calm," "peaceful") with the feeling of relaxation. The client will also incorporate the breathing retraining exercise (see Chapter 8) after relaxing each muscle group. After all muscle groups have been relaxed, you will instruct the client to imagine a pleasant scene. Emphasize the following important points when discussing the rationale for relaxation:

- Anxiety and tension are learned responses.
- Relaxation is a skill.
- To learn this skill, practice is required.
- During relaxation, it is normal to experience unusual physiological and psychological changes.
- Intrusive memories about the assault or other experiences may occur when the client is relaxing. Encourage her to let these thoughts drift away and refocus on the particular muscle group that is being relaxed.
- The client may experience a loss of control. Suggest that it is OK if she occasionally opens her eyes to orient herself to the surroundings, but she should immediately return to the state of relaxation.
- Choose a cue word that the client feels comfortable associating with relaxation.
- Incorporate slow breathing exercises and pleasant imagery into relaxation.

An audiotape will be made of the deep muscle relaxation session to aid her in relaxation at home.

Presenting a Rationale for Deep Muscle Relaxation

Give the client the following rationale for learning deep muscle relaxation:

Today you are going to learn a new skill to help you manage your anxiety and tension. This technique is called "deep muscle relaxation." You will learn to sequentially tense and relax various muscle groups in your body, while you pay attention to the feelings associated with tension and relaxation. In addition to learning how to relax, you will also learn how to recognize tension in your muscles. I am going to ask you to produce tension in your muscles and then release the tension all at once. This allows the muscles to become even more relaxed when you release this tension. It's like a pendulum: If you push it, it will go to the other side, but if you pull it back and then let it go, it goes over further. Also, in order to reduce the tension in your muscles, you must first no-tice it. By tensing and relaxing muscle groups, you will be able to notice the contrast between these two states and will be able to detect the early stages of tension when it is easier to do something about it.

Do you remember what it was like for you when you were first learning to ride a bike or drive a stick-shift car? It was difficult to remember when to do everything and in what order.

Use one of the following examples to illustrate that a very difficult task can become automatic with practice.

EXAMPLE 1: LEARNING TO DRIVE A STICK-SHIFT CAR

Remember when you were learning how to drive a stick-shift car? You had to say to yourself, "OK, my right foot is on the brake pedal, and my left foot is on the clutch. My left hand is on the wheel, and my right hand is moving the gear shift into first gear. Now to get the car moving, I have to take my right foot off the brake pedal and put it on the gas pedal, and so on."

EXAMPLE 2: LEARNING TO RIDE A BICYCLE

Remember when you were learning how to ride a bicycle? First you had to concen-trate on maintaining balance. You started by holding the handlebars of the bike with your hands; you had both feet on the ground on either side of the bike; and you sat on the seat of the bike. Then you had to tell yourself, while you continued to hold the handlebars, to lift your left foot up and place it on the left bike pedal, then to raise your right foot quickly and place it on the right pedal, and then to rotate the left pedal with your left foot while maintaining your balance on the bicycle, and so on.

Now continue with the rationale as follows:

You had to walk yourself through these steps very slowly. At first these new tasks didn't feel comfortable to you, and you might have felt that you could never learn to drive or ride a bike; but eventually with persistence and practice you mastered these skills, and you can probably do them now automatically. Relaxation is a skill that requires practice, as do other skills. You can know what to do, but you may not be any good at it unless you practice. If you practice every day, you will find that you are able to relax very easily and almost automatically when you say the word "relax" or "calm" to yourself.

When you are relaxing or tensing, you may experience some unusual feelings such as a floating sensation, heat in your muscles, tingling in your fingers, or very heavy muscles and limbs. These are signs that your body is beginning to relax and your muscles are loosening up. It is also important that you go with the process, and that you do not fight what your body may be feeling. However, sometimes it happens that women who have been assaulted have intrusive thoughts when they are relaxing. If this happens to you, try to keep your eyes closed, let the thoughts pass through your mind, and refocus on the muscle group you are tensing and relaxing. If you are feeling too distressed, open your eyes to orient yourself, and then close your eyes again when you are feeling more comfortable.

Preparing for Deep Muscle Relaxation Training

In preparation for deep muscle relaxation training, first check on the physical setting of the therapy room:

1. The noise level should be low.
2. The illumination in the room should be dim, although not dark.
3. A comfortable chair should be available for the client.
4. A tape recorder should be available for recording the session. (Remember, the tape recorder should have a cassette in it!)

Relaxation can be more easily achieved with closed eyes. However, if the client refuses to close her eyes, allow her to begin deep muscle relaxation training with her eyes open. Tell the client to find a quiet place for practicing deep muscle relaxation at home. Optimal times during the day to practice are in the morning before getting out of bed, in the afternoon or upon return from work, in the early evening while relaxing after supper, or at bedtime. Initially your client should be discouraged from listening to the relaxation tape before bedtime, since she may fall asleep and fail to learn deep muscle relaxation skills. Once she has learned to relax, she can use this as a strategy to facilitate sleep.

Inform the client that she will be relaxing a number of muscle groups in her face, neck, shoulders, arms, hands, legs, and toes. Before you begin the training, it is important for you to inquire whether she has any injuries, whether she cramps easily, or whether she wears contact lenses. If she has injuries, suggest that she try to relax the injured muscles without doing any tensing. If she cramps easily (usually in the feet or lower leg), tell her to cease tensing if she feels a cramp beginning. Instruct her to focus on the muscles and allow them to go limp and relaxed. If the client wears contact lenses, she may wish to remove them or open her eyes once in a while to relieve any discomfort. Finally, you should ask whether the client has certain muscles in her body that feel particularly tense (e.g., back, shoulders, neck, or jaw). Extra attention can be directed to these muscle groups during training.

Before demonstrating the muscle groups that will be tensed and relaxed, tell the client that it is important that she does not strain her muscles during the exercise. Instruct her to tense *only* the muscle group being focused on at each step; in addition, tell her to tense her muscles so that she feels the tension, but does not strain the muscle. Each muscle group will be tensed and relaxed twice. Finally, remind the client that you will be audiotaping the session so she can take the tape home for practice; this also means that she does not have to memorize what you're doing—just enjoy it.

Demonstrating the Tension–Relaxation Procedure for Each Muscle Group

Next, demonstrate the muscles to be relaxed, explaining each movement verbally and illustrating it with your body. First, say this to the client:

I am going to show you the muscle groups that you are going to be tensing and relaxing. Sometimes people feel uncomfortable about these exercises, especially when they are doing the face exercises, because they are afraid they look strange or funny. I am going to be doing the exercises right along with you, so we can look funny together.

Now proceed through the muscle groups in order, demonstrating tension and relaxation for each group. (See Table 13.1 for a list of muscle groups.) Begin as follows:

Just allow yourself to relax as much as you would like, and focus on each muscle group as we proceed. Now focus your attention on your right fist. Clench your right fist. *Hold it* [use a firm and moderately loud, but not aversive, voice with the client], feeling the tension—hold it, hold it—and *Relax* [say this with a soothing voice]. Let go further and further, noticing the difference between tensing and relaxing, allowing all of the tension to flow out of these muscles, as if it's flowing out of your fingertips. Say to yourself the word "calm" or "relax." Now let's do that again. Repeat, and then continue with other muscle groups.]

Allow about 10 seconds for the tension phase and 30 seconds for the relaxation phase for each muscle group. After each major muscle group has been completed (e.g., all neck muscles), instruct the client to use the breathing retraining exercise (see Chapter 8) to deepen the state of relaxation. As the speech above suggests, it is helpful to make statements during the relaxation phase to encourage the client to relax, such as the following:

- "Allow your muscles to relax."
- "Let go further and further."
- "Notice the difference between tensing and relaxing."
- "Say the world 'calm' [or 'relax,' or whatever the client's cue word is] to yourself."
- "Let yourself relax as much as you feel comfortable."
- "This is your time to relax. You will not be hurried."

TABLE 13.1. List of Muscle Groups for Deep Muscle Relaxation

- Clench fists.
- Bend hands backward at wrists.
- Flex biceps muscles.
- Push shoulders back into chair.
- Hunch shoulders up toward ears.
- Tilt head to left shoulder.
- Tilt head to right shoulder.
- With head down, tuck chin toward chest.
- Press head back against chair.
- Breathe air in deeply through lungs, and hold for a few seconds.
- Tense stomach by contracting muscles as if hit in stomach.
- Wrinkle up forehead and brow.
- Close eyes tightly.
- Open mouth wide.
- Purse lips.
- Bear down slightly on back teeth.
- Tense buttocks.
- Arch back.
- Stretch out right leg and bend toes back.
- Stretch out left leg and bend toes back.
- Stretch out right leg and point toes away from body.
- Stretch our left leg and point toes away from body.
- Curl up toes in shoes.

Adding Pleasant Imagery

After you have completed the tension–relaxation procedure for all muscle groups, ask the client to describe a scene that she finds very pleasant, using the following questions:

- "Can you think of a scene that is particularly pleasant for you to imagine?"
- "Can you describe that scene to me?"

You can offer the client examples if she has difficulty coming up with a pleasant scene—for example, walking or sitting on a beach, sitting in front of a roaring fire, walking through the woods, or listening to music. Once the client has selected a scene, continue as follows:

Please imagine this scene as vividly as possible, bringing in the smells, sounds, colors, and textures that are around you as you imagine it. I want you to stay with that image in your private sanctuary and allow your muscles to go limp and relax. I will ask you to breathe slowly until I speak to you again. This is your time to relax. You will not be hurried. I want you to keep your eyes closed and imagine your pleasant scene. Go to that private sanctuary and see the colors around you, inhale the pleasant scents, listen to the sounds, and relax, further and further. [Pause for 3–5 minutes.] In a moment, I will count backward from 4 to 1. On the count of 4, I'd like you to move your legs and your feet. On the count of 3, move your arms and your hands. On the count of 2, move your head and your neck, and on the count of 1, open your eyes, feeling refreshed and relaxed. Take your time opening your eyes. You have been relaxing, and there is no need to rush.

When the client opens her eyes after imagining the pleasant scene, ask her for her feedback. How did she like it? Did she have any difficulty with any of the muscle groups? Offer her encouragement for completing the exercise.

Cue-Controlled Relaxation

The goal of cue-controlled relaxation is to teach the client to identify tension in her body and to use it as a cue for implementing breathing exercises and relaxation. You should again review breathing retraining with the client, and tell her that this skill can be used for tension in daily stressful situations.

Presenting a Rationale for Cue-Controlled Relaxation

Present the following rationale to the client:

Now I am going to teach you another relaxation strategy, called "cue-controlled relaxation." Cue-controlled relaxation can be used daily to reduce tension, especially in situations that remind you of the assault. When you feel stressed out or anxious, which of your muscles are first effected? [Elicit from the client the muscle groups in which she first notices tension—e.g., neck, jaw, shoulders.] This week, pay attention to which muscles in your body feel tense, and use this tension as a cue to use breathing retraining and relaxation. For example, let's say you have had a difficult day at work because you were unable to concentrate, and you notice that you are clenching your jaw. This will be your cue to start your breathing exercises and to say your cue word (e.g., "calm" or "relax") to help you reduce your tension. Do you notice any muscle group in which there is tension right now, or not as relaxed as the rest?

Practicing Relaxation on Cue

Elicit from the client the area of tension currently in her body, and have her use this as the area for practicing cue-controlled relaxation. Have the client practice breathing, using her cue word, and allowing her muscles in that area to go limp and relax for about 5 minutes.

Differential Relaxation

Presenting a Rationale for Differential Relaxation

After you have taught cue-controlled relaxation to the client, give her the following rationale for differential relaxation (see also Bernstein & Borkovec, 1973):

Now I'd like to review a skill called "differential relaxation." We call it "differential relaxation" because you will be learning to relax specific muscle groups that are not essential for the activity you engage in when you are tense. You may notice that your muscles are feeling tense much of the day. This is because you are anxious and overly alert a good deal of the day. In actuality, when you engage in various activities, you only need to contract those muscle groups directly related to that activity. For example, if you are sitting and watching television, there is no need to have tension in the muscles in your face, arms, legs, stomach, and buttocks. However, in order to sit upright, you need to tense the muscles in your neck and torso slightly. Does this makes sense to you?

Demonstrating Differential Relaxation

Continue as follows:

Let's run a couple of experiments to demonstrate this principle. First, I'd like you to focus on the amount of tension that you feel in your muscles as you sit in the chair. What muscles are feeling tense right now? [Encourage the client to respond.] What are the essential muscle groups that you need to sit in the chair? [Elicit these from the client.]

Even when we are using muscles for an activity, we do not need a high degree of tension—say, the amount when we are tensing the muscles during deep muscle relaxation. Try to keep the minimal amount of tension required for that activity. Now try to reduce the degree of tension that you feel in the muscle groups that are essential for you to sit in the chair, and try to allow the other muscles to relax completely. Do you notice a difference? [Encourage the client to respond.]

Next, give the client a piece of paper and a pencil. Ask her to write her name, using only the muscle groups she needs for this activity. Ask her the following:

- "What muscles are you able to relax while you are writing?"
- "What are the muscle groups that you need to write your name?"

If the client is unable to identify the essential muscle groups involved in her writing, explain to her that only the muscles in her hand and lower arm are tense when writing.

Proceed with another example by asking the client to stand up and notice the muscle groups she needs to maintain her balance and posture. Stand up with the client and model a relaxed stance. Ask her:

- "What muscles are you able to relax while you are standing there?"
- "What are the muscle groups that you need to maintain your balance?"

If the client is unable to identify the essential muscle groups involved in standing, point out that only the muscles in her shoulders, back, and legs are tense when she stands. Note that this tension is minimal and that it is not necessary to tense other muscles, such as those in her arms, buttocks, or face, to stand.

Finally, ask the client to walk around the room and notice what muscle groups are essential for her to walk and maintain her balance. Ask her questions similar to the ones above. If the client is unable to identify the essential muscle groups involved in walking around the room, you will point out that it is only necessary to tense the muscles in her shoulders, back, hips, and legs. Note that this tension is minimal and that she does not need to tense the muscles in her arms or face, for example, to walk around the room.

Practice and Homework

After you have demonstrated and practiced the various relaxation exercises with the client, make sure she understands the purpose of and knows how to perform each of the different forms of relaxation. Ask her to practice deep muscle, cue-controlled, and differential relaxation twice daily. Also, ask her to write down any questions or problems for you to discuss together next session.

14

Role Play and Covert Modeling

Role Play

Role playing consists of acting out behaviors, rehearsing lines and actions, and pretending to be in a specific set of circumstances. Role playing is a way to learn new behaviors and words for old ways of doing things; it is a chance to practice before the event occurs. As a dress rehearsal does, the repeated practice of a behavior reduces anxiety and makes it more likely that a new behavior will be used. During role-play training, you and the client will actually act out scenes in which the client confronts a disturbing situation. Begin with non-assault-related situations before role-playing those that are assault-related.

In each role-play exercise, you should first play the client's role and demonstrate the appropriate social and assertion skills. Then roles are reversed, and the client plays herself. After each role play, encourage the client to critique both your and her performance, pointing out positive aspects first, and then pointing out areas for improvement. After the client's self-critique, you should offer your own feedback. Again, always emphasize the positive aspects first. Each role play is repeated until the client performs the behaviors satisfactorily or reaches a plateau (rarely more than five times).

Overview of Steps for Teaching Role Play

1. Present the rationale for role play.
2. Demonstrate assertive (as opposed to aggressive or passive) interaction, using appropriate eye contact, body language, tone of voice, and expressions of affect that are congruent with statements.
3. Elicit from your client non-assault-related situations that cause her distress, and choose one situation for role play.

4. Play the client's role (model) in the chosen situation.
5. Reverse roles, with the client playing herself.
6. Elicit positive feedback from the client about her performances, and then elicit suggestions for improvement. Next, offer the client positive feedback first, and then make suggestions for refining her skills.
7. Continue to practice until the interaction is performed satisfactorily by the client.
8. Elicit from your client assault-related situations that cause her particular distress. Select one assault-related situation for role play, and repeat Steps 4–7.
9. Continue to offer the client feedback and praise between role plays.

Presenting a Rationale for Role Play

Offer the client the following rationale for using role play:

Today I'm going to teach you a way to learn new behaviors and words for situations that make you anxious. This requires us to use a technique called "role play." Have you ever had the experience of role playing before? Could you describe that to me? [Encourage the client to respond.] Role playing is like a dress rehearsal. If you practice what you want to say before you enter a stressful situation, your anxiety will decrease, and you will have a better chance to obtain your goal.

First I'm going to show you how to engage in a conversation using assertive statements and gestures. Then we're going to pick a non-assault-related situation that bothers you and role-play it. First I'll play you and you'll play the other person, and then you'll play yourself and I'll play the other person. Once you've gotten to the point where you feel comfortable about how you'll do in the future in that situation, we'll do the same thing with an assault-related situation. Do you have any questions at this point?

Defining and Demonstrating Assertive Behavior

It is usually helpful to define assertive versus aggressive or passive behavior so that the client can learn to discriminate among these behavioral styles, especially if you think that she is behaving aggressively or passively. Say something like the following:

One important point is that assertion is not the same as aggression. Think about assertion skills as the golden mean or average between passivity and aggression. If a person is passive all the time and lets people walk all over her, she may become angry and explode over inconsequential incidents. This isn't a helpful way to interact with family, friends, or coworkers. On the other hand, if a person is aggressive with others, she may initially get what she wants, but in the long run people may start avoiding her. Let's talk about the difference between aggressive, nonassertive, and assertive behaviors. [See also Sank & Shaffer, 1984.]

"Aggressive behavior" is denying other people their rights and feelings through blaming, name calling, or using other behaviors that are designed to hurt them or make them feel defensive. "Nonassertive behavior" or "passive behavior" is denying your own rights by not standing up for yourself or not expressing your feelings. It can also include indirect communication that is easy to misinterpret. "Assertive behavior" does not violate your rights or someone else's rights. It is expressing your feelings and preferences in a direct, honest, and appropriate manner. Assertive behavior conveys respect for other people's feelings and facilitates two-way communication. It often involves making compromises. Being assertive involves using specific words, behaviors, and body postures. I'd like to demonstrate some assertive, nonassertive, and aggressive behaviors to you so you can see what I am talking about, and then I'm going to give you a handout to help you learn the differences.

Now act out examples of each of the three types of behavior for the client, taking care to illustrate as many of the points in the Assertive Behaviors handout (Figure 14.1) as possible. Next, give the client a copy of the handout and go over the points with her.

Choosing Situations for Role Plays

Now that you have described and demonstrated assertive behavior for the client, ask her to name some non-assault-related situations in daily life that upset or distress her, and choose one of these as a basis for role play. As noted earlier, you will act out this situation (first with you playing the part of the client, and then with the client playing herself) until it is being performed to the client's and your satisfaction. Next, ask the client to name some assault-related situations in everyday life that are particularly upsetting for her, and select one of these for role play. If the client has difficulty naming examples of situations in either category, you can ask her to choose one from the following lists:

Examples of Non-Assault-Related Situations for Role Play
- Talking to your boss
- Requesting time off work from your boss
- Using assertive behaviors to make a point at work
- Asking significant others to assist you with *in vivo* exposure exercises
- Calling a friend to ask if you can borrow something
- Saying "no" to an authority figure

Assertive Behaviors

The following is a list of helpful hints when you are trying to communicate an important message to someone.

1. Maintain eye contact, and when you take breaks, move your eyes to the side.
   - Moving eyes up makes you look bored.
   - Moving eyes down makes you look shy or insecure.
2. Keep your facial expression appropriate to the message that you are sending (e.g., don't smile when telling someone that you are upset).
3. Maintain an erect, not rigid or slumped, body posture.
   - Sit up straight.
   - Keep your hands and arms by your side.
   - Do not cross your arms or wring your hands.
   - Face your listener.
4. Your voice tone should be even, and your inflection and volume should be normal.
   - Don't yell, scream, or speak too loudly.
   - Don't speak too softly.
   - Don't cry.
5. The content of your statements should be brief and to the point.
   - Do not accuse, blame, or be defensive.
   - It is helpful to tell the listener what you expect him or her to do (e.g., "I would like to talk with you about something very important, and then I would like to hear your feedback," or "I am hoping that you will be able to help me with something").
6. Find the right moment to talk.
   - Don't catch someone who is running off somewhere.
   - Don't interrupt a conversation.
   - Don't demand to speak to someone immediately.
7. When you are telling someone something that is hard for you to say or may be hard for him or her to hear, it is helpful to use the following four "parts":
   - Start with something positive (e.g., "Honey, you know that I love you").
   - Say exactly what it was that the other person did (e.g., "When you come up behind me and surprise me by hugging me . . . ").
   - Say exactly what the effect on you is (e.g., "It startles me and leaves me very rattled").
   - Say exactly what you would like from them in the future (e.g., "I would appreciate it if you could warn me before you hug me from behind, so I don't get startled").

FIGURE 14.1. Assertive Behaviors handout.

Examples of Assault-Related Situations for Role Play
- Telling a family member about the assault
- Walking in a calm and confident manner
- Asking for an escort to walk you to your car in the parking garage
- Saying "no" to a sexual interaction
- Saying "no" to a request to go on a date at night with an unfamiliar man

- Telling a man who approaches you and talks that you don't want to talk to him

Two case examples illustrating the use of role play follow.

Case Example: Role Play of a Non-Assault-Related and an Assault-Related Situation

This example illustrates how role play was taught to a 25-year-old architect named Marie, who had been raped in her bedroom one night by an intruder. (The case is described in more detail by Veronen & Kilpatrick, 1983.)

Marie reported that she often felt as if she was being put down by people. She described experiences during which she felt dismissed by the men with whom she worked at building sites. Marie felt that a particular male building contractor with whom she was working did not take her seriously; so she deferred to her partner, a male architect, with whom she was working.

To demonstrate the role-play skill to Marie, the therapist first played Marie, and Marie pretended that she was the building contractor. Next, Marie played herself, and the therapist acted the role of the building contractor. After one role play, Marie was able to comment on her performance and receive feedback from the therapist. The feedback that Marie received from the therapist focused on the following:

- Her "nonverbals," including her tone of voice, her posture, and her facial expression.
- Her "verbals," or the words that she used.

Marie continued to role-play the scene three more times, each time becoming more confident in her requests. Her homework assignment was to go to work the next day and tell the building contractor what she wanted him to do.

During the next role play, Marie role-played staying alone by herself at night (an assault-related situation). Marie pretended that she was alone and role-played herself doing some cleaning, talking on the phone, writing a letter, and reading a book. The therapist also assigned Marie the following homework: to stay alone for a few hours by herself during the afternoon (a behavioral approximation of staying home alone at night).

Case Example: Assertive Role Play of an Assault-Related Situation

Carla was a 34-year-old married woman who was raped at knifepoint in her car after being forced to drive the assailant from the mall to an abandoned lot.

Her husband tried to be supportive and clearly loved Carla, but he had a difficult time with the idea of the assault, particularly the notion that another man had "violated" his wife. Carla felt that he didn't want to hear anything about the assault; in fact, he would change the subject or encourage her "to forget about it" if she did bring it up. Besides the fact that Carla felt the need to talk about it herself, her husband's reaction made Carla uncomfortable and led her to feel dirty and guilty. Carla brought this issue up when discussing role play. She decided she would like to talk to her husband about it, but she wasn't sure how. First, the therapist played Carla and had Carla play her husband:

THERAPIST (as Carla): Lou, do you have a few minutes now?

CARLA (as her husband): Sure, honey. What's up?

THERAPIST (as Carla): Lou, you know I love you, and I think you're a great husband. You've tried to take care of me after this whole rape thing, and I appreciate it.

CARLA (as her husband): Aw, do we have to talk about that again?

THERAPIST (as Carla): Just bear with me a minute. This is hard for me.

CARLA (as her husband): OK, sorry.

THERAPIST (as Carla): I know the rape was hard on you, too. And I know you don't like to talk about it. But when you change the subject when I bring it up, or when you get so uncomfortable when it comes up, it makes me feel even worse, like you can't even look at me and think what happened to me. It makes me feel dirty and alone, and like you wish you weren't married to me any more. [Carla had said these things to the therapist.]

CARLA (as her husband): It's just that I can't stand to think what that scum did to you.

THERAPIST (as Carla): I know, but just not thinking about it doesn't make it go away. I need to talk to you about it, and I need for you to feel more comfortable hearing and talking about it.

CARLA (as her husband): I don't know how to do that.

THERAPIST (as Carla): We can start by just talking more about it, even when it gets uncomfortable. And I'd like it if you let me talk about it when I bring it up. And I'd love it if you could talk about it more and tell me what you're feeling and thinking. What do you think of this?

CARLA (as her husband): I'm willing to try, if you think it will help you.

Carla and the therapist then discussed things that the therapist said and did that Carla liked. She liked the words the therapist used, and she liked how the therapist didn't drop it when the husband tried to change the subject. Carla also liked the therapist's nonverbal signals; she thought that the therapist's facial expression and posture gave the message that she wasn't going to back down, and this was important. The therapist then asked Carla for feedback on things to improve. Carla felt that her husband would respond positively to her request to allow her to talk, but she didn't know how he would respond to her request for him to share his feelings; still, she decided it was worth a try to ask him anyway. Carla and the therapist then reversed roles, with Carla playing herself and the therapist playing Carla's husband. Carla had some difficulty at first, especially in getting out what she wanted to say and using appropriate nonverbal signals. After two repetitions, Carla "had it down." She felt comfortable and confident, and was determined to go home and have this conversation that evening, which she did.

Covert Modeling

Covert modeling is the imaginal analogue of role playing: It helps the client cope with distressing situations through the rehearsal of coping strategies in her imagination. Many clients cannot even imagine themselves getting through certain situations successfully, and if they cannot imagine it, it will be harder to accomplish. Covert modeling helps them to picture getting through situations successfully, thereby increasing the odds that this will happen in reality.

Teaching this technique is similar to teaching role play. That is, you and the client will first identify a non-assault-related anxiety-provoking situation. Obtain information from her about problems that she encounters in this situation, and incorporate these thoughts, feelings, and behaviors into the scene. You and the client together then imagine someone other than the client in the situation; verbalize the images for the client, and demonstrate how this person exhibits successful coping strategies. Next, ask the client to imagine the same situation and to visualize herself coping successfully with it. After a non-assault-related example has been practiced, you will move to an assault-related example. The imaginal scenes to be used for covert modeling may be the same as those used for role play. In general, however, conversations that are easily acted out are more amenable to role playing; situations that involve only the client (e.g., going places or encountering crowds) are better for covert modeling.

Overview of Steps for Teaching Covert Modeling
1. Provide a rationale for covert modeling.
2. Explain the technique for covert modeling.
3. Select a non-assault-related example.
4. Demonstrate for the client how someone else might cope successfully with the situation; verbalize images and coping strategies out loud.
5. Have client visualize herself in the situation and coping with distress.
6. Select an assault-related situation and repeat Steps 4–5.

Presenting a Rationale for Covert Modeling

Introduce the technique with the following rationale:

I'm going to work with you on another coping skill today that is somewhat similar to role play. This technique is called "covert modeling," which is just a fancy name for "role play in your imagination." It is "covert," or imagined, rather than "overt," or out in the open, like role plays. And it involves "modeling," or picturing someone else going through the situation first. The reason I want to teach you this technique is that it will help you manage situations in which you feel anxious and uncomfortable. The goal is to bring up a problem here that you can visualize in your imagination, and first picture someone else going through it successfully. Then pull the other person out and substitute yourself going through it just the way he or she did. In other words, you practice coping so when this situation or a similar one comes up, you will have successfully practiced dealing with it. The technique is a bit different from role playing because you will first imagine someone else coping with the stressor, then imagine yourself doing the same—not rehearsing it by interacting with me.

Some people can't even imagine themselves doing something, or doing it again after the assault. For example, one woman couldn't even imagine getting through a job interview. When I asked her if she had a friend she *could* picture getting through a job interview, she recalled a friend who she was sure could do it. Together, when we imagined her friend doing it first, we could delineate all of the steps involved and what would be required for a successful outcome. Then it was easier for her to pluck her friend out of the picture and imagine herself doing what was necessary to do it. This is similar to positive visualization, like when a golfer pictures the ball going into the hole before she putts it. First we'll agree on a non-assault-related example to rehearse; then I'll model the technique for you; and then I'll ask you to practice it. After that, we will move on to an assault-related example. Do you have any questions before we begin?

Practicing Covert Modeling in Different Situations

As with all other SIT skills, practice covert modeling first with a non-assault-related example, then an assault-related example. Ask the client to generate a non-assault-related example. Ask her to picture someone she knows going through the situation successfully. Have the client close her eyes to enhance the vividness of imagery. However, if she does not feel comfortable closing her eyes, allow her to keep them open. Tell her to go through each step of the situation and to describe in detail how her "model" would cope with each step. Make sure the client includes all of the relevant steps—especially their stressful aspects—and describes how the other person would respond at each step. If she skips an important step, prompt her with a question. When the client has completed all the steps, ask her to open her eyes (if they were closed) and discuss the process and the situation she chose. Then tell her to include *all* of the same steps and coping responses, but while picturing herself doing it rather than this other person. If she does not follow her previous example, correct her. If the client has trouble naming examples of situations in either category, you can suggest that she choose one from the following lists:

Examples of Non-Assault-Related Situations for Covert Modeling
- Attending a neighborhood party
- Attending a baby or bridal shower
- Going on a job interview
- Entertaining your mother-in-law
- Taking a test

Examples of Assault-Related Situations for Covert Modeling
- Being on a date and the man makes sexual advances
- Being on a date and being anxious in the man's presence
- Walking home from the train station or bus stop
- Leaving work to go to where the car is parked
- Going to public places (e.g., grocery store, mall, restaurant, movie theater)
- Having a sexual interaction with a partner
- Telling someone about the assault
- Talking with coworkers who are making jokes about a woman who was raped

Case Example: Covert Modeling

Joan reported that she had been unable to go shopping alone since she had been assaulted 3 years earlier. This interfered seriously with her daily functioning, since she had to depend on her spouse and friends to transport her. The therapist modeled for Joan a trip to the mall and the use of coping skills as follows:

I am walking in the parking lot and looking all around me. I see an unfamiliar man, and I start to feel anxious. I can feel my heart beating. I take a couple of breaths and say the word "calm" to myself. I keep walking toward the entrance of the mall and say to myself, "One step at a time. You can do it. It's daylight, and there are plenty of people around who could help if I get into trouble." I enter the mall, and my anxiety decreases. I am starting to feel good. All of a sudden, I see a male walking toward me who looks like the man who raped me. I have a flashback; I feel shaky, faint, and nauseated. My heart is beating rapidly, and I think to myself, "This guy is going to rape me." Then I ask myself, "What is the evidence that this is true?", and respond, "This is not the assailant. He may look like the man who raped me, but the man who raped me is in jail. I am in the middle of a mall, and people will help me if he attacks me." I start feeling better, and I am able to go shopping. Now I am feeling great, and I say to myself, "Good job." I buy myself a pair of earrings to reward myself for being able to go to the mall successfully.

After the therapist modeled this situation, Joan closed her eyes and visualized going to the mall by herself and coping with her anxiety successfully. Part of her homework assignment was then to go to the mall by herself, which she was able to accomplish.

15

Common Problems, Termination, and a Full Case Example

Common Problems and Complications

Avoidance/Resistance

Clinical practice suggests that some assault victims with PTSD may be resistant to engaging emotionally during imaginal exposure. There are several reasons for this resistance. First, their trauma was an interpersonal injury caused by an intentionally malicious act that another person directed at them; therefore, their trust in fellow humans can be expected to be greatly diminished. Second, they have a tendency to use avoidant coping mechanisms during exposure treatment. An assault victim is asked to perform two extremely difficult tasks: to expose herself intentionally to the very memories she has been actively avoiding, and to trust you as her therapist to assist her throughout this difficult and challenging experience. The difficulty of trusting, combined with the strong efforts on the part of many assault victims with PTSD to avoid emotional engagement with the traumatic memories, results in reluctance to engage emotionally during reliving sessions. Even when a victim is recounting the details of her assault, she may be emotionally distancing herself, appearing to tell someone else's story rather than her own. This reluctance to engage emotionally is a serious problem, since, as noted in Chapter 5, studies have demonstrated a relationship between emotional responses during imaginal reliving of the trauma and benefit from treatment.

The third issue pertinent to imaginal exposure therapy with rape victims stems from the intimate nature of the rape trauma, which results in enhanced difficulty in disclosing the details of the assault. It is less embarrassing to discuss an attack by a dog than to discuss details of being raped. On the one hand, you should make special efforts to encourage disclosure by asking more probing questions; on the other hand, this inquiry should be conducted with extra sensitivity to the intimate material being presented.

Actual Risk

Another issue specific to the treatment of assault victims is the extreme care that must be exercised when selecting situations for *in vivo* self-exposure. Although such care is exercised in *in vivo* exposure treatment for other anxiety disorders, the careful assessment of the realistic probability for harm during *in vivo* exposure seems especially important in the treatment of assault-related PTSD. Indeed, in some environments assaults are quite frequent. The reality of a victim's fear was demonstrated with one of our clients, who was attacked again during her treatment. Some of our clients were continually threatened or harassed by their assailants. In such a case, it may be necessary to help the client involve the police and obtain a restraining order mandating no more contact. The first obligation is to ensure the client's safety. A shelter or temporary residence may also be considered, although this can be disrupting as well.

Tolerance for Exposure

In deciding how to conduct imaginal or *in vivo* exposure treatment, you must use sensible clinical judgment. For example, although you may structure imaginal exposure to last for 45 minutes with the hope that this will be sufficient time for habituation, it is highly desirable for the client to experience some decrease in distress at the end of the exposure. If a gradual decrease in distress does not occur spontaneously, coping statements such as "But you know you are going to survive" may be introduced in the last 15 minutes of reliving.

Decision-making guidelines for the use of exposure therapy for PTSD have been established; these take into account such client variables as tolerance for extreme arousal, imagery ability, and compliance (Jaycox & Foa, 1996). Clearly, women who are experiencing extreme distress when remembering their assault, or show extreme avoidance of situations, objects, or thoughts that remind them of it, will profit from exposure therapy. However, for some assault victims the memories are excruciatingly painful, resulting in resistance to complying with exposure instructions. In these extreme cases, you may be well advised to take a more gradual approach or to begin therapy with the SIT techniques before instituting exposure.

Compliance

We have experienced more "no-shows" or cancellations with PTSD assault victims than in any other population we have treated. The importance of keeping regular appointments, even when a client is inclined to avoid them, must be highlighted. We do allow somewhat more flexibility in scheduling assault survivors than in scheduling other populations. We have developed a "three strikes" policy for appointments: We reschedule three times after a missed or canceled appointment, but after the third consecutive missed appointment, we stop scheduling. Clients in danger of "striking out" are notified ahead of time.

Compliance can also be a problem in homework practice. The treatment programs we have presented in this book require considerable time from the client outside of the therapy session. In the PE/SIT program (Program 3) in particular, the client must practice SIT skills several times daily, and expose herself imaginally and *in vivo* daily as well. If she is not practicing as prescribed, you should gently inquire as to the reasons. Try to problem-solve with her. If she doesn't seem to have the time to practice between work and taking care of home and the family, go through her day with her. Help her see where she can grab some time for herself. This may require help from a partner or a support person to take up her slack (e.g., by watching the kids after supper while Mom practices). The SIT techniques are all skills that must be practiced to be mastered and used effectively, and exposure requires repeatedly listening to the tape of imaginal exposure and practicing *in vivo* exercises to allow the necessary changes to take place. Therefore, if you discover that the client is not being compliant with homework practice, this *must* be dealt with early in treatment.

If noncompliance continues as a problem and all efforts to remedy it have failed, it may be appropriate to terminate treatment. If this is necessary, it should be done therapeutically, not punitively. You may want to advise the client:

Timing is very important. When it is the right time to deal with a problem, things seem to click. When it is not the right time, even potentially effective techniques don't work, and people get frustrated. I don't know what may make it the right time for you, but it appears that this may not be the right time for you to be in this treatment right now, because you do not find time to give priority to treatment demands. I would prefer that you stop early, knowing you did not have a complete trial, rather than plod along and be unhappy with the results and feel nothing will help. The bottom line is that I don't think you are going to achieve all that you could the way you are going now, so I think it is best to stop treatment at this point and come back to it later, when you are able to devote more time and energy to it. I'm not planning on going anywhere, and you know what's involved with treatment, so when you do feel it is the right time for you, I hope you will call me. If, when you're ready, you think you might like to try again but with a different therapist, I'd be happy to help you find someone. What do you think of this?

Lack of Outside Support for the Client

Many clients will require outside support to enter into and complete a treatment program. This includes emotional support and encouragement to do something as scary as treatment can be. It also includes logistical support (e.g., child care) to make it possible for a client to attend sessions and complete homework. If the client's partner is not supportive, it can greatly interfere with therapy. Often the partner or other significant persons (relatives, etc.) may not understand PTSD and its treatment, and/or may not think it is important. In such a case, it is helpful to educate these persons. With the client's permission, they may be educated by being asked to read the Common Reactions to Assault handout (see Chapter 8) or by having a session with you. Although we do not encourage partners to listen to imaginal exposure tapes, some clients find it helpful. Explaining to the partner the client's reactions and need for treatment may be role-played, so that the client can gain the necessary assertiveness skills to communicate this. Also, you may want to inquire about possible support groups for partners of rape survivors in your area, and to let your client and her partner know that this resource is available. Even if you become very frustrated with interference in treatment by a partner, be sure to remain unbiased about it with your client. This is the person she has chosen to commit herself to, and she needs your help, not criticism of her choice.

It is also important to be aware of another way in which a partner can sabotage treatment. We have heard several accounts of clients' marrying their "knights in shining armor" who rescued and protected them following the assault. In such a case, the entire relationship may be built on the client's having her needs met by her partner and being dependent on him. If she starts getting more independent, adventuresome, and confident, she may no longer need him in the same ways. At the very least, their relationship will change. This may be very threatening and needs to be addressed. Partners can be directed to grow together rather than apart. You may need to make a referral for couple therapy, or have the client bring her partner in to see you so that the three of you can discuss these issues together.

Comorbid Symptoms

Many assault survivors suffer from other psychological problems in addition to PTSD. Substance abuse is particularly common in PTSD sufferers. Many PTSD sufferers use drugs and alcohol to self-medicate themselves, in order to reduce the emotional pain associated with the trauma. It is quite clear in such cases that the substance abuse needs to be addressed before the PTSD, because the substance abuse will inhibit the necessary emotional processing. We usually require at least 90 days of sobriety before treating assault-related issues. Even then, it must be approached cautiously, with tremendous support from the substance use treatment providers.

Many PTSD assault survivors are mildly to moderately depressed. If it is determined that a client is suffering from a severe major depression, the depression should be treated before the PTSD, because severe depression would reduce the client's ability to profit from cognitive-behavioral interventions. Antidepressant medications, psychosocial treatments, or inpatient hospitalization may be indicated. Mild depression should not pose a problem and can be expected to respond favorably to the treatment techniques outlined in this book.

The possible interference of other disorders must be assessed on a case-by-case basis. The client's problems must be prioritized, with the most severe, threatening, and disruptive ones being addressed first. Suicidal tendencies obviously take priority. We have found our treatment programs to be quite effective and manageable with clients suffering from Major Depression and personality disorders. However, your clinical skills must guide you in making decisions affecting a client's welfare.

Determining Whether the Client Needs More Sessions

At the end of Session 8, administer the PDS to the client. Calculate the percentage of improvement in the PTSD symptom picture by comparing this score to the PDS score obtained during the pretreatment evaluation. We suggest that clients who have not improved at least 70% from their pretreatment PTSD severity level can be offered three additional treatment sessions. You will use this information in reviewing the client's progress in the program later in this session and in Session 9. If there are clear reasons why the client has not improved more that are continuing to exert an effect (e.g., if she is in the middle of the criminal trial for the rape or is receiving threatening phone calls), and if you think additional sessions would not be useful at this time, you may want to terminate now. You can also discuss this with the client and offer her additional sessions in the future, when she may be able to profit more from them. Another possibility is to switch modes to provide support during this difficult period and resume cognitive-behavioral work at a later point. In any case, we feel that additional sessions should only be offered if you think they will help. There is a point of diminishing returns, and we are not simply advocating that you keep treating the client with the same methods until she responds.

Begin this conversation as follows:

We have been working together for 8 weeks. The next session will be Session 9. What I would like to do today is to review your progress in the program and decide together if you would like to meet for three additional sessions after Session 9, to continue to work in the same fashion on your reactions to the assault.

Then continue with some of these questions.

- "I think you have made some really nice progress in the program [if true]. How are you feeling about your progress?"

- "How are you feeling now compared to when you began the program?"
- "What have you learned during the last 8 weeks?"
- "What were the most helpful things that we did?"
- "Was there anything that you didn't find very helpful?"
- "Are there any skills that you think you need to continue to practice?"

On the basis of the client's answers to these questions, decide whether or not you think the client could use additional sessions. If you think so, say the following:

- "I think it would be helpful for us to meet for three more sessions to continue to work on_____. How do you feel about this?"

The following session (Session 9) will focus either on treatment planning for additional sessions or on treatment termination. (If Session 9 is the final session, it will include a more detailed review of progress in all the skills learned in treatment; see below.) The client should be prepared for whether her next session will be her last or not. Therefore, we recommend deciding together at the end of Session 8 whether you will offer her additional sessions, and communicating this clearly to the client at this time.

Termination

The process of terminating treatment is extremely important and sensitive. We suggest that the following issues be raised and discussed:

Termination: Agenda for the Final Session
1. Review all of the techniques used in the treatment, and ascertain how each was (or wasn't) helpful.
2. Review the client's progress in detail.
3. Discuss the client's plans for after treatment. Does she feel she needs more treatment? For what issues? Is referral appropriate?
4. Elicit information about stresses or difficulties anticipated in the future, and discuss ways the client can manage these.
5. Schedule follow-up appointments.
6. Say goodbye.

Reviewing All Treatment Techniques

The first step is to review all the techniques you have employed in therapy and to ascertain how helpful each technique was. Depending on the program you chose for your client, you will address any of the following techniques you have employed during therapy:

- Imaginal and *in vivo* exposure: How helpful have these techniques been in making the client feel more comfortable when she thinks about the assault, or when she confronts situations and objects that remind her of the assault?
- Cognitive restructuring: How much has the client utilized this technique to challenge negative thoughts and dysfunctional beliefs that cause her intense negative emotions, and to replace them with more realistic ones?
- Breathing retraining and deep muscle, cue-controlled, and differential relaxation: How much have these techniques been helpful in relaxing the client and controlling her anxiety?
- Thought stopping: How much has this technique helped the client in controlling ruminations about the assault at times when exposure exercises cannot be implemented?
- Guided self-dialogue: How much has this technique helped the client manage her negative self-talk in regard to a stressful event?
- Role play and covert modeling: Have these techniques helped the client behave as she desires in stressful situations? In particular, have they helped promote her assertiveness?

Review briefly how much the client liked each technique, what techniques she has found useful and not useful, and what techniques she thinks will be helpful to her in the future. Encouraging feedback from the client about the usefulness of the treatment and its components can be useful to both the client and the therapist. Try to be open and nondefensive if her feedback includes suggestions for changes. It is also advisable to share with the client the reasons why you chose a particular treatment program for her, and what its benefits are over different programs that she might have preferred. If the client has questions about any other aspect of treatment, you can address these at this time as well. For example, at the end of treatment, one patient said she wished her therapist had talked more about herself. She wanted to know whether she was married, had children, was a rape survivor, and so forth. Rather than answer all of these personal questions, the therapist explained that she was certainly not trying to hide anything, but that it was important to devote all the focus of therapy to helping the client and addressing her difficulties. Also, she had made a conscious decision *not* to talk more about herself in therapy. If she did, some clients might feel slighted and believe that the therapist was dominating therapy time to talk about herself. In general, we suggest that you not engage in sharing personal information, and that you avert personal questions tactfully. Clients vary greatly in their reactions to such information, especially information regarding whether you are a rape survivor or not. Also, some clients may encourage you to talk about yourself as a way to avoid talking about the assault and their own issues.

Reviewing the Client's Progress, Discussing Future Plans, and Anticipating Difficulties

After the review of all techniques employed in treatment, say this to the client:

I'd like to know how you are feeling now about your trauma and the difficulties that you have experienced as a result of it. What parts of the treatment did you find helpful or not helpful? What additional skills do you need to learn? And what are your plans for the near future?

Ask the client the following questions:

- "Have you noticed any changes in your thoughts or feelings as a result of the treatment and learning the skills? Specifically, what are those?"
- "What have you noticed about your level of anxiety or discomfort in certain situations?"
- "What skills have you found most helpful to manage anxiety and discomfort?"
- "Are there any problems that you are still concerned about?" (If so, discuss your professional recommendation for the client.)

After talking over these issues with the client, continue the discussion according to the following stages:

1. A recap of the client's symptom picture, based on the PDS (as determined and discussed in Session 8).
2. An evaluation of the client's skill development.
3. Encouragement and praise.

Next, discuss the client's plans for after treatment. Does she feel she needs more treatment? If so, for what types of issues? If yes, does she need a referral, or can you help her with the remaining problems? If not, schedule follow-up appointments (see below) and discuss those. In addition, elicit information about potential difficulties or stressful situations that may arise in the future, and discuss ways to manage them effectively. For example, a client who knows that her assailant is due to be released from prison a year following termination might expect to experience increased symptoms when this happens. You and the client can plan for this event by choosing which skills might be most helpful, and by making specific plans for the client to continue practicing the skills for use when needed.

Discussing Follow-Up

Make formal or informal arrangements for follow-up with the client. We have found it helpful to maintain infrequent contact for 1 year after therapy ends. This may mean meeting briefly every 3 or even 6 months, or even checking in by phone. It is helpful for the client to keep you and therapy in mind, and to feel you are there if she needs you. It is also important to urge the client to continue to practice the skills that she has learned during treatment.

Saying Goodbye

Although in general we do not encourage physical contact between clients and therapists, many clients like to hug goodbye at their last session; we feel that this is appropriate, as long as the client initiates it and you feel comfortable with it.

As a basic rule, we treat all of our clients as people worthy of respect and show them that respect. It's important to remember that although you probably have many clients, most of your clients only have one therapist. In that way, you are an important person in each client's life. Often, the relationship between a rape victim and her therapist becomes very intimate. She has probably discussed matters with you that she has with no one else. It will help to imagine how you would like such an important relationship to end.

When you are saying goodbye to the client, it is important that you find something positive to say to her. The following is a list of possible statements:

- "I have enjoyed working with you and wish you much luck in the future."
- "It's evident that you are feeling much better, and although you were skeptical, it seems that your hard work paid off."
- "You had some difficult weeks there, but you persisted with courage and patience, and it is obvious that your efforts paid off for you."
- "You mentioned that you were disappointed that you had not made more progress in the program. I'd like to tell you that it is not unusual for clients to express the same feelings, and then discover that they feel much better as time goes on."
- "It takes time to digest and process what happened in treatment. You may continue to feel better as time goes on, especially if you continue to use the skills and techniques that you have learned."

- "I want to tell you that you have put a lot of hard work into your treatment, and you have made a lot of [some] gains."
- "I know this program was difficult for you to complete. In fact, there were a few days [weeks] when you wanted to discontinue your treatment. But you stuck with the program and made progress."
- "When we first started working together, you were having difficulties with _____. Since that time, I've noticed that you are feeling much better."

You can offer examples here of how the client's symptom pattern and behaviors changed, as well as any other feedback for her.

Case Example: Betsy

In this section, we present the case example of Betsy, who was treated with the PE/SIT program. Although we recommend PE alone as a first line of treatment, we present a case example utilizing the PE/SIT program because it is more complicated to administer.

Betsy was raped as a college student, by a stranger who forced her from a grocery store into a nearby parking garage. She presented for treatment about 3 years following the assault. She was still in college, but her functioning had been severely disrupted. Prior to the assault, she had been socially active, friendly, assertive, and an average student. At the time she presented for treatment, she was having difficulty with her courses and had not been able to graduate on schedule. She had become socially withdrawn, tentative, and extremely fearful. She did not want others to know about the assault, fearing they would think badly of her. She had never reported it to the police or sought medical attention. The only people she had told were her boyfriend at the time, Kenneth, and her sister; she had sworn both to secrecy. She described wanting to tell her parents, in part to help explain her troubled college performance, but it was too difficult and embarrassing to talk about. She often responded with excessive anger when her parents tried to talk to her about college or what might be troubling her. She had broken up with Kenneth, partly because she no longer desired a sexual relationship and she felt that this wasn't fair to him. They frequently talked as friends even after the breakup, however.

Kenneth gave Betsy an article from the newspaper describing PTSD and giving information on our treatment programs. She reportedly kept it for several months before gathering the courage to call. As noted above, she was treated with the PE/SIT program.

In the first session, Betsy and her therapist discussed the assault and its aftermath, using the AIHI (Appendix). Betsy cried often, gave brief answers, and had to be prompted for more information. The therapist tried to be very patient and understanding, which Betsy responded well to. The therapist briefly summarized the treatment program, emphasizing the skills that would help Betsy in the areas where it was clear she was having difficulty. At the end, Betsy was taught the brief breathing retraining to counter anxiety that was clearly elicited by discussion of the assault, and the therapist gave her the accompanying handout with instructions to practice for homework. Betsy seemed to respond well to the breathing, clearly relaxing her body, which had been extremely tense during the interview. She had some difficulty holding her breath for the count of 4 at first, but adapted and found it comfortable by the end. She commented at the end that she was glad the session was over, but that it hadn't been as bad as she was afraid it would be.

The therapist praised Betsy for returning for Session 2, commenting that she knew Session 1 was difficult for her. Betsy admitted she had had some thoughts of not returning, but decided in the end that it was "kinda like going to the dentist: I know it won't feel great while I'm there, but I know I need to go anyway." The therapist told Betsy about the agenda for that session and then proceeded discussing the normal reactions to assault, bringing in much of what Betsy had told her and giving her the Common Reactions to Assault handout (Chapter 8). The therapist urged her to read it daily and to share it with anyone she felt she wanted to. The overall treatment program was outlined next, and the rationale for it was discussed. Betsy agreed, noting that it made sense to her, but that she wasn't sure she would be able to do all the exposure. Together, Betsy and the therapist then constructed the following hierarchy for *in vivo* exposure:

SUDs	Item
50	Going back to that grocery store alone
60	Letting Kenneth see the Common Reactions to Assault handout
70	Discussing the Common Reactions to Assault handout and her reactions with Kenneth
80	Discussing the assault and the handout with her sister
90	Telling her best friend and current roommate, Lucinda, about the assault
100	Discussing the assault and the handout with her parents

In Session 3, Betsy reported that she had gone ahead and sent a copy of the handout to Kenneth with a short note, but had not talked to him yet. The therapist praised this effort, especially since it had not even been assigned yet. Betsy was then given the rationales for deep muscle, cue-controlled, and differential relaxation, and was taught these techniques. She responded well to all, but found it difficult to relax her neck and shoulders completely. She also described frequent tension headaches and some jaw clenching. The therapist discussed how to apply the techniques to these problems, as well as the need to practice. Next, thought stopping was discussed and taught. Betsy chose to think about what she would do after graduation as her distraction. She was instructed to practice this technique as well.

In Session 4, Betsy described practicing breathing retraining religiously, but only having done the deep muscle relaxation a few times. She indicated good results when she did practice, but noted that it was hard to find time for it. This was discussed, and it was decided that she would go to bed 30 minutes earlier to practice deep muscle relaxation, which also might help since she often had difficulty falling sleep. The rationale for imaginal exposure was then discussed, and Betsy became tenser as the discussion continued. Here is the transcript of her first lengthy imaginal exposure session:

THERAPIST: OK, go ahead. Where are you now?

BETSY: I'm in my apartment, near campus.

THERAPIST: OK. Periodically, I'm going to ask you where you are on the 0-to-100 scale.

BETSY: Oh, OK.

THERAPIST: OK. Go ahead.

BETSY: Um, I'm in my dorm room and I'm talking to my roommate, and she was going out to dinner across the street with her friends . . . and . . . I'm telling her that I need to go get groceries, and she says, "Well, that's fine, and I'll see you later." And so I went and I caught the—I go and I catch the bus; it comes right outside by our apartment. And . . . it's probably about a 10- or 15-minute bus ride, just because we have to stop at one of the bus stops and wait for the other bus so that people can transfer . . . and . . .

THERAPIST: I want you to go through it as if it's happening now, OK?

BETSY: And uh, well, I get—I'm at the grocery store and I'm shopping, and one of my friends works next door, so I was looking around to see if she was there before I went—before I go in the store and . . . she's not there, so I just go ahead in. And I'm getting my groceries and I look outside and I see . . . just a group of people . . . more guys than girls; there were maybe one or two girls with the group. And they're just out there talking and I thought—I think that maybe my friend's out there, so I look and I don't see her, and I go back to shopping. And . . . it's starting to get dark and I wanted to get on the bus and get back to my apartment before it got completely dark . . . so . . . I start walking outside . . . and I'm walking towards the bus stop, which is down the block a little ways and . . . I guess the group is gone; I don't hear the noises of lots of people talking any more, so I don't even bother to turn around and see if my friend is near, and I just keep walking. And all of a sudden, this man . . . grabs my arm, and he tells me to keep walking and not to say anything . . . and I didn't—I don't know what to do. I can't scream, I can't . . . I can't say anything at all.

THERAPIST: Where are you now on the scale of 0 to 100?

BETSY: 70.

THERAPIST: OK.

BETSY: And . . . and so I keep—I just walk and . . .

THERAPIST: I'm walking . . .

BETSY: I'm scared, I don't know what's going to happen . . . and we go— the library is right across the street from where I had just been shopping . . . and at first I thought we were going to go up the steps, but instead we go down to the garage . . . and, uh . . .

THERAPIST: He's taking me to the garage . . .

BETSY: He's—he's taking me to the garage . . . and . . . and . . . I still don't know if maybe he's—he's just going to put me in his car or—or I don't know what's going to happen . . . and . . .

THERAPIST: What are you seeing?

BETSY: I—I just—it's dark down there, and I see some cars, and I don't hear any noises . . . the door hadn't opened and I can't hear anything at all . . . and it's—it's just really dark and there's some cars, and we walk towards the end . . . away from the doors and away from . . . from the . . . the lamp, down into the garage. And he—all of a sudden, he just starts yelling at me and—and telling me that—that all—all women are bitches and that every-thing is—is a woman's fault, and that I should be blamed, and that I need to be punished, and things like that. And . . . I was wearing a skirt, 'cause even though it was winter it was . . . it was a warm day, and . . . he leaned me up against the car . . .

THERAPIST: He's leaning . . .

BETSY: He's leaning me up against the car and bending me over . . . and he—he just raped me, and then I don't—I remember. I had thrown my stuff on the ground . . . where he had knocked it out of my hands and . . . torn my blouse open. And when he was leaving, he ran and he picked up . . . some of my stuff that had scattered . . . on the floor of the garage . . . and . . . he just left. It didn't last very long, but I just tried to blank out while . . . it was going on, and then—then he left. And I sat there, and I was too shocked to cry or really do anything, so I just tried to get myself together and . . . and go to the bus stop. And uh . . . when I got on the bus, people were looking at me 'cause— I knew I probably looked a mess. And, uh . . . I couldn't go back to my apart-ment or I—I don't want to go back to my apartment—yet, so I go to my boyfriend's apartment and I knock on the door. And he didn't hear me at first, so I knocked a little harder and he came and he answered the door. And he could tell something had happened, and I just told him . . . and . . .

THERAPIST: I'm telling him. Remember, stay in the present.

BETSY: And—and he's telling me that . . . you know, everything's going to be OK, and not to worry about it, and . . . if I wanted to go to the doctor, or if I wanted him to take me to the hospital, or anything. And I told him, "No, no." I was still saying that I didn't want to go anywhere and I just wanted to stay there . . . and I didn't want to go back to my room 'cause I didn't want my roommate to know. And so he . . . he just told me that I could sleep on the sofa, or I could sleep on the bed and he'd sleep on the sofa. And . . . he asked me if I wanted to call my parents, and I said, "No." I . . . just told him I didn't want anybody to know . . . and . . . he told me that if I needed to get some help or if I needed someone to talk to that he'd stay up and talk with me, but I just wanted to go to bed. And . . . I went . . . and I took a shower . . . and he gave me one of his shirts to sleep in and I just went to bed. And . . . I just tried not to think about it for a long time, but then I just . . . feel like things are slipping away and . . . I just . . . I finally started getting some counseling at—uh . . . at school; it was group counseling.

THERAPIST: But that was a while later. What happened right afterwards? The next day when you got up, after . . . did you sleep?

BETSY: Yeah, I slept. I was just tired and I wanted to go to sleep, so I slept . . . and I woke up really early, though I . . . probably woke up around . . . 3 or 4 and I just couldn't get back to sleep. So I stayed up and . . . I had a 9:00 class and . . . I said I was going to go, but I just couldn't—I couldn't get up and leave, so I just walked . . . back to my apartment. I waited until my roommate left for her class . . . and . . . I always get home before she does, so I knew she wouldn't think anything of it if I was there when she got back . . . so I just went back to my room and . . . I just laid on my bed, and read, and stared out the window, and cried. And I didn't know what to do. I didn't know . . . if I could talk to anybody or—or anything . . . and it went on for . . . (sigh) a week, 2 weeks before . . . I started . . . just trying to get up . . . a little bit, at least, instead of just staying in my room all the time. I would go across the street to the gym and go swim or something, 'cause I . . . found that if I swam, it would take my mind off of what happened.

THERAPIST: What are you feeling right now? On the 0-to-100 scale?

BETSY: About 100 . . . I've never thought that anything like that . . . was going to happen to me, and I didn't know how to respond, or how to react, or what I should do . . .

Imaginal exposure was repeated two more times that session, with her SUDs level coming down to 70 at the end.

In Session 5, Betsy described having listened to the tape of the imaginal exposure daily, as instructed. She indicated that it was hard for her, and that she was feeling more "on edge" and was thinking more about the assault lately. She reported using the relaxation methods to try to relax, especially when she was uptight about the assault, especially before bed. She also indicated that Kenneth had received the Common Reactions to Assault handout and had called her. They got together, and she discussed it, her reactions, and the treatment with him. She reported that she was nervous, but that it wasn't as bad as she had expected, and that he was very kind and understanding and encouraging. She indicated that she was glad she had talked to him about it. She also discovered that he had not wanted to break up with her at the time, but since she had initiated it, he wanted to "give her space" if that was what she needed. The therapist discussed all of this and her reactions with Betsy, using generous praise for her display of courage as well as for following her homework instructions. Betsy asked to go ahead and do the imaginal exposure first, which was done. She was able to add more details of the actual rape and reached a SUDs level of 80 the first time, decreasing this to 70 the second time.

Next, Betsy was instructed in cognitive restructuring. She grasped the concept well, and realized that her thinking had changed after the assault. The first, non-assault-related example of a negative thought involved an incident with her current roommate, Lucinda, in which Betsy was scared Lucinda didn't like her any more and wanted her to move out after Betsy left dirty dishes in the sink overnight, breaking a "rule" that had been established when they first moved in together. Betsy was easily able to see that the evidence did not support such a conclusion, and agreed with the endpoint statement that "It would be preferable if I hadn't left dirty dishes in the sink overnight, but it doesn't mean Lucinda doesn't want to be my roommate any more."

Cognitive restructuring was more difficult for Betsy to apply to an assault-related example of a negative thought. She chose to work on her belief that Kenneth saw her as "dirty" since the assault. She was able to provide ample evidence against this and concluded that rationally, she was sure he didn't think she was dirty, and he didn't ever treat her as if she were dirty. However, she reported that although she understood she didn't need to be responding as if he thought she was dirty, she still felt it a little. She was then instructed to use the thought-stopping technique to help her get rid of thoughts she had decided weren't rational or logical. She was able to apply thought stopping successfully, and indicated she knew she'd be better off if she just stopped thinking that way, because she and the therapist had just "proven" it wasn't true. As usual, she was instructed to practice all of the techniques, to listen to the imaginal exposure tape, and to engage in *in vivo* exposure for homework. She discussed with the therapist *in vivo* exposure items to work on; she agreed that she could go shopping at that grocery store, and could send the Common Reactions to Assault handout to her sister and talk with her about it.

Betsy appeared for Session 6 very talkative. She indicated doing very well with her homework, having gone to the grocery store alone where she had been before she was assaulted without too much anxiety. She was happy because she had always liked that store, and now she felt she could use it again. She reported being hypervigilant before she went in and when she came out, looking around in case she might see the assailant again, but indicated that her anxiety level was not too high. She said it helped to have her own car now and not to have to wait for the bus. She also indicated having spoken with her sister over the phone. She said her sister had been wanting to talk with her about the assault, but hadn't wanted to bring it up for fear she would upset Betsy. Betsy indicated that her sister really didn't have an idea what she had been going through, but it was clear to Betsy that her sister cared deeply for her and wanted to be there for her. She said she felt her sister could "handle" it, too, which she had doubted previously. She appeared to be greatly relieved. During imaginal exposure, she was able to include even more details, with her SUDs level coming down to 50 at the highest. She was then instructed in guided self-dialogue, using an upcoming test in a subject she wasn't doing well in as her non-assault-related example and going shopping at that grocery store again as her assault-related example. She reported that she was already trying to tell herself some of the things included on the Guided Self-Dialogue Examples handout (see Chapter 12), so it fit well with her personal strategies.

Session 7 began with Betsy recounting the details of a recent *in vivo* exposure item—telling Lucinda about the assault. She said it had basically gone OK, but that it didn't go as well as when she had talked with Kenneth or her sister. She indicated that Lucinda was nice and supportive and didn't appear to be judgmental, but that the conversation wasn't very long and Lucinda didn't appear to know what to say after a certain point. She added that Lucinda wasn't a big talker, so it had probably gone as well as it could have. The therapist discussed ways others' reactions can affect us, times when our hopes aren't met by reality, and the fact that we sometimes have to forgive others' responses when we know they really mean well and just don't know how to handle the situation.

Imaginal exposure was then conducted, with Betsy reporting a SUDs level of 30. Role play was taught next; it focused first on asking Kenneth over for dinner, then on telling her parents about the assault. She indicated that she was planning on going home this coming weekend and hoped to disclose to her parents then, but she was apprehensive. During role play, she was able to find the right words to tell them. She and the therapist discussed her parents' likely reactions: She anticipated that her mother would cry and hug her, and that her father might get mad that she didn't tell them at the time and report it to the police. This scene was practiced four times, until Betsy felt she at least had the words to start with.

During Session 8, Betsy reported that she had gone home that weekend and did tell her parents. She felt bad that she had started to cry as she told them, and that this did make her mother cry. She was surprised that her father had cried too, but that he didn't seem mad at all; he had wanted to know how she was now, and said that this explained why she hadn't been doing well in school. She indicated that it was hard for all of them, but that she thought it was the right thing to do. She reported that her parents didn't want her to leave on Sunday to go back to school, and that in fact it was hard for her to go. She was still a little teary-eyed in the session, and cried more during imaginal exposure than in the previous session, although she reported a highest SUDs level of 15. She indicated that she was remembering her parents listening to this tape, and that this upset her. Covert modeling was then taught, using the examples first of taking a test and next of going on a date with Kenneth. The PDS was administered, and Betsy's PTSD symptoms were found to be greatly reduced. She and the therapist discussed the option of three more sessions, but both felt that Betsy had improved greatly and that she could continue to practice the skills on her own. Therefore, it was decided that Session 9 would be the last.

Below is the transcript of Betsy's last session of prolonged imaginal exposure. Notice that the level of detail surrounding the actual rape was increased, that her self-reported anxiety was decreased, and that she did a better job of staying in the present tense without as much prompting from the therapist.

THERAPIST: Where are you now on the 0-to-100 scale?

BETSY: Zero.

THERAPIST: OK. Why don't you go ahead and close your eyes and begin?

BETSY: OK . . . Um . . . I'm in the grocery store and I'm waiting to be checked out—my groceries to be checked out. And . . . while I'm waiting, I'm looking out—I'm looking next door at the restaurant to see . . . if my friend is working. And . . . I . . . can't seem to find her right now, so I'm looking across the street . . . and there's a fairly large . . . group of people just standing around talking and laughing . . . and there's one guy in the group stands out . . . in particular, because he's so much taller . . . than everybody else in the group. And . . . he appears to be the ringleader, because as he's talking, everybody else is . . . kinda laughing and . . . "Yeah, ha, that's right, I've heard that before," and . . .

THERAPIST: So you can actually hear what he's saying?

BETSY: You—you—I mean you can just kind of read—read lips and see that people are just laughing and . . . just having a good time, and you can kind of figure out what they're saying or their reactions . . .

THERAPIST: OK.

BETSY: . . . and what you think they might be saying. And, um . . . at one point . . . he . . . turns his—he's turning his head to talk to the person . . . standing next to him and . . . just . . . because I'm . . . still looking at him, I notice that his nose is really . . . sharp and it's one of the really . . . flat bridges and it comes to a . . . rather sharp point at the end. And, um . . . at that point I was just—I'm just looking, seeing . . . you know, I'm just noticing what everybody has on, and . . . I notice that . . . he's wearing just a pair of regular . . . blue jeans, a—a T-shirt, and some running shoes . . . and, uh . . . other than that, I'm not really—I'm not . . . really concentrating on . . . any particular look or anything. I can . . . see that he has sandy—sandy blondish-brownish hair; it's more brown . . . than anything else, with just streaks of blonde in it . . . and . . .

he looks like he's been on . . . vacation or maybe he's . . . been to a tanning salon or something, 'cause . . . he has a . . . pretty decent tan for . . . the middle of winter . . . and his—I don't really notice the color of his eyes from . . . far away, and I didn't have my—I don't have my glasses on, so I can't . . . make any clear distinction of the color of his eyes, but they appear to be . . . kind of . . . brownish. But, um . . . when I see him later, I notice they're . . . they have a bit of hazel, kinda green flecks in 'em . . . and . . . um . . . that's . . . about all I notice of him for right now. And when I'm done with my groceries, I'm . . . walking down the street towards the bus stop . . . and he . . . comes up behind me and he's grabbing my arm . . . and he's telling me to smile and . . . just . . . kind of look friendly and look like I'm with him. And . . . at this point was when I turn around . . .

THERAPIST: I'm turning around . . .

BETSY: I'm turning around to see . . . who's grabbed onto my arm, and that's . . . when I notice that it—it's the guy that . . . I had seen from the grocery store. And . . . I'm noticing that . . . now his eyes had more . . . color than just brown to 'em, they have . . . little flecks of green and hazel in them, and . . . his nose is really sharp and pointed. And . . . when he's grabbing my arm, I don't feel . . . any bushy arm hair or anything . . . like that rubbing up against . . . my arm; it's more just . . . skin, smooth skin. Um, his hands . . . are . . . kind of rough. They're not . . . they're not soft, but they're not really . . . hard— hard . . . but I can feel . . . kind of a few calluses on his hands when he's holding onto my arm. And as we're walking, he's . . . swinging his other arm and as he's swinging, it . . . passes by my side and . . . I glance down at his hand . . . and I notice a—uh . . . a watch, just like a black leather band with a gold face. I can't . . .

THERAPIST: Where are you now on the 0-to-100 scale?

BETSY: Zero. I can't notice the, um . . . I don't notice the, um . . . the maker of the watch—whether it really was . . . it really is an expensive watch or—or what. Um . . . and . . . I had noticed before that he's . . . he's tall, he's . . . um, but he has a . . . very athletic build, not . . . not . . . big and muscular, but you can still see the . . . the muscles in arms through his T-shirt. And he looks like he . . . works out daily or . . . just like he takes good care of himself. And . . . um . . . we're walking . . . down into the garage, and as we're walking down into the garage, he's mumbling things that . . . I can't really understand, I . . . don't understand at this point. And I'm starting . . . to get . . . scared. I was already a little frightened because I wasn't sure . . . what was going to happen. I'm not sure whether . . . we're walking up the steps into the library, or what. And . . . when he starts leading me down . . . into the . . . garage, I'm really starting to get . . . scared. I'm still . . . not sure what's going to happen. I'm . . . thinking maybe . . . we're going to his car or that . . . we'll be going through one of the . . . doors in the library that leads to the lower levels. But instead of . . . going through any doors, or getting in any car . . . in the front of the garage, we're . . . walking towards the back. We — it's really dark, there's no light from . . . the ramp we walked down or . . . the ramp on the other side . . . of the garage. And . . . when . . . we get to . . . this car, he . . . starts saying that . . . women have — women have hurt him, and . . . women deserve to be punished, women are bitches, women have . . . done . . . this thing to him and that. And he . . . I can catch the word "women," and . . . some other sentence, and in the other sentences, he's just . . . mumbling, but . . . he seems to have . . . great hostility for women. And . . . that's when he . . . says that, you know women . . . deserve — when he says, "Women deserve to be punished," I was really — that . . . just really scared me I wasn't sure . . . what he was going to do. Um . . . when he starts — he's starting to . . . unbutton my blouse now and he can't . . . get all of the buttons unbuttoned, so he's tugging at the ends trying to pull the buttons off . . . and they start popping off and they're — I can hear them falling on the . . . garage floor. And . . . I'm really scared now, I'm really frightened.

THERAPIST: Where are you now on the 0-to-100 scale?

BETSY: Zero. Um . . . he's turning me around; I wasn't, I'm not really . . . facing him — facing him, I'm kind of at an angle. And now he's turning me around and he's . . . putting my face into the hood of the car and he's putting his . . . palm in the middle of my back to . . . hold me in place, and I can feel the pressure . . . of his palm in the middle of my back. And . . . I'm . . . beginning to . . . block things out, I'm beginning to . . . to go . . . numb a little bit. I'm just . . . I'm still not exactly sure what's going to happen but I have . . . a fairly good idea, and so I'm beginning to let myself go numb. And . . . he — as he tries — he's fiddling with my skirt and he's . . . trying to see if it would be easier for him to pull it down, I suppose, because he's tugging at it and as he's tugging at it . . . he's — he's making rips in the fabric. And . . . I . . . suppose it was too hard for him to tug down, so he's slipping the — the back of . . . my skirt up. And . . . he . . . pulled my — he's pulling my underwear down around my ankles, and . . . as he's entering me, it is very painful. Um . . . it hurts a lot, but . . . now I'm just — I'm really blocking everything out of my mind and I'm really just . . . going numb and . . . trying not to let myself feel anything. And . . . when he's finished — I'm not sure . . . how long the whole thing lasted; I had lost track of time. It didn't seem like very long, but . . . I'm not sure how long it really was. Um . . . as he's getting ready . . . to leave, I'm not — there's one point he still has his hand; his hand is still in the middle of my back . . . but . . . he's bending over and I'm not sure whether he's . . . pulling up his jeans, or . . . if he's picking up my groceries — some of my groceries that had . . . fallen on the ground. But I'm . . . not really paying attention to that. I don't care . . . um . . . I'm still just bent over the hood of the car . . . and . . . after a while I don't feel . . . I can't feel the pressure . . . of anybody's hand in my back. And, um . . . . I'm starting to slide off the hood of the car, and I just . . . turn around, and I'm putting my head on the bumper of the car . . . and I'm just . . . I'm crying and I'm shaking . . . and I'm . . . starting to look for the buttons to my blouse.

THERAPIST: Where are you now?

BETSY: Zero. I can't find all of them, so I just—I say, "Forget it," and I put my head back . . . up against the car . . . up against the—the bumper. And I'm trying to . . . pat my hair down and . . . button what I can of my shirt up and tuck in my skirt. And my eyes are . . . they're really puffy from crying, and I'm—I've been shaking, I'm shaking now. I'm . . . really frightened, I'm scared, I . . . don't know what to do, other than I know I want . . . to go home. I know I don't . . . want to talk to anybody about what's happened. And . . . I'm sitting there, and I'm gathering my groceries . . . and I'm looking for my other groceries, but I can't find them, so I assume that he's taken them. And . . . I'm . . . walking up the other ramp and I'm getting on the bus . . . and . . . as I'm getting on the bus, people are—people are kind of staring at me, you know. My eyes are really puffy, and I'm sure my hair is . . . still a mess. My skirt is torn in . . . some places, and you can . . . kind of tell that . . . my blouse doesn't have all its buttons, but . . . it's not . . . all that noticeable . . . um . . . but I'm trying not to concentrate on what . . . the people on the bus are thinking. I don't really care . . . I'm just . . . really, I'm still really numb. I'm still . . . blocking everything out of my mind, I'm . . . still a little . . . shaky . . . but . . . I'm just—I'm—want to get home. So I'm getting off the bus at my boyfriend's, and . . . I'm . . . knocking on his door until he answers it. I'm—he's asking me, "What happened? Why are you crying? Why were you crying? Why are your eyes puffy?" And . . . I'm just—I'm telling him . . . I was raped and all I want to do is . . . take a shower and go to bed. I don't want to talk to anybody, I don't . . . want to go to the hospital, I don't want to report it to the police, or anything. And . . . he lets me, and I go—I'm going to sleep. And . . . the next morning . . . I'm . . . walking back to my room, and I'm sitting in my room . . . all day and not doing anything. I'm not going out . . . I'm just staying in there watching people go back and forth to class and . . . reading my books . . . I'm not really . . . interacting with anybody. I don't want to . . . and . . . I'm mainly concentrating on trying to block the rape out of my mind, but every now and then . . . I'm . . . I'm thinking about it, and I'm . . . thinking, you know, "How—how could I have let this happen? Why—why did I let it happen? Is it my fault? And . . ."

THERAPIST: Where are you now on the 0-to-100 scale?

BETSY: Zero.

THERAPIST: Why don't you go over now any kind of—if they're not "hot spots," "warm spots"?

BETSY: Um, for the first—almost month after the rape . . . um . . . I'm really concerned about whether or not the rape occurred, whether or not it was my fault, whether or not I brought it on, and . . .

THERAPIST: Where are you on the 0-to-100 scale when you think of that?

BETSY: Um, now it's 0, but at the time around 100.

THERAPIST: I mean now.

BETSY: Zero.

THERAPIST: Is there any part of imagery bothering you?

BETSY: His face doesn't bother me as much as . . . I'm still unsure of what my reaction would be if I saw him just . . . even at a glance, whether he was following me, whether he saw me or not . . . just what my reaction is—will be if I see him again. Um . . . and I'm still . . .

THERAPIST: How much anxiety does that give you? When you think that you might bump into him?

BETSY: Around a 15. Um . . . I'm not that scared of seeing him again. It's just—I don't know, whether or not I'm going to run into him, and say something to him, or whether or not I'm just going to acknowledge that he's there and walk on and just let that be the end of it, or if I'm going to—to call the police and let them know that I've seen him.

THERAPIST: So that's the meaning of your concern about seeing him? Seeing him at another time? Can you bring that up OK?

BETSY: Yes.

THERAPIST: And how much anxiety does that cause?

BETSY: None.

THERAPIST: OK, go ahead.

BETSY: Um, I'm not sure what my reaction is going to be to seeing him . . . um, not sure . . . about going to the other side of campus. I know that whether I'm going to exercise for this or to go shopping, that I'm going to have to go over there sooner or later. But I'm still a little—I'm nervous about going over there. And I'm still—I'm not sure—I know I can go out at night around here, but I'm . . . not—a little unsure of going out at night again on campus, because I haven't been on campus at night for a long time.

Betsy and the therapist then discussed Betsy's progress in treatment (which both felt was substantial), the various techniques and which ones worked best for her, and what she needed to continue to work on. Betsy felt that the imaginal exposure was the most important component for her, especially because she had so much difficulty talking about the assault. She was generally pleased with having discussed it with the people she had chosen, and wished now that she had told her parents at the time. She liked the breathing and differential relaxation techniques, but indicated that she rarely found the time for the deep muscle or cue-controlled relaxation. She used thought stopping and cognitive restructuring to help with her thoughts, but she didn't find role play useful because she was embarrassed to ask anyone to role-play with her. She indicated liking covert modeling, but not using the guided self-dialogue the therapist taught much, because she already tended to use coping self-statements.

At a follow-up appointment 3 months later, Betsy was in good spirits. Her PTSD had nearly disappeared; she was going to graduate in the spring; she was dating Kenneth again, but "they were taking it slow"; and she was planning for her future. She still felt uncomfortable with sex, but was happy that her desire had returned, and she felt that Kenneth was being patient and supportive. She said she felt like the person she had been before the assault, and she hadn't thought that was possible.

It is our sincere wish that you and all of your clients find these treatment interventions as helpful as Betsy did. Good luck!

APPENDIX

Assault Information and History Interview (AIHI)

Subject # _____   Date _____
Date of Assault _____   Therapist _____

Say to client: Our purpose in meeting today [tonight] is to talk about the assault and about how you have been feeling since that time. I understand that much of what we will discuss may be quite difficult for you to talk about. If there is anything I can do to make our conversation less difficult for you, please let me know. We may want to take a break at some point. Do you have any questions before we begin? [If no, proceed with interview.]

_____ 1. Age
_____ 2. Gender   1 - Male 2 - Female
_____ 3. Race
              1 - Black   4 - Asian-American
              2 - White   5 - Native American
              3 - Hispanic   6 - Other
_____ 4. Relationship status
              1 - Single   4 - Divorced or separated
              2 - Married   5 - Widowed
              3 - Cohabiting   6 - Other (specify) _____
_____ 5. Sexual orientation
              1 - Heterosexual   2 - Homosexual
              3 - Bisexual
_____ 6. Number of children
_____ 7. What is your current religious identification?
              1 - Catholic
              2 - Protestant [which sect? _____]

3 - Jewish

4 - Other [which one? _____]

5 - None

_____ 8. What is your employment status now?

0 - Not working

1 - Working part-time

2 - Working full-time (more than 30 hours per week)

3 - On disability

4 - Student

_____ 9. What was your employment status at the time you were assaulted?

0 - Not working

1 - Working part-time

2 - Working full-time (more than 30 hours per week)

3 - On disability

4 - Student

_____ 10. What is your job? [If unemployed, what was last job?]

Specify: _____

1 - Professional (i.e., physician, lawyer, psychologist, social worker, nurse, accountant, architect, engineer, teacher)

2 - White-collar (i.e., clerk, secretary, salesperson, bookkeeper, middle manager)

3 - Blue-collar (i.e., technician, laborer, mechanic, food service worker, child care worker)

4 - Student

5 - Homemaker (and/or full-time child caretaker)

6 - Unemployed and without previous occupation

_____ 11. What is your highest educational degree? [What was the last grade you completed in school?]

1 - PhD, MD, or equivalent   5 - AA or some college

2 - MA/MS or equivalent   6 - High school graduate

3 - Some graduate school   7 - Some high school

4 - BA/BS or equivalent   8 - Grammar school
                                      (eighth grade or less) _____

_____ 12. With whom do you live?

0 - Alone

1 - Spouse/partner

2 - Children

3 - Spouse/partner and children

4 - Parents or relatives

5 - Parents or relatives and children

6 - Parents/relatives and spouse/partner and children

7 - Roommate(s)

_____ 13. What is your current household income?

  1 - $50,000 and up   5 - $15,001–$20,000
  2 - $40,001–$50,000   6 - $10,001–$15,000
  3 - $30,001–$40,000   7 - $5,001–$10,000
  4 - $20,001–$30,000   8 - $5,000 or less

_____ 14. How many persons are dependent on this income [indicate number]?

Preassault Information

Say to client: The next series of questions relate to stressful events that you might have experienced before the assault. [Take notes on relevant assaults.]

_____ 15. Has anyone, including family members or friends, ever attacked you with the intent to kill or seriously injure you?

  0 - No   1 - Yes

_____ 16. If yes, did they use a weapon (gun, knife, etc.)?

  0 - No   1 - Yes   (N/A if not applicable)

_____ 17. If yes, how old were you at the time [of worst incident]? (N/A if not applicable)

_____ 18. As a child, did you ever see or hear violence take place between members of your family? This might include things such as seeing your brothers or sisters seriously beaten, or seeing your parents hit each other.

  0 - No   1 - Yes

_____ 19. If yes, how old were you at the time [age range]? (N/A if not applicable)

_____ 20. Were you ever seriously beaten as a child [up to age 17] by a parent or caretaker?

  0 - No   1 - Yes

_____ 21. If yes, how old were you at the time [age range]? (N/A if not applicable)

_____ 22. Before you were 13, did anyone 5 years or more older than you have sexual contact with you? When we say "sexual contact," we mean any sexual contact between someone else and your sexual organs, or between you and someone else's sexual organs.

  0 - No   1 - Yes

_____ 23. If yes, how old were you at the time [worst incident, or age range]? (N/A if not applicable)

_____ 24. Since age 13, has anyone ever used pressure, coercion, or nonphysical threats to make you have unwanted sexual contact with them?

  0 - No   1 - Yes

_____ 25. If yes, how old were you at the time [worst incident]? (N/A if not applicable)

_____ 26. Has anyone ever used physical force or the threat of physical force to make you have some type of unwanted sexual contact with them?
0 - No   1 - Yes

_____ 27. If yes, how old were you at the time? (N/A if not applicable)

_____ 28. Have you had any other traumatic experiences in your lifetime? [Use this space to take notes on other traumas that may be relevant to treatment.]

Postassault Information

_____ 29. Since the assault that we are focusing on now, has anyone tried to sexually assault you or rape you? [Check most severe case if more than one occurred.]
0 - No
1 - Exposure of genitals
2 - Yes, kissed or held, rubbed, restrained against will
3 - Yes, genitals rubbed or fondled
4 - Attempted rape
5 - Rape (coitus) or other sex act completed
6 - Other (specify) _____

_____ 30. How old were you when this happened? [Indicate age at most severe trauma.] (N/A if not applicable)

_____ 31. Have you been beaten by anyone since the assault?
0 - No   3 - Yes, repeatedly
1 - Yes, once   4 - Yes, repeatedly and to the
2 - Yes, 2–3 times   point of needing medical care

Assault Information

Say to client: Could you tell me briefly what happened the night [day] you were assaulted? What were you doing just before you were assaulted? What happened during the incident itself?

_____

_____

_____

_____

_____

_____

_____ 32. How many people participated in the assault?

_____ 33. What time of day did the assault occur?
1 - Day   2 - Night

_____ 34. Where did the assault occur?
    1 - My residence
    2 - Assailant's residence
    3 - Other residence
    4 - Alley, street, or abandoned building
    5 - Car or vehicle
    6 - Other (specify) _____

_____ 35. What was the race of the assailant?
    1 - Black   3 - Hispanic
    2 - White   4 - Other

_____ 36. What was the age of the assailant?
    1 - Under 12   4 - 25–39
    2 - 13–17   5 - 40–55
    3 - 18–24   6 - over 55

_____ 37. Who was the assailant?
    1 - Stranger   7 - Ex-lover
    2 - Acquaintance 8 - Ex-husband or estranged husband
    3 - Coworker   9 - Spouse
    4 - Friend   10 - Brother
    5 - Date   11 - Other relative
    6 - Lover   12 - Other (specify) _____

_____ 38. Had you ever had a sexual relationship with the assailant before the assault?
    0 - No   1 - Yes

_____ 39. Do you think the assailant was under the influence of drugs or alcohol?
    0 - No   1 - Yes   2 - Unsure

_____ 40. Were you under the influence of drugs or alcohol at the time of the incident?
    0 - No   1 - Yes

_____ 41. At the time of the incident, did you think you would be killed or seriously injured?
    0 - No   1 - Yes

_____ 42. How long did the episode last [record in minutes]?

_____ 43. Was anyone else with you?
    0 - No   1 - Yes

_____ 44. Did the assailant display a weapon?
    0 - No
    1 - Yes, a potentially harmful weapon (specify) _____
    2 - Yes, a clear weapon (specify) _____

_____ 45. Did the assailant imply that he had a weapon but not show it?
    0 - No   1 - Yes

_____ 46. Did the assailant verbally threaten you?
    0 - No   1 - Yes

_____ 47. Did he restrain you with his body [arms, legs, etc]?
    0 - No   1 - Yes

_____ 48. Did he restrain you in any other way [e.g., tie you up]?
        0 - No   1 - Yes

_____ 49. Did he reassure you in any way [e.g., tell you that he would not harm you]?
        0 - No   1 - Yes

_____ 50. Did he hit you with his fist?
        0 - No   1 - Yes

_____ 51. Did he hit you with an object?
        0 - No   1 - Yes (specify) _____

_____ 52. Did the assailant hold a gun to your head or a knife to your throat?
        0 - No   1 - Yes

_____ 53. Were you shot or cut during the assault?
        0 - No   1 - Yes

_____ 54. Did the assailant choke you or attempt to choke you?
        0 - No   1 - Yes

_____ 55. Did the assailant try to harm you in any other way [e.g., force you to take drugs]?
        0 - No   1 - Yes

_____ 56. At the time of the assault, did you think you would be killed or seriously injured?
        0 - No   1 - Yes

_____ 57. Were you abducted (e.g., driven in a car)?
        0 - No   1 - Yes

_____ 58. Did you escape the situation on your own, or did someone come to your assistance?
        0 - Didn't escape/assailant[s] left
        1 - Escaped on my own
        2 - Escaped with assistance
        3 - Rescued while unconscious
        4 - Unsure

What acts did the assailant perform?

_____ 59. Vaginal intercourse   0 - No   1 - Yes

_____ 60. Oral intercourse   0 - No   1 - Yes

_____ 61. Anal intercourse   0 - No   1 - Yes

_____ 62. Other sexual act _____ 0 - No   1 - Yes

_____ 63. Simple assault   0 - No   1 - Yes

_____ 64. Aggravated assault   0 - No   1 - Yes

_____ 65. Robbery   0 - No   1 - Yes

_____ 66. Other nonsexual act _____ 0 - No   1 - Yes

In considering the sexual acts performed, was this the first experience you ever had with:

_____ 67. Vaginal intercourse   0 - No   1 - Yes   (N/A if not applicable)

_____ 68. Oral intercourse   0 - No   1 - Yes   (N/A if not applicable)

_____ 69. Anal intercourse   0 - No   1 - Yes   (N/A if not applicable)
_____ 70. Other sexual act _____ 0 - No   1 - Yes   (N/A if not applicable)
_____ 71. How many persons had sexual contact with you?
_____ 72. How many persons had nonsexual criminal contact with you [excluding those counted in previous question]?

Say to client: Next, I am going to ask you why you think the assault occurred. [_Important:_ Assure the client that you are not suggesting that she should or should not think any of these statements, but that you are asking whether she agrees or disagrees with them. Read statements to client and answer each item.]

_____ 73. I was not careful enough.
          0 - No   1 - Yes
_____ 74. I did not realize how dangerous the situation was.
          0 - No   1 - Yes
_____ 75. My behavior contributed to it [e.g., I was drunk].
          0 - No   1 - Yes
_____ 76. His behavior wasn't predictable; he was acting crazy.
          0 - No   1 - Yes
_____ 77. I was just in the wrong place at the wrong time.
          0 - No   1 - Yes
_____ 78. How much do you think your actions contributed to the incident?
          0 - I don't think my actions made any difference.
          1 - I think my actions made things a little better.
          2 - I think my actions made things a lot better.
          3 - I think my actions made things a little worse.
          4 - I think my actions made things a lot worse.
_____ 79. How much do you blame yourself for what happened?
          0 - Not at all   3 - Very much
          1 - A little   4 - Completely
          2 - Some
      80. Sometimes people try to figure out why bad events happen. How much do you blame each of the following factors for the assault? Please designate a percentage of blame for each factor, for a total of 100%.
          _____ Myself
          _____ Assailant[s]
          _____ Other people
          _____ Environment
          _____ Chance
      81. To the extent that you blame yourself, how much was due to each of the following factors, so that the overall assignment of blame totals 100%?
          _____ My behavior (what I did or did not do)
          _____ My character or personality (who I am)

PTSD Symptoms and Related Reactions

Say to client: The next set of questions is about why you think you currently have symptoms of PTSD. [Assure the client again that these are not ways she should or should not think.] Indicate the degree to which you agree that each statement is contributing to your symptoms.

> 1 - Not at all agree
> 2 - Somewhat agree
> 3 - Very much agree

_____ 82. The assault was just too stressful for me to handle.

_____ 83. My symptoms developed because of simple bad luck.

_____ 84. Changes in my body chemistry caused my symptoms.

_____ 85. I learned to be more afraid.

_____ 86. I am unconsciously still reacting to the assault.

_____ 87. Do you feel you are experiencing any unusual fears or phobias as a direct result of the incident? [Examples: fear of darkness, being alone, certain houses or buildings, etc.]
> 0 - No   1 - Yes

_____ 88. Do you feel that repetitious behaviors [rituals, compulsive acts] have come about as a direct result of the assault? [Examples: repetitive bathing, or repetitive checking of locks on doors and windows.]
> 0 - No
> 1 - Yes, somewhat; a minor problem
> 2 - Yes, very definitely; a major problem

_____ 89. Do you feel guilty about the occurrence of the assault or about the way you behaved during it?
> 0 - No
> 1 - Yes, somewhat, occasional guilt feelings
> 2 - Yes, much guilt, frequent guilt feelings

_____ 90. Do you feel ashamed about the occurrence of the assault or about the way you behaved during it?
> 0 - No
> 1 - Yes, somewhat, occasional feelings of shame
> 2 - Yes, much shame, frequent feelings of shame

Other Mental Health Problems since Asssault

_____ 91. How has your overall mood been since the assault?
> 1 - Good
> 2 - Fair
> 3 - Poor

_____ 92. Since the assault, how often have you thought that life is not worth living, or thought seriously about suicide?

0 - Never
1 - Once
2 - Twice
3 - Three times
4 - Four or more times (use four as maximum)

_____ 93. Have you gone so far as to make a careful plan as to how you would kill yourself? Selected a location or date? Bought a gun? Obtained pills?

0 - No
1 - Once
2 - Twice
3 - Three times
4 - Four or more times (use four as maximum)

_____ 94. Have you made a suicide attempt since the incident?

0 - No
1 - Once
2 - Twice
3 - Three times
4 - Four or more times (use four as maximum)

_____ 95. Have you sought psychiatric or psychological help as a result of the assault, other than at a crisis center? [Do not include *this* treatment.]

0 - No   1 - Yes

_____ 96. Have you been to the hospital *since the assault* for a nervous condition? Suicide attempt? Alcohol or drug addiction?

0 - No   1 - Yes

[If yes:] Tell me why you were hospitalized. _____

Alcohol and Drug Use

Say to client: Since the assault, how often have you used the following drugs?

0 - None
1 - Once in the past month
2 - Twice in the past month
3 - About once a week
4 - Twice a week or more/not daily
5 - Daily

_____ 97. Prescription medications (specify):

_____ 98. Street drugs (specify):

_____ 99. Over-the-counter medications (specify):

_____ 100. Since the assault, on the average, about how many alcoholic drinks do you have per day? [Consider one drink to be a 12-ounce can of beer, one cocktail, or a 4-ounce glass of wine.]
   0 - I never drink
   1 - Rare use of alcohol: 1–2 drinks per month
   2 - Occasional use: 1–2 drinks per week
   3 - One drink per day or less (not to excess)
   4 - Two or three drinks per day; binges rarely or occasionally
   5 - Binges to excess 2–3 times per week
   6 - Daily heavy use (>3 drinks per day)
_____ 101. Have you ever had legal, social, or employment problems because of your alcohol or drug use?
   0 - No   1 - Yes
_____ 102. Do you consider yourself to have a drinking or drug problem?
   0 - No   1 - Yes

Gynecological Problems

Say to client: Gynecological problems and injuries may occur as a result of an assault. I'd like to ask you some questions about any injuries that you may have received from the assault, or problems you are having now. [If client suffered a nonsexual assault only, enter N/A for this section.]

_____ 103. Were you given a gynecological exam after the assault?
   0 - No   1 - Yes
_____ 104. Were you given an HIV test after the assault?
   0 - No   1 - Yes
_____ 105. Are you HIV-positive as a result of the assault?
   0 - No   1– Yes
_____ 106. Are you worried that you are HIV-positive as a result of the assault?
   0 - No   1– Yes
_____ 107. Were you pregnant, and did you have a miscarriage because of the assault?
   0 - No   1– Yes
_____ 108. Did you get pregnant as a result of the assault?
   0 - No   1– Yes

_____ 109. If yes, did you have a D&C or an abortion to terminate the pregnancy?
     0 - No   1– Yes

_____ 110. Did you contract any other sexually transmitted diseases as a result of the assault [e.g., herpes, pelvic inflammatory disease, or vaginal warts]?
     0 - No   1– Yes

111. As a result of the assault, have you had any of the following injuries [circle any of the following items that apply to victim]:
    1 - Vaginal bruises or trauma
    2 - Genital or rectal lacerations
    3 - Pain and discomfort in vaginal or anal area
    4 - Burning sensations in vaginal or anal area
    5 - Itching in vaginal or rectal area
    6 - Bloating
    7 - Abnormal or unusual bleeding
    8 - Pain or burning during urination
    9 - Pain or burning during elimination
    10 - Rectal bruises or trauma

_____ 112. How has your general physical health been?
    1 - Good, no complaints
    2 - Okay, usual problems
    3 - Marginal, unusual problems
    4 - Poor, significant problems (specify) _____

Life Changes and Legal Activity

Say to client: Now I'm going to ask some questions about changes you've made in your life since the assault, and about any legal activity you might be involved with. Since the assault, what changes have you made *due to the assault?*

_____ 113.	Moved	0 - No	1 - Yes
_____ 114.	Changed phone number	0 - No	1 - Yes
_____ 115.	Divorced or separated	0 - No	1 - Yes
_____ 116.	Broke up with a lover	0 - No	1 - Yes
_____ 117.	Increased security	0 - No	1 - Yes
_____ 118.	Carry a weapon	0 - No	1 - Yes
_____ 119.	Changed job	0 - No	1 - Yes
_____ 120.	Quit/transferred school	0 - No	1 - Yes

_____ 121. How many people have you confided in about the assault [enter number]?

_____ 122. How difficult has it been confiding about the assault?
    0 - Not difficult
    1 - Moderately difficult
    2 - Very difficult
    (N/A if not applicable)

_____ 123. Did you report the assault to the police?
      0 - No   1 - Yes
_____ 124. Did you press charges [Are you pressing charges]?
      0 - No   1 - Yes
      [If no, the next nine questions are N/A; go to question 133.]
_____ 125. Did you identify the assailant?
      0 - No
      1 - Yes, in person
      2 - Yes, in a book
      (N/A if not applicable)
_____ 126. If the assailant has been caught, was he arrested?
      0 - No   1 - Yes   (N/A if not applicable)
_____ 127. Have you attended a preliminary hearing?
      0 - No   1 - Yes   (N/A if not applicable)
_____ 128. How many times has your hearing been postponed? (N/A if not applicable)
_____ 129. What was the result of the hearing?
      0 - Released
      1 - Out on bail, pending trial
      2 - In jail, pending trial
      (N/A if not applicable)
_____ 130. Have you been to your trial?
      0 - No   1 - Yes   (N/A if not applicable)
_____ 131. How many times has the trial been postponed? (N/A if not applicable)
_____ 132. What was the outcome of the trial?
      0 - Not guilty
      1 - Guilty
      2 - Mistrial
      (N/A if not applicable)
_____ 133. Was the sentence appropriate?
      0 - No   1 - Yes   (N/A if not applicable)
_____ 134. Have you had any contact with the assailant?
      0 - No
      1 - Yes, on the phone
      2 - Yes, in person (publicly)
      3 - Yes, in person (privately)
_____ 135. Has the assailant threatened you?
      0 - No   1 - Yes
_____ 136. Has anyone associated with the assailant threatened you?
      0 - No   1 - Yes
_____ 137. Has the assailant physically harmed you since the assault?
      0 - No   1 - Yes

References

American Psychiatric Association (APA). (1980). *Diagnostic and statistical manual of mental disorders* (3rd ed.). Washington, DC: Author.

American Psychiatric Association (APA). (1987). *Diagnostic and statistical manual of mental disorders* (3rd ed., rev.). Washington, DC: Author.

American Psychiatric Association (APA). (1994). *Diagnostic and statistical manual of mental disorders.* (4th ed.). Washington, DC: Author.

Amir, N., Foa, E. B., & Cashman, L. (1996). *Predictors of posttraumatic stress disorder: A propective study of rape and nonsexual assault victims.* Manuscript submitted for publication.

Anisman H., & Sklar, L. S. (1979). Catecholamine depletion in mice upon reexposure to stress: Mediation of the escape deficits produced by inescapable shock. *Journal of Comparative and Psychology, 93,* 610–625.

Armstrong, K., O'Callahan, W., & Marmar, C. R. (1991). Debriefing Red Cross disaster personnel: The Multiple Stressor Debriefing Model. *Journal of Traumatic Stress, 4*(4), 581–593.

Atkeson, B., Calhoun, K., Resick, P., & Ellis, E. (1982). Victims of rape: Repeated assessment of depressive symptoms. *Journal of Consulting and Clinical Psychology, 50,* 96–102.

Bart, P. (1975, May). *Unalienating abortion, demystifying depression, and restoring rape victims.* Paper presented at the 128th Annual Convention of the American Psychiatric Association, Anaheim, CA.

Baum, A., Gatchel, R. J., & Schaeffer, M. A. (1983). Emotional, behavioral, and physiological effects of chronic stress at Three Mile Island. *Journal of Consulting and Clinical Psychology, 4,* 565–572.

Baum, M. (1970). Extinction of avoidance responding through response prevention (flooding). *Psychological Bulletin, 74,* 276.

Beck, A. T. (1976). *Cognitive therapy and the emotional disorders.* New York: International Universities Press.

Beck, A. T., Emery, G., & Greenberg, R. L. (1985). *Anxiety disorders and phobias: A cognitive perspective.* New York: Basic Books.

Beck, A. T., Rush, A. J., Shaw, B. F., & Emery, G. (1979). *Cognitive therapy of depression.* New York: Guilford Press.

Beck, A. T., Ward, C. H., Mendelson, M., Mock, J., & Erbaugh, J. (1961). An inventory for measuring depression. *Archives of General Psychiatry, 4,* 561–571.

Becker, J. V., & Abel, G. G. (1981). Behavioral treatment of victims of sexual assault. In S. M. Turner, K. S. Calhoun, & H. E. Adams (Eds.), *Handbook of clinical behavior therapy* (pp. 347–379). New York: Wiley.

Becker, J. V., Skinner, L. J., Abel, G. G., & Treacy, E. C. (1982). The incidence and types of sexual dysfunctions in rape and incest victims. *Journal of Sex and Marital Therapy, 8,* 65–74.

Bell, J. L. (1995). Traumatic event debriefing: Service delivery designs and the role of social work. *Social Work, 40*(1), 36–43.

Bernstein, D. A. & Borkovec, T. D. (1973). *Progressive relaxation training.* Champaign, IL: Research Press.

Bernstein, E. M., & Putnam, F. W. (1986). Development, reliability and validity of a dissociation scale. *Journal of Nervous and Mental Disease, 174,* 727–734.

Birkhimer, L. J., DeVane, C. L., & Muniz, C. D. (1985). Posttraumatic stress disorder: Characteristics and pharmacological response in the veteran population. *Comprehensive Psychiatry, 26,* 304–310.

Blake, D. D., Weathers, F. W., Nagy, L. M., Kaloupek, D. G., Klauminzer, G., Charney, D. S., & Keane, T. M. (1990). A clinician rating scale for assessing current and lifetime PTSD: The CAPS-1. *The Behavior Therapist, 18,* 187–188.

Blanchard, E. B., & Abel, G. G. (1976). An experimental case study of the biofeedback treatment of a rape induced psychophysiological cardiovascular disorder. *Behavior Therapy, 7,* 113–119.

Blanchard, E. B., Kolb, L. C., Gerardi, R. J., Ryan, D., & Pallmeyer, T. P. (1986). Cardiac response to relevant stimuli as an adjunctive tool for diagnosing posttraumatic stress disorder in Vietnam veterans. *Behavior Therapy, 17,* 592–606.

Blanchard, E. B., Kolb, L. C., Pallmeyer, T. P., & Gerardi, R. J. (1982). A psychophysiological study of post-traumatic stress disorder in Vietnam veterans. *Psychiatric Quarterly, 54,* 220–229.

Bleich, A., Siegel, B., Garb, R., & Lerer, B. (1986). Post-traumatic stress disorder following combat exposure: Clinical features and psychopharmacological treatment. *British Journal of Psychiatry, 149,* 365–369.

Boudewyns, P. A., & Hyer, L. (1990). Physiological response to combat memories and preliminary treatment outcome in Vietnam veterans PTSD patients treated with direct therapeutic exposure. *Behavior Therapy, 21,* 63–87.

Boudewyns, P. A., Hyer, L., Woods, M. G., Harrison, W. R., & McCranie, E. (1990). PTSD among Vietnam veterans: An early look at treatment outcome using direct therapeutic exposure. *Journal of Traumatic Stress, 3,* 359–368.

Boudewyns, P. A., Stwertka, S., Hyer, L., Albrecht, W., & Sperr, E. (1993). Eye movement desensitization for PTSD of combat: A treatment outcome pilot study. *The Behavior Therapist, 16,* 29–33.

Bowen, G. R., & Lambert, J. A. (1986). Systematic desensitization therapy with post-traumatic stress disorder cases. In C. R. Figley (Ed.), *Trauma and its wake* (Vol. 2, pp. 280–291). New York: Brunner/Mazel.

Bravo, M., Rubio-Stipec, M., Canino, G. J., Woodbury, M. A., & Ribera, J. (1990).

The psychological sequelae of disaster stress prospectives and retrospectives evaluated. *American Journal of Community Psychology, 5,* 661–680.

Bremner, J. D., Southwick, S., Brett, E., Fontana, A., Rosenheck, R., & Charney, D. (1992). Dissociation and posttraumatic stress disorder in Vietnam combat veterans. *American Journal of Psychiatry, 149,* 328–332.

Breslau, N., & Davis, G. C. D. (1987). Posttraumatic stress disorder: The stressor criterion. *Journal of Nervous and Mental Disease, 175,* 255–264.

Breslau, N., Davis, G. C. D., Andreski, P., & Peterson, E. (1991). Traumatic events and posttraumatic stress disorder in an urban population of young adults. *Archives of General Psychiatry, 48,* 218–222.

Brom, D., Kleber, R. J., & Defres, P. B. (1989). Brief psychotherapy for posttraumatic stress disorders. *Journal of Consulting and Clinical Psychology, 57,* 607–612.

Bromet, E. J., & Schulberg, H. C. (1986). The Three Mile Island disaster: A search for high-risk groups. In J. H. Shore (Ed.), *Disaster stress studies: New methods and findings* (pp. 1–19). Washington, DC: American Psychiatric Press.

Burgess, A. W., & Holmstrom, L. L. (1974a). The rape trauma syndrome. *American Journal of Psychiatry, 131,* 981–986.

Burgess, A. W., & Holmstrom, L. L. (1974b). *Rape: Victims of crisis.* Bowie, MD: R. J. Brady.

Burgess, A. W., & Holmstrom, L. L. (1976). Coping behavior of the rape victim. *American Journal of Psychiatry, 133,* 413–418.

Burgess, A. W., & Holmstrom, L. L. (1978). Recovery from rape and prior life stress. *Research in Nursing and Health, 1,* 165–174.

Burns, D. D. (1980). *Feeling good: The new mood therapy.* New York: Morrow.

Burstein, A. (1985). Posttraumatic flashbacks, dream disturbances, and mental imagery. *Journal of Clinical Psychiatry, 46*(9), 374–378.

Burstein, A., Ciccone, P. E., Greenstein, R. A., Daniels, N., Olsen, K., Mazarek, A., Decatur, R., & Johnson, N. (1988). Chronic Vietnam PTSD and acute civilian PTSD: A comparison of treatment experiences. *General Hospital Psychiatry, 10,* 245–249.

Butler, G., Fennell, M., Robson, P., & Gelder, M. (1991). Comparison of behavior therapy and cognitive behavior therapy in the treatment of generalized anxiety disorder. *Journal of Consulting and Clinical Psychology, 59,* 167–175.

Butler, R. W., Braff, D. L., Rausch, J. L., Jenkins, M. A., Sproch, J., & Geyer, M. A. (1990). Physiological evidence of exaggerated startle response in a subgroup of Vietnam veterans with combat related PTSD. *American Journal of Psychiatry, 147,* 1308–1312.

Cairns, E., & Wilson, R. (1984). The impact of political violence on mild psychiatric morbidity in Northern Ireland. *British Journal of Psychiatry, 145,* 631–635.

Calhoun, K. S., Atkeson, B. M., & Resick, P. A. (1982). A longitudinal examination of fear reactions in victims of rape. *Journal of Counseling Psychology, 29,* 655–661.

Cardeña, E., & Spiegel, D. (1993). Dissociative reactions to the San Francisco Bay Area earthquake of 1989. *American Journal of Psychiatry, 150*(3), 474–478.

Charney, D. S., Deutch, A. Y., Krystal, J. H., Southwick, S. M., & Davis, M. (1993). Psychobiologic mechanisms of posttraumatic stress disorder. *Archives of General Psychiatry, 50*(4), 294–305.

Clark, D. M. (1986). A cognitive approach to panic. *Behaviour Research and Therapy*, 24, 461–470.

Clark, D. M. (1989). Anxiety states: Panic and generalized anxiety. In K. Hawton, P. Salkovskis, J. Kirk, & D. M. Clark (Eds.), *Cognitive behaviour therapy for psychiatric problems: A practical guide*. Oxford: Oxford University Press.

Cooper, N. A. & Clum, G. A. (1989). Imaginal flooding as a supplementary treatment for PTSD in combat veterans: A controlled study. *Behavior Therapy*, 20, 381–391.

Courtois, C. (1988). *Healing the incest wound: Adult survivors in therapy*. New York: Norton.

Cryer, L., & Beutler, L. (1980). Group therapy: An alternative treatment approach for rape victims. *Journal of Sex and Marital Therapy*, 6, 40–46.

Dancu, C., Rothbaum, B. O., Riggs, D., & Foa, E. (1990, November). *The relationship between dissociation and PTSD*. Poster presented at the 23rd Annual Convention of the Association for Advancement of Behavior Therapy, San Francisco.

Davidson, J. R. T., Hughes, D., Blazer, D. G., & George, L. K. (1991). Post-traumatic stress disorder in the community: An epidemiological study. *Psychological Medicine*, 21, 713–721.

Davidson, J. R. T., Kudler, H. S., Smith, R. D., Mahoney, S. L., Lipper, S. L., Hammett, E., Saunders, W. B., & Cavenar, J. O. (1990). Treatment of posttraumatic stress disorder with amitriptyline and placebo. *Archives of General Psychiatry*, 47, 259–266.

Davidson, L. M., & Baum, A. (1986). Chronic stress and post-traumatic stress disorders. *Journal of Consulting and Clinical Psychology*, 54, 303–308.

Davis, R. C., Brickman, E. R., & Baker, T. (1991). Effects of supportive and unsupportive responses of others to rape victims: Effects on concurrent victim adjustment. *American Journal of Community Psychology*, 19, 443–451.

Ellis, A. (1977). The basic clinical theory and rational–emotive therapy. In A. Ellis & R. Grieger (Eds.), *Handbook of rational–emotive therapy* (pp. 3–34). New York: Springer.

Ellis, E. M., Atkeson, B. M., & Calhoun, K. S. (1981). An assessment of long-term reaction to rape. *Journal of Abnormal Psychology*, 90, 263–266.

Ellis, E. M., Calhoun, K. S., & Atkeson, B. M. (1980). Sexual dysfunction in victims of rape. *Women and Health*, 5, 39–47.

Epstein, S. (1991). Impulse control and self-destructive behavior. In L. P. Lipsitt & L. L. Mitnick (Eds.), *Self-regulatory behavior and risk taking: Causes and consequences* (pp. 273–284). Norwood, NJ: Ablex.

Evans, H. I. (1978). Psychotherapy for the rape victim: Some treatment models. *Hospital and Community Psychiatry*, 29, 309–312.

Fairbank, J. A., Gross, R. T., & Keane, T. M. (1983). Treatment of posttraumatic stress disorder: Evaluation of outcome with a behavioral code. *Behavior Modification*, 7, 557–568.

Famularo, R., Kinscherff, R., & Fenton, T. (1988). Propranolol treatment for childhood posttraumatic stress disorder, acute type. *American Journal of Diseases of Children*, 142, 1244–1247.

Feldman-Summers, S., Gordon, P. E., & Meagher, J. R. (1979). The impact of rape on sexual satisfaction. *Journal of Abnormal Psychology, 88,* 101–105.

Fesler, F. A. (1991). Valproate in combat-related posttraumatic stress disorder. *Journal of Clinical Psychiatry, 52,* 361–364.

Fisher, C. (1943). Hypnosis in treatment of neuroses due to war and to other causes. *War Medicine, 4*(6), 565–576.

FitzGerald, M. L., Braudaway, C. A., Leeks, D., Padgett, M. B., Swartz, A. L., Samter, J., Gary-Stephens, M., & Dellinger, N. F. (1993). Debriefing: A therapeutic intervention. *Military Medicine, 158*(8), 542–545.

Foa, E. B., Cashman, L., Jaycox, L. H., & Perry, K. (in press). The validation of a self-report measure of PTSD: The PTSD Diagnostic Scale (PDS). *Psychological Assessment.*

Foa, E. B., Feske, U., Murdock, T. B., Kozak, M. J., & McCarthy, P. R. (1991a). Processing of threat-related information in rape victims. *Journal of Abnormal Psychology. 100,* 156–162.

Foa, E. B., Franklin, M. E., Perry, K. J., & Herbert, J. D. (1996). Cognitive biases in generalized social phobia. *Journal of Abnormal Psychology, 105*(3), 433–439.

Foa, E. B., Hearst-Ikeda, D. E., & Perry, K. (1995a). Evaluation of a brief cognitive-behavioral program for the prevention of chronic PTSD in recent assault victims. *Journal of Consulting and Clinical Psychology, 63,* 948–955.

Foa, E. B., & Jaycox, L. H. (in press). Cognitive-behavioral treatment of posttraumatic stress disorder: Theory and practice. In D. Spiegel (Ed.), *Psychotherapeutic frontiers: New principles and practices.* Washington, DC: American Psychiatric Press.

Foa, E. B., & Kozak, M. J. (1985). Treatment of anxiety disorders: Implications for psychopathology. In A. H. Tuma & J. D. Maser (Eds.), *Anxiety and the anxiety disorders* (pp. 421–452). Hillsdale, NJ: Erlbaum.

Foa, E. B., & Kozak, M. J. (1986). Emotional processing of fear: Exposure to corrective information. *Psychological Bulletin, 99,* 20–35.

Foa, E. B., & Kozak, M. J. (1991). Emotional processing: Theory, research, and clincial implications for anxiety disorders. In J. D. Safran & L. S. Greenberg (Eds.), *Emotion, psychotherapy, and change* (pp. 21–49). New York: Guilford Press.

Foa, E. B., & Kozak, M. J. (1996). Psychological treatment for obsessive–compulsive disorder. In M. R. Mavissakalian & R. F. Prien (Eds.), *Long-term treatments of anxiety disorders* (pp. 285–309). Washington, DC: American Psychiatric Press.

Foa, E. B., & Meadows, E. A. (1997). Psychosocial treatments for post-traumatic stress disorder: A critical review. In J. Spence, J. M. Darley, & D. J. Foss (Eds.), *Annual review of psychology* (Vol. 48, pp. 449–480). Palo Alto, CA: Annual Reviews.

Foa, E. B., Molnar, C., & Cashman, L. (1995b). Change in rape narratives during exposure therapy for PTSD. *Journal of Traumatic Stress, 8*(4), 675–690.

Foa, E. B., & Riggs, D. S. (1993). Post-traumatic stress disorder in rape victims. In J. Oldham, M. B. Riba, & A. Tasman (Eds.), *American Psychiatric Press review of psychiatry* (Vol. 12, pp. 273–303). Washington, DC: American Psychiatric Press.

Foa, E. B., & Riggs, D. S. (1995). Posttraumatic stress disorder following assault:

Theoretical considerations and empirical findings. *Current Directions in Psychological Science, 4*(2), 61–65.

Foa, E. B., Riggs,, D. S., Dancu, C. V., & Rothbaum, B. O. (1993). Reliability and validity of a brief instrument for assessing post-traumatic stress disorder. *Journal of Traumatic Stress, 6,* 459–473.

Foa, E. B., Riggs, D. S., & Gershuny, B. S. (1995c). Arousal, numbing, and intrusion: Symptom structure of PTSD following assault. *American Journal of Psychiatry, 152*(1), 116–120.

Foa, E. B., Riggs, D. S., Massie, E. D., & Yarczower, M. (1995d). The impact of fear activation and anger on the efficacy of exposure treatment for PTSD. *Behavior Therapy, 26,* 487–499.

Foa, E. B., Rothbaum, B. O., & Kozak, M. J. (1989a). Behavioral treatments of anxiety and depression. In P. Kendall & D. Watson (Eds.), *Anxiety and depression: Distinctive and overlapping features* (pp. 413–454). New York: Academic Press.

Foa, E. B., Rothbaum, B. O., & Molnar, C. (1995e). Cognitive-behavioral therapy of post-traumatic stress disorder. In M. J. Friedman, D. S. Charney, & A. Y. Deutch (Eds.), *Neurobiological and clinical consequences of stress: From normal adaptation to post-traumatic stress disorder* (pp. 483–494). New York: Lippincott-Raven.

Foa, E. B., Rothbaum, B. O., Riggs, D., & Murdock, T. (1991b). Treatment of post-traumatic stress disorder in rape victims: A comparison between cognitive-behavioral procedures and counseling. *Journal of Consulting and Clinical Psychology, 59,* 715–723.

Foa, E. B., Steketee, G., & Rothbaum, B. O. (1989b). Behavioral/cognitive conceptualization of post-traumatic stress disorder. *Behavior Therapy, 20,* 155–176.

Foa, E. B., Steketee, G., & Young, M. (1984). Agoraphobia: Phenomenological aspects, associated characteristics and theoretical considerations. *Clinical Psychology Review, 4,* 431–457.

Foa, E. B., Zinbarg, R., & Rothbaum, B. O. (1992). Uncontrollability and unpredictability in post-traumatic stress disorder: An animal model. *Psychological Bulletin, 112,* 218–238.

Forman, B. D. (1980). Cognitive modification of obsessive thinking in a rape victim: A preliminary study. *Psychological Reports, 47,* 819–822.

Fox, S. S., & Scherl, D. J. (1972). Crisis intervention with victims of rape. *Social Work, 17,* 37–42.

Foy, D. W., Sipprelle, R. C., Rueger, D. B., & Carroll, E. M. (1984). Etiology of posttraumatic stress disorder in Vietnam veterans: Analysis of premilitary, military, and combat exposure influences. *Journal of Consulting and Clinical Psychology, 52*(1), 79–87.

Frank, E., Anderson, B., Stewart, B. D., Dancu, C., Hughes, C., & West, D. (1988). Efficacy of cognitive behavior therapy and systematic desensitization in the treatment of rape trauma. *Behavior Therapy, 19,* 403–420.

Frank, E., & Stewart, B. D. (1983). Treatment of depressed rape victims: An approach to stress-induced symptomatology. In P. J. Clayton, & J. E. Barrett (Eds.), *Treatment of depression: Old controversies and new approaches.* New York: Raven Press.

Frank, E., & Stewart, B. D. (1984). Depressive symptoms in rape victims. *Journal of Affective Disorders, 1,* 269–277.

Frank, E., Turner, S. M., & Duffy, B. (1979). Depressive symptoms in rape victims. *Journal of Affective Disorders, 1*, 269–277.

Frank, E., Turner, S. M., & Stewart, B. (1980). Initial response to rape: The impact of factors within the rape situation. *Journal of Behavioral Assessment, 62*, 39–53.

Frank, J. B., Kosten, T. R., Giller, E. L., & Dan, E. (1988). A randomized clinical trial of phenelzine and imipramine for post-traumatic stress disorder. *American Journal of Psychiatry, 145*, 1289–1291.

Gerardi, R. J., Blanchard, E. B., & Kolb, L. C. (1989). Ability of Vietnam veterans to dissimulate a psychophysiological assessment for post-traumatic stress disorder. *Behavior Therapy, 20*(2), 229–243.

Green, B. L., Grace, M. C., Lindy, J. D., Gleser, G. C., Leonard, A. C., & Kramer, T. L. (1990). Buffalo Creek survivors in the second decade: Comparison with unexposed and nonlitigant group. *Journal of Applied Social Psychology, 20*, 1033–1050.

Green, B. L., Koral, M., Grace, M. C., Vary, M. G., Leonard, A. C., Gleser, G. C., & Smithson-Cohen, S. (1991). Children and disaster: Age, gender, and parental effects on PTSD symptoms. *Journal of the American Academy of Child and Adolescent Psychiatry, 6*, 945–951.

Grigsby, J. P. (1987). The use of imagery in the treatment of posttraumatic stress disorder. *Journal of Nervous and Mental Disease, 175*, 55–59.

Grinker, R. R., & Spiegel, J. P. (1943). *War neurosis in North Africa, the Tunisian campaign, January to May 1943.* New York: Josiah Macy Foundation.

Hearst (1969). Aversive conditioning and external stimulus control. In B. A. Campbell & R. M. Church (Eds.), *Punishment and aversive behavior* (pp. 235–277). New York: Appleton-Century-Crofts.

Henderson, J. L., & Moore, M. (1944). The psychoneuroses of war. *New England Journal of Medicine, 230*(10), 273–278.

Hickling, E. J., Sison, G. F. P., & Vanderploeg, R. D. (1986). Treatment of posttraumatic stress disorder with relaxation and biofeedback training. *Biofeedback and Self-Regulation, 11*, 125–134.

Hogben, G. L., & Cornfield, R. B. (1981). Treatment of traumatic war neurosis with phenelzine. *Archives of General Psychiatry, 38*(4), 440–445.

Horowitz, M. J. (1976). *Stress response syndromes.* Northvale, NJ: Jason Aronson.

Horowitz, M. J. (1986). *Stress response syndromes* (2nd ed.). Northvale, NJ: Jason Aronson.

Horowitz, M. J., Wilner, N., & Alvarez, W. (1979). Impact of Event Scale: A measure of subjective distress. *Psychosomatic Medicine, 41*, 209–218.

Horowitz, M. J., Wilner, N. R., Kaltreider, N. B., & Alvarez, W. (1980). Signs and symptoms of posttraumatic stress disorder. *Archives of General Psychiatry, 37*(1), 85–92.

Hudson, J. I., & Pope, H. G. (1990). Affective spectrum disorder: Does antidepressant response identify a family of disorders with a common pathophysiology? *American Journal of Psychiatry, 5*, 552–564.

Hyer, L., O'Leary, W. C., Saucer, R. T., Blount, J., Harrison, W. R., & Boudewyns, P. A. (1986). Inpatient diagnosis of posttraumatic stress disorder. *Journal of Consulting and Clinical Psychology, 54*, 698–702.

Janoff-Bulman, R. (1992). *Shattered assumptions: Towards a new psychology of trauma*. New York: Free Press.

Jaycox, L. H., & Foa, E. B. (1996). Obstacles in implementing exposure therapy for PTSD: Case discussions and practical solutions. *Clinical Psychology and Psychotherapy, 3*(3), 176–184.

Jensen, J. A. (1994). An investigation of eye movement desensitization and reprocessing (EMD/R) as a treatment for posttraumatic stress disorder (PTSD) symptoms of Vietnam combat veterans. *Behavior Therapy, 25*(2), 311–325.

Jiranek, D. (1993). Use of hypnosis in pain management and post-traumatic stress disorder. *Australian Journal of Clinical and Experimental Hypnosis, 21*(1), 75–84.

Johnson, C. H., Gilmore, J. D., & Shenoy, R. Z. (1982). Use of a feeding procedure in the treatment of a stress-related anxiety disorder. *Journal of Behavior Therapy and Experimental Psychiatry, 13*, 235–237.

Keane, T. M., Fairbank, J. A., Caddell, J. M., & Zimering, R. T. (1989). Implosive (flooding) therapy reduces symptoms of PTSD in Vietnam combat veterans. *Behavior Therapy, 20*, 245–260.

Keane, T. M., & Kaloupek, D. G. (1982). Imaginal flooding in the treatment of posttraumatic stress disorder. *Journal of Consulting and Clinical Psychology, 50*, 138–140.

Keane, T. M., Zimering, R. T., & Caddell, J. M. (1985). A behavioral formulation of posttraumatic stress disorder in Vietnam veterans. *The Behavior Therapist, 8*, 9–12.

Kessler, R. C., Sonnega, A., Bromet, E., Hughes, M., & Nelson, C. B. (1995). Posttraumatic stress disorder in the National Comorbidity Survey. *Archives of General Psychiatry, 52*, 1048–1060.

Kilpatrick, D. G. (1988). Rape Aftermath Symptom Test. In M. Hersen & A. S. Bellack (Eds.), *Dictionary of behavioral assessment techniques*. Oxford: Pergamon Press.

Kilpatrick, D. G., Amick, A., & Resnick, H. S. (1988, September). *Preliminary research data on post-traumatic stress disorder following murders and drunk driving crashes*. Paper presented at the 14th Annual Meeting of the National Organization for Victim Assistance, Tucson, AZ.

Kilpatrick, D. G., & Best, C. L. (1984). Some cautionary remarks on treating sexual assault victims with implosion [Letter to the Editor]. *Behavior Therapy, 15*, 421–423.

Kilpatrick, D. G., Best, C., L., Saunders, B. E., Veronen, L. J. (1988). Rape in marriage and in relationships: How bad is it for mental health? *Annals of the New York Academy of Sciences, 528*, 335–344.

Kilpatrick, D. G., Best, C. L., Veronen, L. J., Amick, A. E., Villeponteaux, L. A., & Ruff, G. A. (1985). Mental health correlates of victimization: A random community survey. *Journal of Consulting and Clinical Psychology, 53*(6), 866–873.

Kilpatrick, D. G., Resick, P. A., & Veronen, L. J. (1981). Effects of a rape experience: A longitudinal study. *Journal of Social Issues, 37*, 105–122.

Kilpatrick, D. G., Saunders, B. E., Veronen, L. J., Best, C. L., & Von, J. M. (1987a). Criminal victimization: Lifetime prevalence, reporting to police, and psychological impact. *Crime and Delinquency, 33*, 479–489.

Kilpatrick, D. G. & Veronen, L. J. (1984). Treatment for rape-related problems: Crisis intervention is not enough. In L. Cohen, W. Claiborn, & G. Specter (Eds.), *Crisis intervention* (2nd ed.) New York: Human Sciences Press.

Kilpatrick, D. G., Veronen, L. J., & Resick, P. A. (1979a). Assessment of the aftermath of rape: Changing patterns of fear. *Journal of Behavioral Assessment, 1,* 133–148.

Kilpatrick, D. G., Veronen, L. J., & Resick, P. A. (1979b). The aftermath of rape: Recent empirical findings. *American Journal of Orthopsychiatry, 49,* 658–659.

Kilpatrick, D. G., Veronen, L. J., & Resick, P. A. (1982). Psychological sequelae to rape: Assessment and treatment strategies. In D. M. Dolays & R. L. Meredith (Eds.), *Behavioral medicine: Assessment and treatment strategies* (pp. 473–497). New York: Plenum Press.

Kingsbury, S. J. (1988). Hypnosis in the treatment of posttraumatic stress disorder: An isomorphic intervention. *American Journal of Clinical Hypnosis, 31,* 81–90.

Kinzie, J. D., & Leung, P. (1989). Clonidine in Cambodian patients with posttraumatic stress disorder. *Journal of Nervous and Mental Disease, 177,* 546–550.

Kleinknecht, R. A., & Morgan, M. P. (1992). Treatment of posttraumatic stress disorder with eye movement desensitization. *Journal of Behavior Therapy and Experimental Psychiatry, 23*(1), 43–49.

Kline, N. A., Dow, B. M., Brown, S. A., & Matloff, J. L. (1993, May). *Sertraline for PTSD with comorbid major depression.* Paper presented at the 146th Annual Convention of the American Psychiatric Association, San Francisco.

Kolb, L. C., Burris, B. C., & Griffiths, S. (1987). Propranolol and clonidine in the treatment of post-traumatic stress disorders of war. In B. A. van der Kolk (Ed.), *Post-traumatic stress disorder: Psychological and biological sequelae* (pp. 98–105). Washington, DC: American Psychiatric Press.

Koopman, C., Classen, C., & Spiegel, D. A. (1994). Predictors of posttraumatic stress symptoms among survivors of the Oakland/Berkeley, Calif., firestorm. *American Journal of Psychiatry, 151*(6), 888–894.

Koss, M. P., & Harvey, M. R. (1987). *The rape victim: Clinical and community approaches to treatment.* Lexington, MA: Stephen Greene Press.

Kozak, M. J., Foa, E. B., & Rothbaum, B. O. (1992). *Post-traumatic stress disorder in rape victims: Autonomic habituation to auditory stimuli.* Unpublished manuscript.

Kozak, M. J., Foa, E. B., & Steketee, G. (1988). Process and outcome of exposure treatment with obsessive–compulsives: Psychophysiological indicators of emotional processing. *Behavior Therapy, 19,* 157–169.

Krystal, J. H., Kosten, T. R., Southwick, S. M., Mason, J. W., Perry, B. D., & Giller, E. L. (1989). Neurobiological aspects of PTSD: Review of clinical and preclinical studies. *Behavior Therapy, 20*(2), 177–198.

Lang, P. J. (1979). A bio-informational theory of emotional imagery. *Psychophysiology, 6,* 495–511.

Leung, J. (1994). Treatment of post-traumatic stress disorder with hypnosis. *Australian Journal of Clinical and Experimental Hypnosis, 22*(1), 87–96.

Lindy, J. D., Green, B. L., Grace, M., & Titchener, J. (1983). Psychotherapy with survivors of the Beverly Hills Supper Club fire. *American Journal of Psychotherapy, 4,* 593–610.

Lipke, H. J., & Botkin, A. L. (1992). Case studies of eye movement desensitization and reprocessing (EMDR) with chronic post-traumatic stress disorder. *Psychotherapy, 4,* 591–595.

Litz, B. T. (1992). Emotional numbing in combat-related post-traumatic stress disorder: A critical review and reformulation. *Clinical Psychology Review, 12*(4), 417–432.

Lohr, J. M., Kleinknecht, R. A., Tolin, D. F., & Barrett, R. H. (1995). The empirical status of the clinical application of eye movement desensitization and reprocessing. *Journal of Behavior Therapy and Experimental Psychiatry, 26,* 285–302.

MacHovec, F. J. (1983). Treatment variables and the use of hypnosis in the brief therapy of post-traumatic stress disorders. *International Journal of Clinical and Experimental Hypnosis, 1,* 6–14.

Malloy, P. E., Fairbank, J. A., & Keane, T. M. (1983). Validation of a multimethod assessment of post-traumatic stress disorder in Vietnam veterans. *Journal of Consulting and Clinical Psychology, 51,* 488–494.

Manton, M., & Talbot, A. (1990). Crisis intervention after an armed hold-up: Guidelines for counsellors. *Journal of Traumatic Stress, 3,* 507–522.

Marks, I. M., Boulougouris, J., & Marset, P. (1971). Flooding versus desensitization in the treatment of phobic disorders. *British Journal of Psychiatry, 119,* 353–375.

Marmar, C. R., Horowitz, M. J., Weiss, D. S., Wilner, N. R., & Kaltreider, N. B. (1988). A controlled trial of brief psychotherapy and mutual-help group treatment of conjugal bereavement. *American Journal of Psychiatry, 145,* 209–209.

Marmar, C. R., Weiss, D. S., Schlenger, W. E., Fairbank, J. A., Jordan, B. K., Kulka, R. A., & Hough, R. L. (1994). Peritraumatic dissociation and posttraumatic stress in male Vietnam theater veterans. *American Journal of Psychiatry, 151*(6), 902–907.

Mattick, R. P., Peters, L., & Clarke, J. C. (1989). Exposure and cognitive restructuring for social phobia: A controlled study. *Behavior Therapy, 20,* 3–23.

McCann, I. L., & Pearlman, L. A. (1990). *Psychological trauma and the adult survivor: Theory, therapy, and transformation.* New York: Brunner/Mazel.

McFarlane, A. C. (1986). Long-term psychiatric morbidity after a natural disaster: Implications for disaster planners and emergency services. *Medical Journal of Australia, 145*(11–12), 561–563.

McFarlane, A. C. (1988a). The longitudinal course of posttraumatic morbidity: The range of outcomes and their predictors. *Journal of Nervous and Mental Disease, 176,* 30–39.

McFarlane, A. C. (1988b). The phenomenology of posttraumatic stress disorders following a natural disaster. *Journal of Nervous and Mental Disease, 176,* 22–29.

McNally, R. J., Luedke, D. L., Besyner, J. K., Peterson, R. A., Bohm, K., & Lips, O. J. (1987). Sensitivity to stress-relevant stimuli in posttraumatic stress disorder. *Journal of Anxiety Disorders, 1,* 105–116.

Meichenbaum, D. (1974a). Self-instructional methods. In F. H. Kanfer & A. P. Goldstein (Eds.), *Helping people change*. Elmsford, NY: Pergamon Press.

Meichenbaum, D. (1974b). *Cognitive behavior modification*. Morristown, NJ: General Learning Press.

Mellman, T., & Davis, G. C. (1985). Combat-related flashbacks in post traumatic stress disorder: Phenomenology and similarity to panic attacks. *Journal of Clinical Psychiatry, 46*, 379–382.

Mitchell, J. T., & Bray, G. (1990). *Emergency services stress: Guidelines for preserving the health and careers of emergency services personnel*. Englewood Cliffs, NJ: Prentice-Hall.

Montgomery, R. W., & Ayllon, T. (1994). Eye movement desensitization across images: A single case design. *Journal of Behavior Therapy and Experimental Psychiatry, 25* (1), 23–28.

Mowrer, O. A. (1960). *Learning theory and behavior*. New York: Wiley.

Muse, M. (1986). Stress-related, posttraumatic chronic pain syndrome: Behavioral treatment approach. *Pain, 25*, 389–394.

Nadelson, C. C., Notman, M. T., Zackson, H., & Gornick, J. (1982). A follow-up study of rape victims. *American Journal of Psychiatry, 139*, 1266–1270.

Nader, K., Pynoos, R., Fairbanks, L., & Frederick, C. (1990). Children's PTSD reactions one year after a sniper attack at their school. *American Journal of Psychiatry, 147*(11), 1526–1530.

National Institute of Mental Health (1985). Clinical Global Impression Scale. *Psychopharmacology Bulletin, 21*, 357–362.

Norris, J., & Feldman-Summers, S. (1981). Factors related to the psychological impact of rape on the victim. *Journal of Abnormal Psychology, 90*, 562–567.

Orlando, J. A., & Koss, M. P. (1983). The effects of sexual victimization on sexual satisfaction: A study of the negative-association hypothesis. *Journal of Abnormal Psychology, 92*, 104–106.

Ornitz, E. M., & Pynoos, R. S. (1989). Startle modulation in children with post traumatic stress disorder. *American Journal of Psychiatry, 146*, 866–870.

Ost, L. G. (1987). Applied relaxation: Description of a coping technique and review of controlled studies. *Behaviour Research and Therapy, 25*, 397–409.

Ost, L.-G., Salkovskis, P. M., & Hellstrom, K. (1991). One-session therapist-directed exposure vs. self-exposure in the treatment of spider phobia. *Behavior Therapy, 22*(3), 407–422.

Page, H. (1885). *Injuries of the spine and spinal cord without apparent mechanical lesion*. London: J. & A. Churchill.

Pallmeyer, T. P., Blanchard, E. B., & Kolb, L. C. (1986). The psychophysiology of combat-induced post-traumatic stress disorder in Vietnam veterans. *Behaviour Research and Therapy, 24*, 645–652.

Peebles, M. J. (1989). Through a glass darkly: The psychoanalytic use of hypnosis with post-traumatic stress disorder. *International Journal of Clinical and Experimental Hypnosis, 37*(3), 192–206.

Peniston, E. G. (1986). EMG biofeedback-assisted desensitization treatment for Vietnam combat veterans post-traumatic stress disorder. *Clinical Biofeedback and Health, 9*, 35–41.

Perl, M., Westin, A. B., & Peterson, L. G. (1985). The female rape survivor: Time-limited group therapy with female/male co-therapists. *Journal of Psychosomatic Obstetrics and Gynecology, 4,* 197–205.

Piaget, J. (1954). *The construction of reality in the child.* New York: Basic Books.

Pitman, R. K., Orr, S. P., Altman, B., Longpre, R. E., Poire, R. E., & Macklin, M. L. (1996). Emotional processing during eye-movement desensitization and re-processing therapy of Vietnam veterans with chronic post-traumatic stress disorder. *Comprehensive Psychiatry, 37*(6), 419–429.

Pitman, R. K., Orr, S. P., Forgue, D. F., Altman, B., deJong, J. B., & Herz, L. R. (1990a). Psychophysiologic responses to combat imagery of Vietnam veterans with post-traumatic stress disorder vs. other anxiety disorders. *Journal of Abnormal Psychology, 99,* 49–54.

Pitman, R. K., Orr, S. P., Forgue, D. F., deJong, J. B., & Claiborn, J. M. (1987). Psychophysiologic assessment of post-traumatic stress disorder imagery in Vietnam combat veterans. *Archives of General Psychiatry, 44,* 970–975.

Pitman, R. K., Orr, S. P., Lowenhagen, M. J., Macklin, M. L., & Altman, B. (1991). Pre-Vietnam contents of posttraumatic stress disorder veterans' service medical and personnel records. *Comprehensive Psychiatry, 32* (5), 416–422.

Pitman, R. K., van der Kolk, B. A., Orr, S. P., & Greenberg, M. S. (1990b). Naloxone-reversible analgesic response to combat-related stimuli in posttraumatic stress disorder: A pilot study. *Archives of General Psychiatry, 47*(6), 541–544.

Putnam, F. W. (1985). Dissociation as a response to extreme trauma. In R. P. Kluft (Ed.), *Childhood antecedents of multiple personality* (pp. 65–97). Washington, DC: American Psychiatric Press.

Putnam, F. W., Guroff, J. J., Silberman, E. K., Barban, L., & Post, R. M. (1986). The clinical phenomenology of multiple personality disorder: 100 recent cases. *Journal of Clinical Psychiatry, 47,* 285–293.

Putnam, J. J. (1881). Recent investigations into patients of so-called concussion of the spine. *Boston Medical and Surgical Journal, 109,* 217.

Pynoos, R. S., Frederick, C., Nader, K. Arroyo, W., Steinberg, A., Eth, S., Nunez, F., & Fairbanks, L. (1987), Life threat and posttraumatic stress in school-age children. *Archives of General Psychiatry, 44,* 1057–1063.

Rachman, S. (1980). Emotional processing. *Behaviour Research and Therapy, 18,* 51–60.

Rachman, S. (1989). *Fear and courage* (2nd ed.). New York: W. H. Freeman.

Rado, S. (1942). Pathodynamics and treatment of traumatic war neurosis (traumatophobia). *Psychosomatic Medicine, 42,* 363–368.

Raphael, B., Meldrum, L., & McFarlane, A. (1995). Does debriefing after psychological trauma work? *British Medical Journal, 310,* 1479–1480.

Reist, C., Kauffmann, C. D., Haier, R. J., Sangdahl, C., DeMet, E. M., & Chicz-DeMet, A. (1989). A controlled trial of desipramine in 18 men with posttraumatic stress disorder. *American Journal of Psychiatry, 146,* 513–516.

Renfrey, G., & Spates, C. R. (1994). Eye movement desensitization: A partial dismantling study. *Journal of Behavior Therapy and Experimental Psychiatry, 25*(3), 231–239.

Resick, P. A. (1987). *The impact of rape on psychological functioning.* Unpublished manuscript, University of Missouri, St. Louis.

Resick, P. A. (1988). *Reactions of female and male victims of rape or robbery* (Final Report, NIJ Grant No. 85-IJ-CV-0042). Submitted to the National Institute of Justice, Washington, DC.

Resick, P. A., Calhoun, K. S., Atkeson, B. M., & Ellis, E. M. (1981). Social adjustment in victims of sexual assault. *Journal of Consulting and Clinical Psychology, 49*, 705–712.

Resick, P. A., Jordan, C. G., Girelli, S. A., Hutter, C. K., & Marhoefer-Dvorak, S. (1988). A comparative victim study of behavioral group therapy for sexual assault victims. *Behavior Therapy, 19*, 385–401.

Resick, P. A., & Schnicke, M. K. (1992). Cognitive processing therapy for sexual assault victims. *Journal of Consulting and Clinical Psychology, 60*, 748–756.

Resick, P. A., & Schnicke, M. K. (1993). *Cognitive processing therapy for rape victims: A treatment manual*. Newbury Park, CA: Sage.

Resnick, H. S., Kilpatrick, D. G., Dansky, B. S., Saunders, B. E., & Best, C. L. (1993). Prevalence of civilian trauma and posttraumatic stress disorder in a representative national sample of women. *Journal of Consulting and Clinical Psychology, 61*(6), 984–991.

Resnick, H., Veronen, L. J., Saunders, B., Kilpatrick, D. G., & Cornelison, V. (1989b). *Assessment of PTSD in a subset of rape victims at 12 to 36 months post-assault*. Unpublished manuscript.

Richards, D. A., Lovell, K., & Marks, I. M. (1994). Post-traumatic stress disorder: Evaluation of a behavioral treatment program. *Journal of Traumatic Stress, 7*(4), 669–680.

Rickels, K., & Schweizer, E. (1990). Clinical overview of serotonin reuptake inhibitors. *Journal of Clinical Psychiatry, 51*(Suppl. B), 9–12.

Riggs, D. S., Dancu, C. V., Gershuny, B. S., Greenberg, D., & Foa, E. B. (1992). Anger and post-traumatic stress disorder in female crime victims. *Journal of Traumatic Stress, 5*, 613–625.

Riggs, D. S., Rothbaum, B. O., & Foa, E. B. (1995). A prospective examination of symptoms of post-traumatic stress disorder in victims of non-sexual assault. *Journal of Interpersonal Violence, 2*, 201–214.

Robins, L. N., Helzer, J. E., Croughan, J., & Ratcliff, K. S., (1981). The NIMH Diagnostic Interview Schedule: Its history, characteristics, and validity. *Archives of General Psychiatry, 38*, 381–389.

Ross, R. J., Ball, W. A., Cohen, M. E., Silver, S. M., Morrison, A. R., & Dinges, D. F. (1989a). Habituation of the startle reflex in posttraumatic stress disorder. *Journal of Neuropsychiatry and Clinical Neurosciences, 1*(3), 305–307.

Ross, R. J., Ball, W. A., Sullivan, K. A., & Caroll, S. N. (1989b). Sleep disturbances as the hallmark of post-traumatic stress disorder. *American Journal of Psychiatry, 146*(6), 697–707.

Roth, S., Dye, E., & Lebowitz, L. (1988). Group therapy for sexual-assault victims. *Psychotherapy, 25*, 82–93.

Rothbaum, B. O. (1997). A controlled study of eye movement desensitization and reprocessing in the treatment of posttraumatic stress disordered sexual assault victims. *Bulletin of the Menninger Clinic, 61*, 1–18.

Rothbaum, B. O., & Foa, E. B. (1992b). Exposure therapy for rape victims with posttraumatic stress disorder. *The Behavior Therapist, 15*, 219–222.

Rothbaum, B. O., Foa, E. B., Riggs, D., Murdock, T., & Walsh, W. (1992). A prospective examination of post-traumatic stress disorder in rape victims. *Journal of Traumatic Stress, 5,* 455–475.

Rothbaum, B. O., Ninan, P. T., & Thomas, L. (1996). Sertraline in the treatment of PTSD rape victims. *Journal of Traumatic Stress, 9*(4), 865–871.

Saigh, P. A. (1988). Anxiety, depression, and assertion across alternating intervals of stress. *Journal of Abnormal Psychology, 97,* 338–341.

Sank, L. I., & Shaffer, C. S. (1984). *A therapist's manual for cognitive behavior therapy in groups.* New York: Plenum Press.

Sargent, W. W., & Slater, E. (1940). Acute war neuroses. *Lancet, ii,* 1–2.

Scarvalone, P., Cloitre, M., & Difede, J. (1995, June). *Interpersonal process therapy for incest survivors: Preliminary outcome data.* Paper presented at the Annual Convention of the Society for Psychotherapy Research, Vancouver, British Columbia.

Schindler, F. E. (1980). Treatment by systematic desensitization of a recurring nightmare of a real life trauma. *Journal of Behavior Therapy and Experimental Psychiatry, 11,* 53–54.

Schlenger, W. E., Kulka, R. A., Fairbank, J. A., Hough, R. L., Jordan, B. K., Marmar, C. R., & Weiss, D. S. (1992). The prevalence of post-traumatic stress disorder in the Vietnam generation: A multimethod, multisource assessment of psychiatric disorder. *Journal of Traumatic Stress, 5*(3), 333–363.

Shapiro, F. (1989). Eye movement desensitization: A new treatment for PTSD. *Journal of Behavior Therapy and Experimental Psychiatry, 3,* 211–217.

Shapiro, F. (1995). *Eye movement desensitization and reprocessing: Basic principles, protocols, and procedures.* New York: Guilford Press.

Shestatsky, M., Greenberg, D., & Lerer, B. (1988). A controlled trial of phenelzine in posttraumatic stress disorder. *Psychiatry Research, 24,* 149–155.

Shore, J. H., Tatum, E., & Vollmer, W. M. (1986). Psychiatric reactions to disaster: The Mt. St. Helen's experience. *American Journal of Psychiatry, 143,* 590–595.

Silver, S. M., Brooks, A., & Obenchain, J. (1995). Treatment of Vietnam war veterans with PTSD: A comparison of eye movement desensitization and reprocessing, biofeedback, and relaxation training. *Journal of Traumatic Stress, 8*(2), 337–342.

Smith, E. M., Robins, L. N., Przybeck, T. R., Goldring, E., & Solomon, S. D. (1986). Psychosocial consequences of a disaster. In J. H. Shore (Ed.), *Disaster stress studies: New methods and findings* (pp. 49–76). Washington, DC: American Psychiatric Press.

Solomon, Z., & Mikulincer, M. (1988). Psychological sequelae of war: A two year follow-up study of Israeli combat stress reaction (CSR) casualties. *Journal of Nervous and Mental Disease, 176,* 264–269.

Solomon, Z., Mikulincer, M., & Benbenishty, R. (1989). Locus of control and combat-related post-traumatic stress disorder: the intervening role of battle intensity, threat appraisal and coping. *British Journal of Clinical Psychology, 28*(2), 131–144.

Spiegel, D. (1988). Dissociation and hypnosis in post-traumatic stress disorders. *Journal of Traumatic Stress, 1,* 17–33.

Spiegel, D. (1989). Hypnosis in the treatment of victims of sexual abuse. *Psychiatric Clinics of North America, 12*(2), 295–305.

Spiegel, D., & Cardeña, E. (1991). Disintegrated experience: The dissociative disorders revisited. *Journal of Abnormal Psychology, 100*(3), 366–378.

Spiegel, D., Hunt, T., & Dondershine, H. E. (1988). Dissociation and hypnotizability in posttraumatic stress disorder. *American Journal of Psychiatry*, 145(3), 301–305.

Spielberger, C. D., Gorsuch, R. L., & Lushene, R. E. (1970). *Manual for the State–Trait Anxiety Inventory (self-evaluation questionnaire)*. Palo Alto, CA: Consulting Psychologists Press.

Spitzer, R. L., Williams, J. B. W., & Gibbon, M. (1987). *Structured Clinical Interview for DSM-III-R (SCID)*. New York: Biometrics Research Department, New York State Psychiatric Institute.

Stampfl, T. G., & Levis, D. J. (1967). Essentials of implosive therapy: A learning-theory-based psychodynamic behavioral therapy. *Journal of Abnormal Psychology*, 72(6), 496–503.

Stern, R. S., & Marks, I. M. (1973). Brief and prolonged flooding: A comparison in agoraphobic patients. *Archives of General Psychiatry*, 28, 270–276.

Suinn, R. (1974). Anxiety management training for general anxiety. In R. Suinn & R. Weigel (Eds.), *The innovative therapy: Critical and creative contributions*. New York: Harper and Row.

Thompson, J. A., Charlton, P. F. C., Kerry, R., Lee, D., & Turner, S. W. (1995). An open trial of exposure therapy based on deconditioning for post-traumatic stress disorder. *British Journal of Clinical Psychology*, 34, 407–416.

Tolin, D. F., Montgomery, R. W., Kleinknecht, R. A., & Lohr, J. M. (1995). An evaluation of eye movement desensitization and reprocessing (EMDR). In L. Vande-Creek, S. Knapp, & T. L. Jackson (Eds.), *Innovations in clinical practice: A source book* (Vol. 14). Sarasota, FL: Professional Resources Press.

Torrie, A. (1944). Psychosomatic casualties in the Middle East. *Lancet, i*, 139–143.

Trandel, D. V., & McNally, R. J. (1987). Perception of threat cues in post-traumatic stress disorder: Semantic processing without awareness? *Behaviour Research and Therapy*, 25(6), 469–476.

Turner, S. M. (1979). *Systematic desensitization of fears and anxiety in rape victims*. Paper presented at the Annual Convention of the Association for Advancement of Behavior Therapy, San Francisco.

Ullman, S. E. (1995). Adult trauma survivors and post-traumatic stress sequelae: An analysis of reexperiencing, avoidance, and arousal criteria. *Journal of Traumatic Stress*, 8(1), 179–188.

van der Kolk, B. A. (Ed.). (1987). *Post-traumatic stress disorder: Psychological and biological sequelae*. Washington, DC: American Psychiatric Press.

van der Kolk, B. A., Dreyfuss, D., Michaels, M., Shera, D., Berkowitz, R., Fisler, R. E., & Saxe, G. N. (1994). Fluoxetine in posttraumatic stress disorder. *Journal of Clinical Psychiatry*, 55(12), 517–522.

van der Kolk, B. A., Greenberg, M. S., Boyd, H., & Krystal, J. (1985). Inescapable shock, neurotransmitters and addiction to trauma: Towards a psychobiology of post-traumatic stress. *Biological Psychiatry*, 20, 314–325.

Vargas, M. A., & Davidson, J. R. T. (1993). Post-traumatic stress disorder. *Psychiatric Clinics of North America*, 4, 737–748.

Vaughan, K., Armstrong, M. S., Gold, R., O'Connor, N., Jenneke, W., & Tarrier, N. (1994). A trial of eye movement desensitization compared to image habituation training and applied muscle relaxation in post-traumatic stress disorder. *Journal of Behavior Therapy and Experimental Psychiatry*, 25(4), 283–291.

ver Ellen, P., & van Kammen, D. P. (1990). The biological findings in post-traumatic stress disorder: A review. *Journal of Applied Social Psychology, 20*(21), 1789–1821.

Veronen, L. J., & Kilpatrick, D. G. (1980). Self-reported fears of rape victims: A preliminary investigation. *Behavior Modification, 4*, 383–396.

Veronen, L. J., & Kilpatrick, D. G. (1982, November). *Stress inoculation training for victims of rape: Efficacy and differential findings*. Paper presented at the 16th Annual Convention of the Association for Advancement of Behavior Therapy, Los Angeles.

Veronen, L. J., & Kilpatrick, D. G. (1983). Stress management for rape victims. In D. Meichenbaum & M. E. Jaremko (Eds.), *Stress reduction and prevention* (pp. 341–374). New York: Plenum Press.

von Moltke, L. L., Greenblatt, D. J., Harmatz, J. S., & Shader, R. I. (1994). Cytochromes in psychopharmacology. *Journal of Clinical Psychopharmacology, 14*, 1–4.

Watson, C. G., Kucala, T., Manifold, V., Vassar, P., & Juba, M. (1988). Differences between posttraumatic stress disorder patients with delayed and undelayed onsets. *Journal of Nervous and Mental Disease, 176*, 568–572.

Watts, F. N. (1979). Habituation model of systematic desensitization. *Psychological Bulletin, 86*(3), 627–637.

Wegner, D. M. (1994). Ironic processes of mental control. *Psychological Review, 101*, 34–52.

Weiss, D. S., Marmar, C. R., Schlenger, W. E., Fairbank, J. A., Jordan, B. K., Hough, R. L., & Kulka, R. A. (1992). The prevalence of lifetime and partial post-traumatic stress disorder in Vietnam theater veterans. *Journal of Traumatic Stress, 5*(3), 365–376.

Wilkinson, C. B. (1983). Aftermath of a disaster: The collapse of the Hyatt Regency Hotel skywalks. *American Journal of Psychiatry, 9*, 1134–1139.

Williams, J. M. G., Watts, F. N., MacLeod, C., & Mathews, A. (1988). *Cognitive psychology and emotional disorders*. New York: Wiley.

Wilson, S. A., Becker, L. A., & Tinker, R. H. (1995). Eye movement desensitization and reprocessing (EMDR) treatment for psychologically traumatized individuals. *Journal of Consulting and Clinical Psychology, 63*(6), 928–937.

Wolff, R. (1977). Systematic desensitization and negative practice to alter the after-effects of a rape attempt. *Journal of Behavior Therapy and Experimental Psychiatry, 8*, 423–425.

Wolpe, J. (1958). *Psychotherapy by reciprocal inhibition*. Stanford, CA: Stanford University Press.

Wolpe, J., & Abrams, J. (1991). Post-traumatic stress disorder overcome by eye-movement desensitization: A case report. *Journal of Behavior Therapy and Experimental Psychiatry, 22*(1), 39–43.

Woolfolk, R. L., & Grady, D. A. (1988). Combat-related posttraumatic stress disorder: Patterns of symptomatology in help-seeking Vietnam veterans. *Journal of Nervous and Mental Disease, 176*, 107–111.

Yalom, I. (1995). *The theory and practice of group psychotherapy* (4th ed.). New York: Basic Books.

Yassen, J., & Glass, L. (1984). Sexual assault survivors groups: A feminist practice perspective. *Social Work, 3*, 252–257.

Index